By the Numbers

Sean Manseau

Photographs by Brian Poon

Additional photos by Greg Saulmon, Liz Greene, and Lisa Hepfer

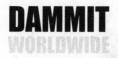
DAMMIT
WORLDWIDE

Library of Congress Cataloging-in-Publication Data

Manseau, Sean. 1970-

    By the Numbers / Sean Manseau

ISBN-13: 978-0692475911 (DAMMIT Worldwide)

ISBN-10: 0692475915

1. By the Numbers Method 2. Fitness Instruction 3. Coaching

This book is for educational purposes. The author and publisher of this instructional manual is not responsible in any manner whatsoever for any adverse effects arising directly or indirectly as a result of the information provided in this book. If not practiced safely and with caution, working out can be dangerous to you and others. It is important to consult with a professional fitness instructor before beginning training. It is also very important to consult with a physician prior to training due to the intense and strenuous nature of the techniques in this book.

The methods and opinions described in this work are solely the Author's and in no way claim to be representative of the practices of and opinions held by the owners and employees of CrossFit®. CrossFit® is a registered trademark of CrossFit, Inc.

TABLE OF CONTENTS

Introduction

Part I: By the Numbers Theory and Concepts

Part II: Teaching and Coaching By the Numbers

Week One

Week Two

Week Three

Week Four

Week Five

Week Six

Week Seven

Week Eight

Part III: Appendices

Introduction
WHAT THIS BOOK DOES (AND DOESN'T DO)

This book is not a CrossFit® manual.

By the Numbers is a guide to teaching exercises commonly utilized in what might be termed Multimodal General Physical Preparedness (MMGPP) training—programs that combine elements of running, rowing, weightlifting, gymnastics, and other disciplines in creative ways. CrossFit is the most popular program of this type, but there are many others, such as Iron Tribe, Gym Jones, Orange Theory, Mountain Athlete, Alpha Training, etc. Each has its own spin on MMGPP, but the ideas in this book can be applied to them all.

I wrote *By the Numbers* to reinforce the standards of performance for the exercises programmed in MMGPP, and to encourage trainers to teach those standards in classroom environments distinguished by copious practice and rigorous correction. It's my attempt to distill seven years of full-time coaching experience into a manual that can aid new trainers in running safe and effective MMGPP classes. Hopefully there will be a few novel approaches and tricks of the trade that experienced instructors can benefit from, as well.

What this Book Does

The book's specific focus is on what I consider to be a MMGPP instructor's number one job: to get people moving well. It explains the principles that underlie the By the Numbers method (BtN), then describes BtN's pedagogical philosophy, a model for progression, a formalized approach to organizing class time, a system for teaching the exercises programmed in "classical" MMGPP, pragmatic fixes for common faults of execution, and an innovative approach to structuring WODs that reduces risk and promotes improvement.

By the Numbers Principles

BtN is based on progression at every scale: micro, meso, and macro. It builds exercises pose-by-pose, movement skill exercise-by-exercise, and tests movement skill with incremental increases in volume, load, and intensity.

A Pedagogical Philosophy

Biomechanically correct, efficient, powerful movement has an intrinsic beauty, and teaching exercises not as gross motor patterns, but as a series of ideal positions, is an attempt to wring beauty out of the everyday. That's a pretty good definition of the artistic quest; thus, By the Numbers invites coaches to treat their vocation as art. And I want athletes to adopt an artist's attitude, as well. Here's what I mean:

In arts that have as their goal a real-time expression of ability, like ballet, or playing the piano, it is accepted that there is a time to practice, and a time to perform. A piano student doesn't walk out on the recital stage to fumble her way through a composition she can "kind of" play, hoping her performance will improve as she goes. Nor would any music teacher worth his salt want her to. Instead, together they choose a piece that will allow the student to show off her current abilities. She carefully prepares. And when it's time, she shines.

A similar approach greatly benefits learning to train with MMGPP. MMGPP metabolic conditioning workouts (colloquially known as "WODs", for "Workout of the Day") should be considered *performance*. WODs are the time to demonstrate movement skill, not develop it; when athletes go hard, BtN insists they use movements they have mastered. No one is allowed to hack, nor is it ever necessary, because if and when fatigue overwhelms an athlete's technical capacities, BtN offers an array of easier-to-perform exercise options that preserve the intended training stimulus. BtN allows you to ensure your athletes have a safe, successful performance every time they take on the WOD.

The flip side of performance is preparation, and so BtN puts a great emphasis on formal practice sessions. These are discussed at length in Chapter Three.

A Model for Progression

BtN organizes the exercises commonly programmed in MMGPP into categories ordered by increasing complexity. These categories are called "Movement Hierarchies". By requiring athletes to master a simple exercise before attempting a more challenging variant, or that they default to the simple exercise when fatigue makes competent execution of its complex version impossible, BtN ensures your athletes will always be getting the most out of their workouts, while taking every possible step to prevent bad habits and/or injury.

Classroom Concepts

From the moment class begins until it is dismissed, you, as an instructor, are (or should be) in constant transaction with your athletes. However, the way you relate with them depends on context. BtN postulates formal classroom modes for teachers and students that describe the various phases of this relationship. These modes, in turn, suggest strategies for more effective teaching.

Teaching Movement By the Numbers

The bulk of the book is dedicated to a system for instructing and coaching forty-five or so exercises that comprise "classical" MMGPP. I've broken each movement into a series of poses. These poses are easy for students to learn and remember, and easy to for you to teach, even to large groups. BtN will enable you to observe an athlete's movements and identify instantly what's right or wrong by comparing their position to an idealized mental image.

Coaching and Correcting By the Numbers

Once athletes have been taught an exercise, By the Numbers offers Positional Drills and corrective techniques that will help them master it. These Positional Drills allow you, the instructor, to make corrections in real time, as opposed to trying to explain to the athlete after the fact what they did wrong. You can drill positions one at a time, or in combination to emphasize certain aspects of execution.

Drilling By the Numbers is a remarkably fast and effective way to ingrain in your athletes correct motor patterns for simple, foundational movements like the air squat, as well as highly technical exercises like the barbell snatch. Further, encouraging athletes to practice movements in terms of key positions also helps them understand the common principles that underlie functional movements. Learning to hip hinge in the good morning, for example, makes it easier for an athlete to learn the deadlift or the kettlebell swing.

BtN's corrective techniques have two goals: to quickly get athletes moving reasonably well, no matter what their individual issues of mobility, and to maintain group cohesion by minimizing the need for separate, remedial instruction for struggling athletes. So at the end of each teaching section in this book, I offer a robust (if not encyclopedic) collection of commonly seen faults and the various cues you might use to address them, as well as battle-tested ways to implement common gym items as corrective orthoses.

Structuring Benchmark Workouts for Logical Progression

MMGPP programming tends to avoid predictability. From day to day, one never knows what's going to show up on the whiteboard—that's part of the fun and adventure. Given the wide variety of exercises utilized in MMGPP, and parameters of load, volume, time domain, etc., a good programmer could spiel out fun, innovative workouts for years without once repeating herself.

But MMGPP programs often claim to be "evidence-based"—that is, claims to efficacy are built on observed, measured, and recorded data regarding power output: what you did (work), and how long it took to do (time). If we never get to repeat a workout, to compare performances over a certain period of time, how can we be sure our fitness is actually increasing? We need metrics.

At the end of each chapter, we'll look at how BtN restructures some representative WODs to make them more accessible for a general population. I believe the approach described here is the programmatic version of BtN's movement progressions: a safe and effective way to ramp up challenge over time.

What This Book Doesn't Do

As MMGPP trainers, we wear many hats: exercise instructor, cheerleader, drill sergeant, amateur psychologist. We're also often the first place our clients turn for information about nutrition, injury diagnosis, fashion advice, etc. However, for the protection of both our clients and ourselves, it's important that we not exceed the scope of our practice. With that in mind, there was a limit on what I could include in this book.

Not an On-Ramp

The movement instruction section of this book, while structured as classes extending over a period of weeks, is not an On-Ramp program*, although it could easily serve as the basis for one. It's more like a thought experiment: given unlimited time, what would be the ideal order in which to teach all of the movements we program? Exercises are introduced only after trainees have had an opportunity to master their constituent fundamentals and pass certain movement screens. This principle applies any time athletes are exposed to new movements, whether in an On-ramp course or in regular classes.

Not a Guide to Programming

Although in Part One's classroom concepts chapter "Are You Mr. Garrison or Mr. Chips?" I offer templates for skill development work, and in the "Benchmarks" sections of Part Two I talk about various strategies for structuring classes and workouts, this book does not delve into the subject of programming for a MMGPP gym. That could be a 500 page book all its own, and I leave it for someone else to write.

No Nutritional Advice

...except for this: if athletes are not following a coherent nutritional strategy (the Zone Diet, Paleo, etc.), they are not doing MMGPP and should not expect to realize the promised

---

* An "On-Ramp" (also known as "Elements" or "Fundamentals") is an introductory course many gyms require prospective members to complete before joining group classes.

results. Period.

No Formal Mobility Prescriptions

It's been my observation that if you continually guide new athletes toward ideal positions, over time their movement dysfunctions—weakness, inflexibility, lack of coordination—tend to resolve. However, many people will have mobility issues severe enough to make certain exercises unsafe or even impossible, at least initially. BtN makes it easy to assign movements within a limited athlete's capability, but in the long term, remedial mobility work and/or physical therapy might be necessary for an athlete to correctly perform even a fundamental movement like the overhead squat.

Diagnosis of mobility issues and prescription for the treatment of same are beyond the purview of this book. Readers are strongly encouraged to purchase and study Kelly Starrett's *Becoming a Supple Leopard*, an indispensable maintenance manual for the human body, so that you have some rehab and prehab techniques to teach your clients. Even once you've familiarized yourself with *BSL*, though, don't take on too much. If your clients have persistent pain or more than moderate limitations, please encourage them to see a licensed physical therapist.

The Goals of By the Numbers

The goals of By the Numbers are threefold: helping instructors of MMGPP to get their athletes moving well, providing athletes with progressions they can use to map their development, and promoting an approach to structuring workouts that is effective in establishing the level of intensity appropriate to a developing athlete's current capacities.

1. "Moving well" means, in BtN terms, meeting standards both technical and aesthetic. It's not enough to hit points of performance. Or maybe a better way to put that is, for athlete and instructor alike, to stop concentrating on movement quality once points of performance are met robs MMGPP training of its potential to serve as a vehicle for self-actualization. The journey toward mastery never ends.

2. The exercise progressions presented in these pages work, but they are by no means the final word on the matter. I'd like them to serve as a starting point for discussion and debate within the MMGPP community. I encourage others to present their ideas; test them against mine, and may be the better progression win! That's how things improve.

3. Benchmark workouts are important part of any MMGPP program. BtN's hypothetical benchmark workouts server as a logical jumping off point for presenting ideas about how to take the guesswork out of "scaling" a given WOD's movements, load, and volume.

As of this writing, By the Numbers is the best (the only?) formal method for working with people of wildly varying abilities all seeking that "entertrainment" that MMGPP training provides. Let me amend that—it's the best method *I've* come up with, and it's a work in progress. I offer By the Numbers to you in the hope you'll take it, teach it, and make it better.

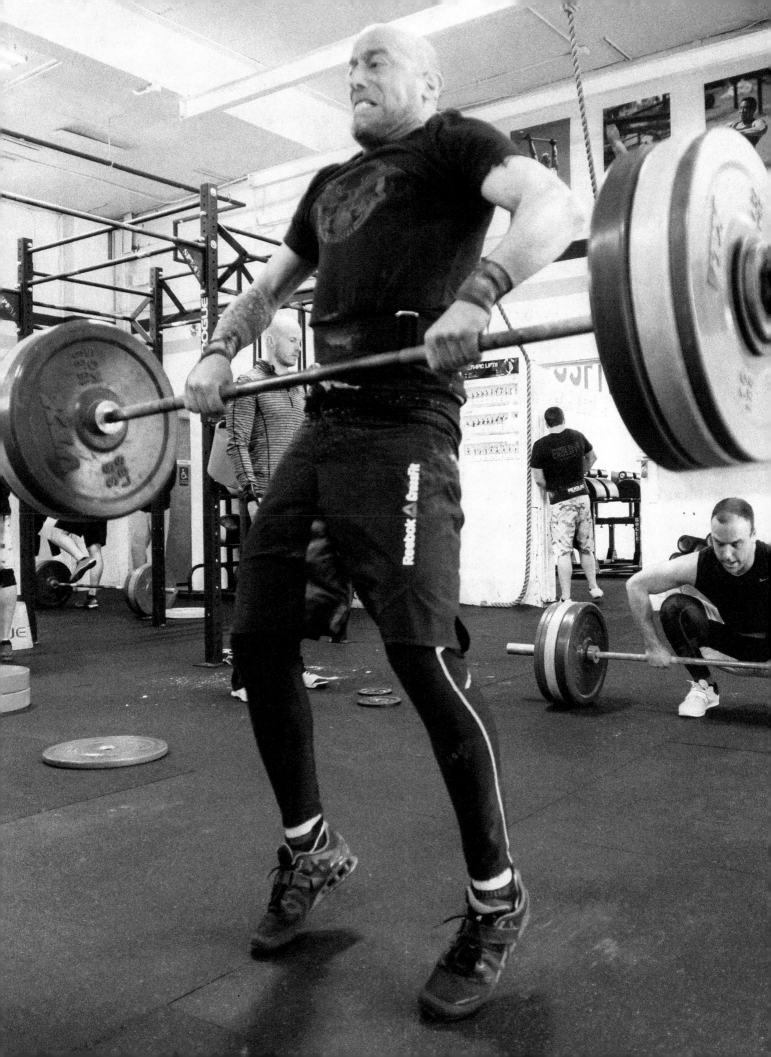

PART ONE:

BY THE

NUMBERS

Theory and Concepts

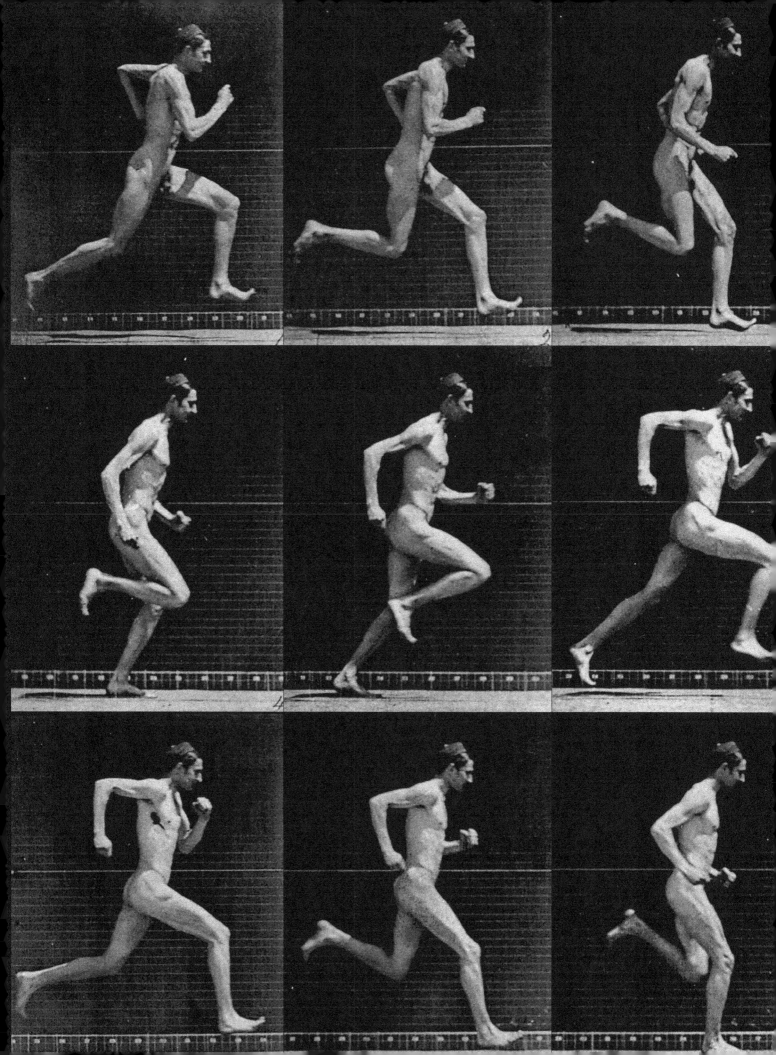

Chapter One
EVERY TRAINER IS AN ARTIST

After the gym I founded in 2007 had grown to the point it was necessary to open a second location, I realized we had a problem: our clients were no longer getting a consistent product. Instructors in our Hadley box taught movements one way, and trainers in our Northampton facility taught them another. Occasionally, contradictory advice would be given, leaving athletes confused. On top of that, our expanded schedule meant our training cadre was teaching more than ever, and in danger of burning out. We needed to standardize instruction, and we needed a method to accelerate the development of our apprentice trainers into fully-fledged instructors.

It was just a fortunate coincidence that around the same time, I had been thinking a lot about the parallels between creating animation and teaching MMGPP.

MMGPP and the Principles of Animation

A couple of careers before owning a gym, I was an animator in the video game industry. Animation, whether hand-drawn (think Disney's *Snow White and Seven Dwarves*), stop-motion (*The Nightmare Before Christmas*), pre-rendered CGI (*Toy Story*) or real-time rendered CGI (*Call of Duty IV*), is the process of creating the illusion of life by playing a series of still images in such rapid succession that the eye of the viewer is fooled into perceiving continuous motion.

The production of animation, no matter what its intended medium, always begins the same way: with an animator carefully analyzing the movement to be depicted. It could be a herd of deer running, a complex song-and-dance number, or an air battle between spaceships and dragons above a forest planet; it makes no difference. The animator must study the action, and then break it down into its most dramatic, or key, poses. Key poses are "used to describe those critical positions of an animated character or an object which depict the extreme points in its path of motion." (Atkinson, 2012)

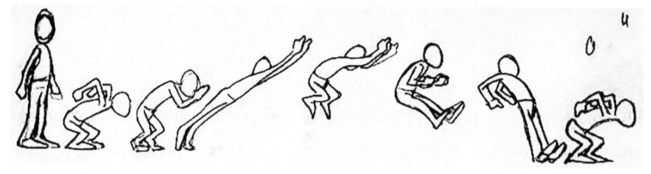

Key poses of a jump-and-land sequence

These key poses are only the bare bones of the animation. Smoothing out the motion between the keys are drawings of transitional states created by a junior animator, or "in-betweener." It might only take one second of screen time for an animated character to jump and land, but that one second represents 24 frames of film—that's 24 individual drawings that must be created, even for such a simple action.

But if what we see on screen doesn't match what we've observed of people and animals running, jumping, and interacting with their environment, then the illusion of life is lost, and all that work will have been wasted. It doesn't take any training to recognize bad animation. It simply doesn't look right.

One part of *looking right* is the aesthetic qualities of the key poses. They must have *energy*, *rhythm*, and *balance*. For characters, this means bodies are depicted as assuming

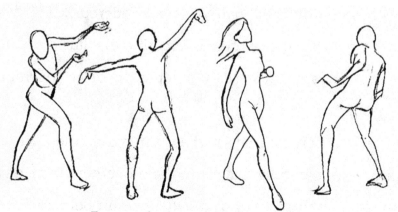

Energy, rhythm, and balance in art

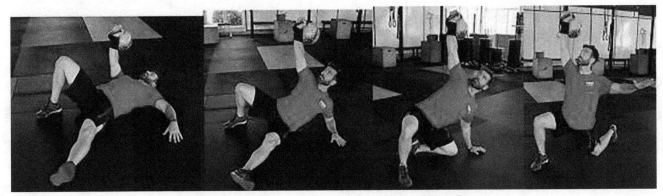

Energy, rhythm, and balance on the gym floor

geometric shapes, rather than organic. Think arms and legs at sharply defined angles... precisely the shapes the body adopts when it is moving most efficiently. You could analyze film of a world-class athlete executing her event and at any point find energy, rhythm, and balance in her positions.*

Just as critical for the succesful creation of the illusion of life is *timing* of the poses. A take-off pose that arrives just a split second too late will be interpreted by the viewer as an impossible violation of physics. Unless the right key pose is in the right place at exactly the right time, it's back to the drawing board.

My *eureka!* moment connecting animation and MMGPP came one day when I was teaching the power clean to a group of athletes. A weightlifter by the name of Tony Blanksteen had shown me a way to break down the clean into a series of positions: floor, hang, pockets, finish, scarecrow, catch. But I was still teaching the clean as one gross motor skill, and trying to make corrections after the fact. "Ready, go! Okay, John, next time, try to open your hips up all the way as you 'finish.' Sue, don't reverse curl the bar, pull your elbows up and keep the bar close to your body in 'scarecrow'."

My athletes' cleans were sloppy, though. They were missing positions, and their timing was all over the place. I was getting frustrated that they weren't getting it. So I started making them do the positions one at a time, holding still as I made corrections to their form. And then it hit me: *These are key poses!*

As an animator I had worked in a virtual environment, adjusting the on-screen actions

---

* Check out the Eadweard Mubridge photos facing the first page of this chapter for more examples of dynamic poses.

of the balrog or the Matrix agent or what have you until they just *looked right*. That day in the gym I was in the real world, but the job at hand was the same: I was breaking down a complex movement into its most important parts, its most dramatic and extreme poses, and making sure the bodies I was working with adopted those exact shapes, at exactly the right time. Five years after leaving the videogame industry, I was animating again.

I started laughing right in the middle of the gym floor, while my athletes stared at me in consternation. I suddenly knew exactly how to standardize the way we taught exercise at PVCF, and how to accelerate the development of our apprentice trainers. I would break down all of the movements of MMGPP into series of discrete positions—exactly the same poses an animator would choose if he or she were to create an animation depicting that exercise. But for simplicity's sake, rather than having special names for each position ("hang, pockets, finish, scarecrow"), I'd just give each position a number.

I did it that day with the power clean: "Okay, set up in 'floor' position. Let's call that 'one.' 'Hang' position will be 'two', 'Pockets', three, and etc. Let's try it. Hit 'one' for me. 'Two.' 'Three'. 'Four.' 'Five.'"

And it worked. It really worked! The individual positions created a kind of road map for the movement, or maybe a better analogy would be the dance-step charts on the floor of an Arthur Murray studio. My athletes practiced the "steps" of the clean slowly and methodically. Once they got comfortable with the individual poses, I had them them blend multiple poses into sequences to work on their timing. Finally, when I had them try the full power clean at speed, their performance was vastly improved. They were in exactly the right places at exactly the right time.

Over the next couple weeks I systematically went through all the movements we commonly programmed, broke them down pose by pose, and numbered the positions. I taught these breakdowns to my instructor cadre, and as we familiarized our members with this new approach, something amazing happened: by teaching and drilling positions one at a time, by insisting each pose have its own energy, rhythm, and balance, and by requiring those poses be mastered before being smoothed into the exercise as usually performed, we turned our everyday clientele into the best moving general population of any gym in the world.

The best moving general population in the world? *Really?* Okay, okay, I'm exaggerating. A little. *Maybe.* But I will claim without reservation that teaching movements as a series of positions to be practiced one-at-time made a startling difference in the quality of our members' athletic development—and they were good to start with.

I've never seen a gym with standards stricter than ours. How could there be? We require our clients to strive for ideal positions in their movements. Will anybody ever reach that ne plus ultra? Probably not. By definition, an ideal is practically unattainable. But that doesn't mean we make our athletes feel nothing will ever be good enough. It doesn't mean we don't praise their efforts as they strive for perfection. It just means we have job security.

The Advantages of Teaching Pose-to-Pose

Teaching pose-to-pose has a number of advantages over the way the exercises MMGPP programs are traditionally instructed:

1. Working pose-to-pose improves athletes' proprioception, as holding a pose gives them time to make sense of the relative positions of limbs and trunk.

2. Holding poses aids in trainees' forming muscle memory, expediting their progress from learning basic mechanics to being able to perform an exercise with consistently good form.

3. Drilling poses allows corrections to be made in real time, while the errors are occurring.

4. Pose-to-pose is a powerful tool for instructing large groups, especially in complex movements like the clean or Turkish get-up. I'll never forget the day we did a "Bring a Buddy" WOD that had 40 people in our gym—20 of our athletes, and 20 people who'd never done any MMGPP. Working with one assistant instructor, by teaching the air squat BtN-style, I was able to get those 20 newbies squatting to standard in about five minutes. It gave me goose bumps!

That was when I knew we were really onto something.

5. Positional training makes learning new movements easier, as athletes come to understand commonalities between exercises.

6. Teaching pose-to-pose standardizes instruction, so all of your trainees are getting the same information, no matter who happens to be teaching.

At my gym, our instructor cadre strives ceaselessly to get our athletes to hit aesthetically pleasing positions in every rep of an exercise. We *will* our athletes into being always in the right place, at always the right time. We're not just trainers, we're artists, we're animators—kinetic sculptors, if you will. Using BtN, you can be one, too.

MMGPP By the Numbers

Over time, By the Numbers has become more than just a way to teach movement. It's now, dare I say, a complete pedagogical method. That method is based on a set of principles that prioritize movement integrity over exercise intensity.

1. Every exercise utilized in MMGPP programming can be placed in a category of movements ordered from least to most complex. For instance, the "Push Object (Vertical)" hierarchy includes the press, push press, push jerk, and split jerk.

2. Every exercise should be introduced in its simplest version (in the above case, the press). Athletes must master each variation before being introduced to the next.

3. Initial movement instruction should emphasize discrete positions, rather than complete motor patterns.

4. Certain poses are common to multiple exercises, as they arise these commonalities should be pointed out. This expedites the learning process. For instance, Front Squat Position 2 (FS 2) is exactly the same as Power Clean Position 7 (PC 7). The hip hinge and torso angle of Deadlift Position 2 (DL 2) is

similar to that of Russian Swing Position 1 (RS 1).

5. In a MMGPP class, there is a time to learn, a time to practice, and a time to perform. Skills-based warm-ups, coaching pairs, and strength training are practice—they develop movement skill. Metabolic conditioning workouts (WODs) are performance—they test (and hopefully prove) movement skill. (We'll leave aside for the moment the idea that WODs develop work capacity.)

6. During practice, execution should be methodical and deliberate, with mistakes addressed immediately.

7. When it's time to perform, make sure your athletes are each doing an exercise appropriate to their level of development, one which preserves the desired training stimulus.

8. During performance, athletes whose technique degrades due to fatigue and are not responsive to correction should default to the next movement down in the hierarchy of complexity.

9. Intensity is movement agnostic. During WODs, always prefer a simple exercise performed well to a more complex movement executed poorly.

In short, BtN promotes virtuosity.

By the Numbers and the Road to Virtuosity

Virtuosity, according to CrossFit founder Greg Glassman, means "doing the common uncommonly well." For athletes, virtuosity is a quality that arises from mastering technique so completely that technique disappears, leaving only beauty.

For coaches, virtuosity is much more humble and homespun. Virtuosic coaching is about insisting on fundamentals. In BtN we teach and coach positionally, because what could be more fundamental than the relationships between limbs and trunk, the shifts of weight, the trajectories of applied force that define each successive stage of a movement?

But we have to take it further than that. We must insist that athletes work their way up to performing the high-skill exercises we program by starting with the simplest of movements, and then gradually learning and mastering more and more complex variants. To become truly proficient athletes, to gain any ground on virtuosity, our athletes have to work their way through the Movement Hierarchies.

Chapter Two
THE GREAT CHAIN OF BEING AWESOME

You know what sucks? A gym full of athletes moving poorly.

You know what's awesome? A gym full of athletes moving well.

You know what makes the difference between the two? Movement Hierarchies.

What are Movement Hierarchies?

On a macro level, the desired training effect of a well-designed MMGPP-style metabolic conditioning workout is always increased work capacity across broad time and modal domains. On a micro level, each exercise that comprises the WOD is also a stimulus of a specific type. For example, in a workout like this...

> *Ten rounds for time of*
> 5 power cleans @ 155/108lbs,
> 6 ring dips
> 7 toes-to-bar

...the prescribed exercises can be classified as 5 repetitions of "Pull Object (ground to shoulder)", 6 reps of "Push Away from Object (vertical)"; and 7 reps of "Hip and Trunk Flexion (hanging, straight leg)". These descriptive types define categories of exercises. In By the Numbers, we refer to these types as **Movement Hierarchies**.

Movement Hierarchies are exercises that all approximate the same stimulus. These exercises are ordered in terms of increasing complexity (required strength, flexibility, balance, coordination, etc). Movement Hierarchies are the road map that can guide an athlete, in a logical fashion, from clumsy newbie status all the way to virtuosic firebreather.

Everyone should squat...but should everyone overhead squat? Everyone should have a technique that allows them to take a load from the ground to a secure position on the shoulder, but should all athletes barbell clean?

I don't think so. Not immediately, anyway. Not everybody has the shoulder flexibility to overhead squat. Nobody who has not mastered the front squat should attempt a clean. Putting a piece of PVC pipe in a beginner's hand and telling them "Just do your best!" doesn't cut it—and I'm speaking as someone who, in the early days of my career, did just that.

The overhead squat and the clean sit at the apex of their respective Movement Hierarchies. For instance, the Squat hierarchy goes like this: box squat, air squat, dumbbell squat, back squat, front squat, overhead squat. Each squat requires a more upright torso, more flexibility of the back and shoulders, and better balance than the last. Each is more challenging. Each is more complex. Athletes must work their way through these progressions during practice, trying and failing, gradually improving. Then, in a WOD, when it's time to test their movement skill and improve their work capacity, both you and they will know exactly which version of an exercise to use: the one they can consistently perform to standard. That's not necessarily the one written on the white board!

For instance, imagine the workout of the day in your box is five rounds for time of a 400m run and 15 overhead squats (95/65lbs). Many people, even experienced athletes, lack the mobility to do them correctly. So when a workout like this comes up in the programming, what do you do with a big, strong guy who can't overhead squat much more than an empty barbell?

Traditionally, the answer was "scale". That meant retaining the movement, but reducing the load. But for someone who hasn't mastered the basic mechanics of an exercise, whether because of inexperience or physical restriction, any intensity is going to have a negative impact on execution, even with a negligible weight. What you end up with is an athlete doing 75 sub-par repetitions.

That's not going to make our big guy better at overhead squats. It's just going to further ingrain bad motor patterns. A better choice is to have him default back through the movement hierarchy to find the most complex movement he can do well.

BtN's rule of thumb is, **during WODs, always prefer a simple exercise performed well to a more complex movement executed poorly**. Can our guy front squat? Awesome! Load him up and let him rip. Or, if he lacks the mobility for decent front squats, drop back one more level in the hierarchy. Let him take the barbell out of the rack for five rounds of runs and back squats.

Which do you think has the superior metabolic conditioning ROI for our strong, experienced, but inflexible athlete: seventy-five piss-poor overhead squats with an empty barbell, or seventy-five good back squats at 135 pounds? This athlete will have a much better workout if you don't allow him to attempt something he's not ready for.

BtN Movement Hierarchies Defined

On the next nine pages you'll find the By the Numbers Movement Hierarchies, first in chart form, and then a bulleted list.

Vertically, the hierarchies start with the simplest movement that preserves a desired training stimulus. Each exercise beneath represents an increase in complexity, in terms of demands on flexibility, balance, coordination, etc.*

Horizontally, the movements are staggered to indicate how more complex exercises are dependent on less complex. For instance, the Turkish get-up is built on the floor press, the sit-up, and the walking lunge, so a trainee should be competent with all three before learning the TGU.

Feel free to alter and embellish these exercise progressions as you see fit. Just make sure you offer your athletes progressions for *everything*.

---

* There are a few exercises listed that would seem to be misfits in their category; for instance, I put the GHD sit-up in the hierarchy "Hip and Trunk Flexion (seated)", even though trunk flexion is exactly what you don't want in that movement. A sit-up's a sit-up, though, and rather than create a whole new category, I crammed it in with the rest.

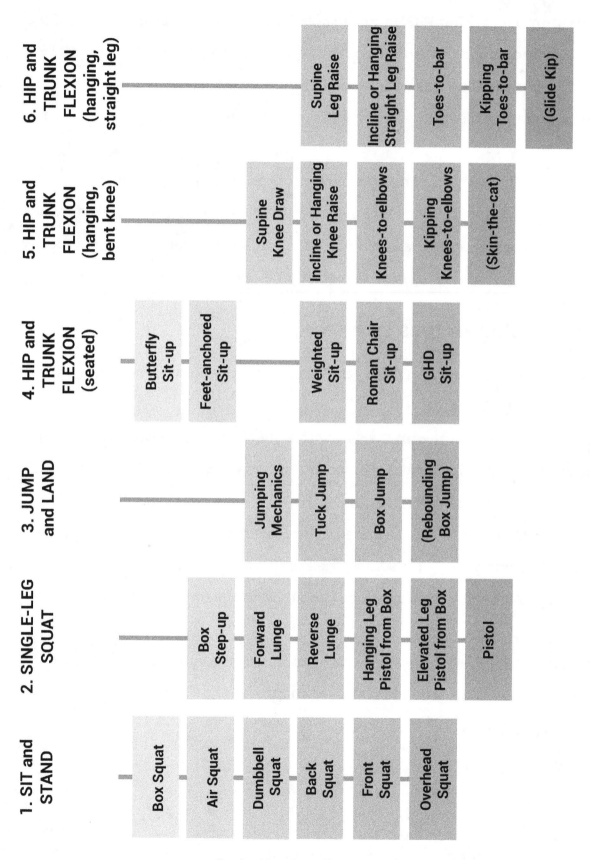

By the Numbers Movement Hierarchies

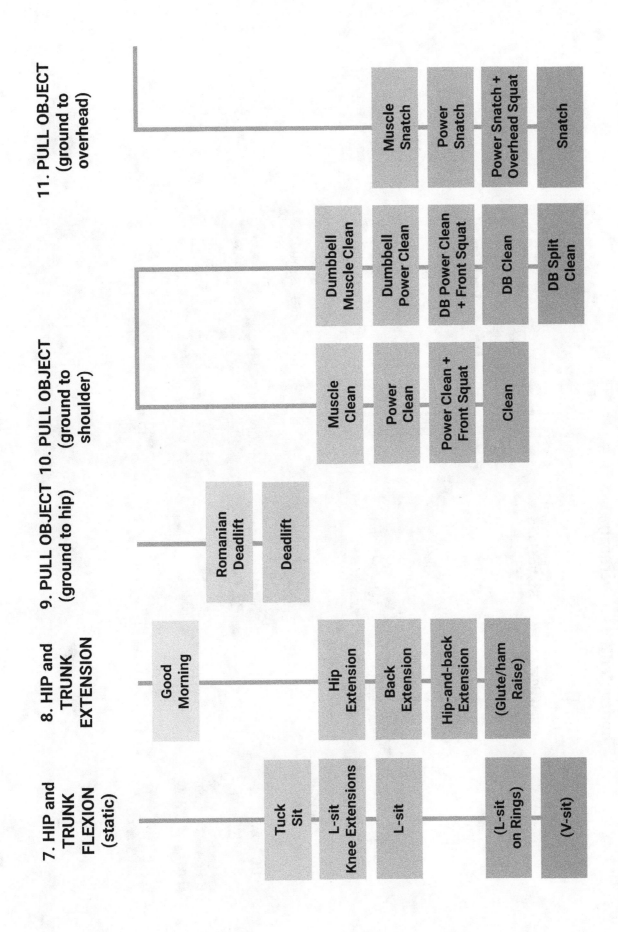

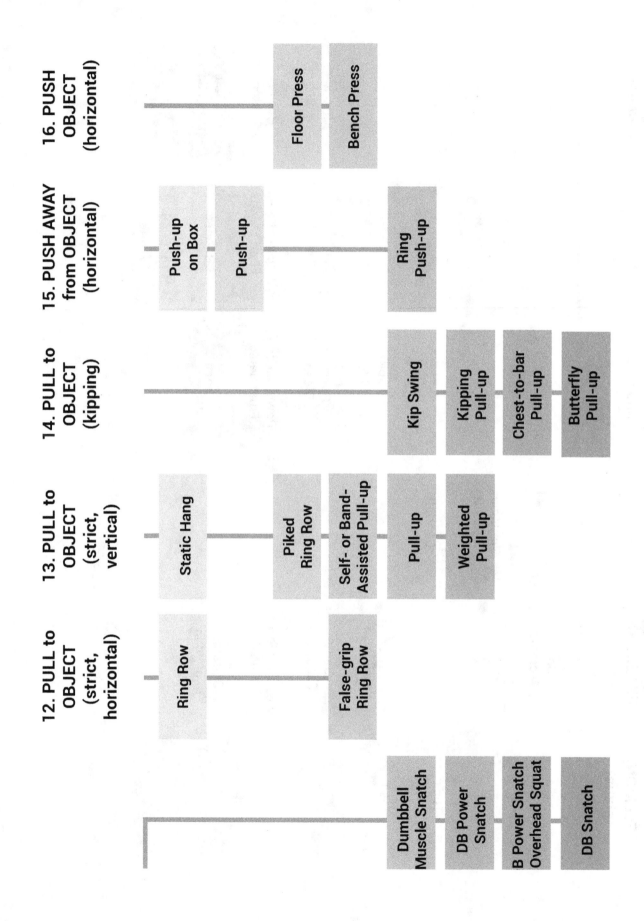

16. PUSH OBJECT (horizontal)
- Floor Press
- Bench Press

15. PUSH AWAY from OBJECT (horizontal)
- Push-up on Box
- Push-up
- Ring Push-up

14. PULL to OBJECT (kipping)
- Kip Swing
- Kipping Pull-up
- Chest-to-bar Pull-up
- Butterfly Pull-up

13. PULL to OBJECT (strict, vertical)
- Static Hang
- Piked Ring Row
- Self- or Band-Assisted Pull-up
- Pull-up
- Weighted Pull-up

12. PULL to OBJECT (strict, horizontal)
- Ring Row
- False-grip Ring Row

- Dumbbell Muscle Snatch
- DB Power Snatch
- DB Power Snatch Overhead Squat
- DB Snatch

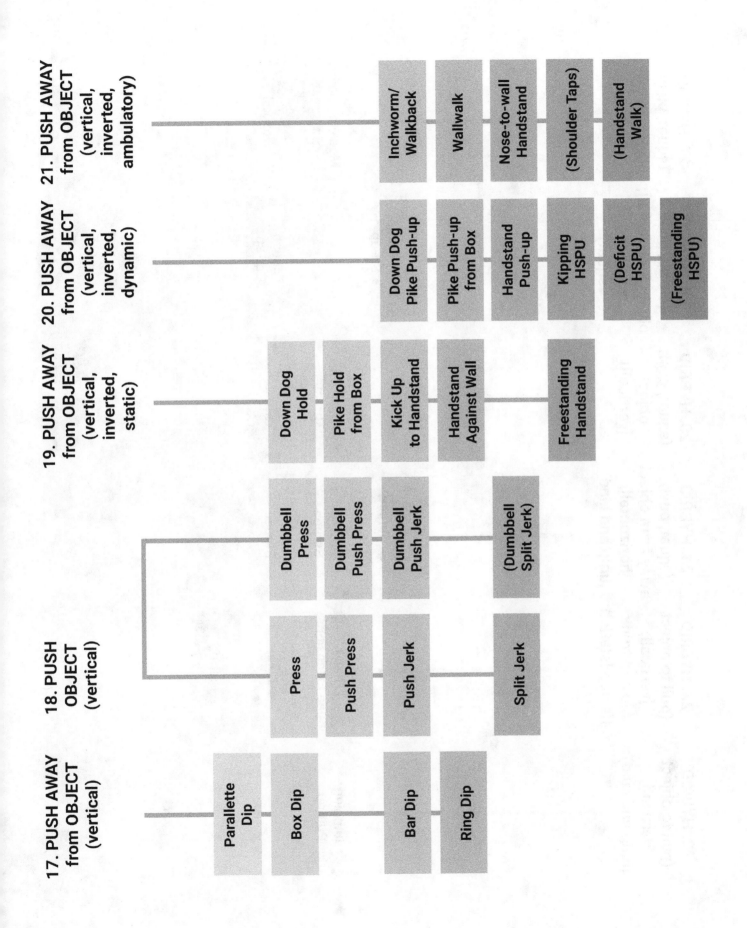

17. PUSH AWAY from OBJECT (vertical)

- Parallette Dip
- Box Dip
- Bar Dip
- Ring Dip

18. PUSH OBJECT (vertical)

- Press
- Push Press
- Push Jerk
- Split Jerk

- Dumbbell Press
- Dumbbell Push Press
- Dumbbell Push Jerk
- (Dumbbell Split Jerk)

19. PUSH AWAY from OBJECT (vertical, inverted, static)

- Down Dog Hold
- Pike Hold from Box
- Kick Up to Handstand
- Handstand Against Wall
- Freestanding Handstand

20. PUSH AWAY from OBJECT (vertical, inverted, dynamic)

- Down Dog Pike Push-up
- Pike Push-up from Box
- Handstand Push-up
- Kipping HSPU
- (Deficit HSPU)
- (Freestanding HSPU)

21. PUSH AWAY from OBJECT (vertical, inverted, ambulatory)

- Inchworm/Walkback
- Wallwalk
- Nose-to-wall Handstand
- (Shoulder Taps)
- (Handstand Walk)

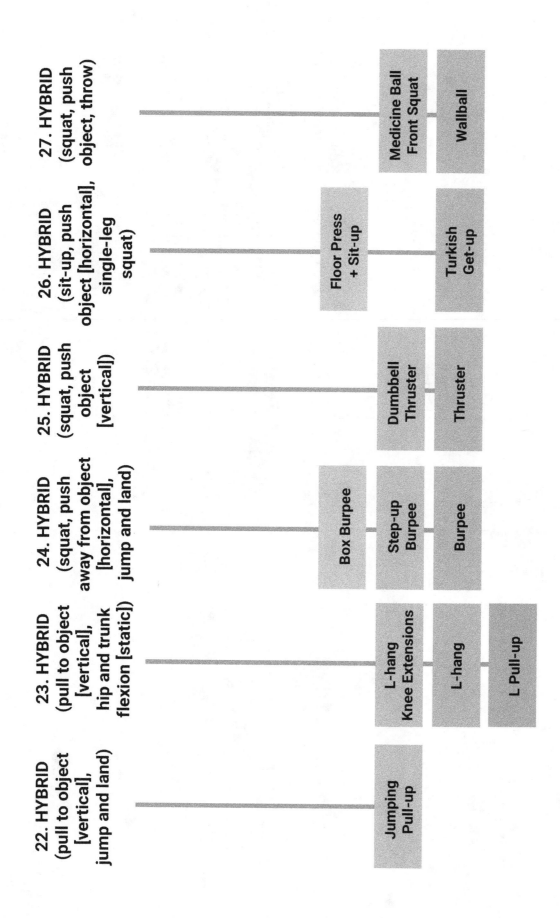

22. HYBRID (pull to object [vertical], jump and land)

Jumping Pull-up

23. HYBRID (pull to object [vertical], hip and trunk flexion [static])

L-hang Knee Extensions

L-hang

L Pull-up

24. HYBRID (squat, push away from object [horizontal], jump and land)

Box Burpee

Step-up Burpee

Burpee

25. HYBRID (squat, push object [vertical])

Dumbbell Thruster

Thruster

26. HYBRID (sit-up, push object [horizontal], single-leg squat)

Floor Press + Sit-up

Turkish Get-up

27. HYBRID (squat, push object, throw)

Medicine Ball Front Squat

Wallball

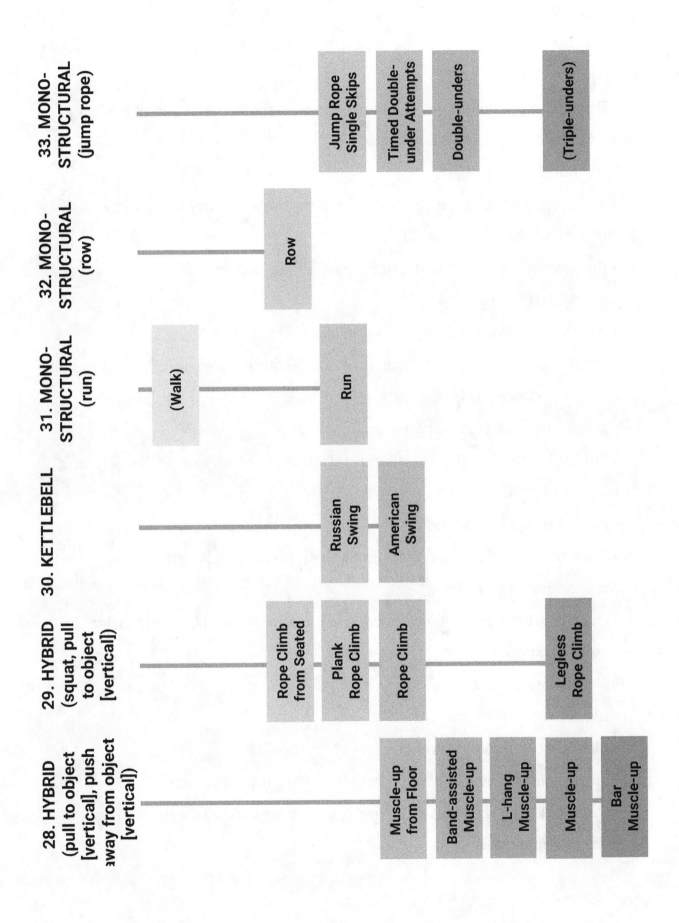

33. MONO-STRUCTURAL (jump rope)
- Jump Rope Single Skips
- Timed Double-under Attempts
- Double-unders
- (Triple-unders)

32. MONO-STRUCTURAL (row)
- Row

31. MONO-STRUCTURAL (run)
- (Walk)
- Run

30. KETTLEBELL
- Russian Swing
- American Swing

29. HYBRID (squat, pull to object [vertical])
- Rope Climb from Seated
- Plank Rope Climb
- Rope Climb
- Legless Rope Climb

28. HYBRID (pull to object [vertical], push away from object [vertical])
- Muscle-up from Floor
- Band-assisted Muscle-up
- L-hang Muscle-up
- Muscle-up
- Bar Muscle-up

1. *Sit and Stand*

   • Box squat, air squat, dumbbell squat, back squat, front squat, overhead squat

2. *Single-leg Squat*

   • Box step-up, forward lunge, reverse lunge, hanging-leg pistol from box, elevated-leg pistol from box, pistol

3. *Jump and Land*

   • Jumping mechanics, tuck jump, box jump, (rebounding box jump)*

4. *Hip and Trunk Flexion (seated)*

   • Butterfly sit-up, feet-anchored military sit-up, weighted sit-up, Roman chair sit-up, GHD sit-up

5. *Hip and Trunk Flexion (hanging, bent knee)*

   • Supine knee draw, incline or hanging knee raise, knees-to-elbows, kipping knees-to-elbows, (skin-the cat)*

6. *Hip and Trunk Flexion (hanging, straight leg)*

   • Supine leg raise, incline or hanging straight leg raise, toes-to-bar, kipping toes-to-bar, (glide kip)*

7. *Hip and Trunk Flexion (static)*

   • Tuck sit, L-sit knee extensions, L-sit, (L-sit on rings)*, (V-sit)*

8. *Hip and Trunk Extension*

   • Good morning, hip extension, back extension, hip and back extension, (glute ham raise)*

9. *Pull Object (ground to hip)*

   • Romanian deadlift, deadlift

10. *Pull Object (ground to shoulder)*

   • Muscle clean, power clean, power clean + front squat, clean

   • Dumbbell muscle clean, db power clean, db power clean + front squat, db clean, db split clean

---

* Exercises in asterisked parentheses are logically implied by their particular movement hierarchy, but aren't covered in this book.

11. *Pull Object (ground to overhead)*

- Muscle snatch, power snatch, power snatch + overhead squat, snatch
- Dumbbell muscle snatch, db power snatch, db power snatch + overhead squat, db snatch

12. *Pull to Object (strict, horizontal)*

- Ring row, false grip ring row

13. *Pull to Object (strict, vertical)*

- Static hang, piked ring row, self- or band-assisted pull-up, pull-up, weighted pull-up

14. *Pull to Object (kipping)*

- Kip swing, kipping pull-ups, chest-to-bar kipping pull-up, butterfly pull-up

15. *Push Away from Object (horizontal)*

- Push-up from box, push-up, ring push-up

16. *Push Object (horizontal)*

- Floor press, bench press

17. *Push Away from Object (vertical)*

- Parallette dip, box dip, bar dip, ring dip

18. *Push Object (vertical)*

- Press, push press, push jerk, split jerk
- Dumbbell press, db push press, db push jerk, db split jerk

19. *Push Away from Object (vertical, inverted, static)*

- Down dog pike hold, pike hold from box, kick up to handstand, wall-assisted handstand, (freestanding handstand)*

20. *Push Away from Object (vertical, inverted, dynamic)*

- Down dog push-up, pike push-up from box, handstand push-up, kipping HSPU, (deficit HSPU) *, (freestanding HSPU)*

21. *Push Away from Object (vertical, inverted, ambulatory)*

- Inchworm/walkback, wallwalk, nose-to-wall handstand, (shoulder taps)*,

(handstand walk)*

22. *Hybrid (pull to object [vertical], jump and land)*

   • Jumping pull-up

23. *Hybrid (pull to object [vertical], hip and trunk flexion [static])*

   • L-hang knee extensions, L-hang, L pull-up

24. *Hybrid (squat, push-up, jump and land)*

   • Box burpee, step-up burpee, burpee

25. *Hybrid (squat, push object)*

   • Dumbbell thrusters, thrusters

26. *Hybrid (sit-up, push object, single-leg squat)*

   • Floor press and sit-up, Turkish get-up

27. *Hybrid (squat, push object, throw)*

   • Medicine ball front squats, wallballs

28. *Hybrid (pull to object [vertical], push away from object [vertical])*

   • Muscle-up from floor, band-assisted muscle-up, L-hang muscle-up, muscle-up, bar muscle-up

29. *Hybrid (squat, pull to object [vertical])*

   •Rope climb from seated, plank rope climb, rope climb, legless rope climb

30. *Kettlebells*

   • Russian swing, American swing

31. *Monostructural (run)*

   • (Walk)*, run

32. *Monostructural (row)*

   • Row

33. *Monostructural (jump rope)*

   • Rope skips, timed double-under attempts, double-unders

Movement Hierarchies Applied Pedagogically

Introducing New Movements

All athletes should be introduced to a new movement beginning with the simplest exercise in its Hierarchy.

Imagine you've got a group of five athletes of varying ability just entering your program. It's Day 1, and you need to teach them how to squat. You *could* start them with the air squat—definitely a universal motor pattern.

However, more likely than not, there's going to be at least one member of your group who will have trouble with even this seemingly most basic of exercises. The cause might be tight hamstrings, a weak lower back, hip impingement, missing ankle dorsiflexion... you name it! And no matter how fine your instruction is, no matter how you cue, that person is not going to be able to do an acceptable air squat—not today, anyway. You're going to spend an inordinate amount of time trying to get them moving decently and then, when you realize it's futile, you're either going to let it slide—"Okay, that's the best we're going to get"—or you're going to go get them a box or whatever other orthosis they need to approximate good positions. Either way, at some level, that athlete, acutely self-conscious that they are not keeping up with the group, will feel embarrassed and alienated.

Needless to say, this is not how you want someone to start out in your program! Many people coming into a MMGPP class for the first time are intimidated and anxious, if not outright terrified. Especially early on, they need to feel like they can succeed in this "extreme" endeavor. Setting them up for success is critical. In this instance, the way you do that is with the box squat.

Anyone who can use the toilet by themselves can box squat. If you give everyone in your group of five a 12" box with three Abmats stacked on it, every one of your new trainees will be able to sit down on the top pad, and then stand back up. (If they can't, their ability to participate in a MMGPP program, at least in a group context, is in serious question.) If one of your trainees has some form trouble—rounds his back, shifts his weight onto the balls of his feet—that athlete can keep working to three Abmats, while you have everyone else take away a mat to increase range-of-motion. As you progress the rest of the group toward a full box squat, your needs-a-little-extra-help trainee will not feel on the spot or left out. He's just working at the appropriate level of challenge.

This same approach will be used as the group is gradually, over the course of several weeks, introduced to the rest of the exercises in the squat hierarchy. Each new squat builds on the last, adding an additional layer of challenge to your athletes' strength, flexibility, and balance. Only when athletes demonstrate competence in a given movement (say, by doing ten reps with good form) should they be taught the next movement in the chain.

Some gyms have attempted to implement protocols like Gray Cook's Functional Movement Screen to formally determine who might have problems performing certain exercises. If you have the bandwidth to apply the FMS to every individual who wants to join your program, more power to you! But I believe that the simple exercises at the base of each Movement Hierarchy serve as convenient, accurate, and most importantly, efficient screens in themselves. As they are introduced to new exercises, everyone in the group is screened at once; athletes identified as having motor control and/or flexibility issues will stay at the level that challenges their competence. For the trainer running a program based on groups, rather than individual training, this is invaluable.

Teaching More Complex Variations to a Group of Varied Ability

Regular MMGPP classes are very heterogeneous, with athletes ranging from nervous newbs just out of Fundamentals, to old salts who have PRs for many benchmark WODs. No matter what their level of experience, they *all* need coaching if they want to improve.

The best way to help athletes realize this goal is to regularly program technique review sessions based on a specific movement hierarchy, followed by a period of deliberate practice or coaching pairs (which will be discussed in the next chapter).

Suppose the topic of the day is the clean. You are working with a dozen athletes, each of them at different stages of competence with that challenging movement. Here's how you could structure your session:

1. Begin with a demonstration and explanation of the muscle clean, segueing into a group Positional Drill in which the athletes adopt, at your command, the various poses of the exercise. They hold these positions while you make any necessary corrections. This serves as both technique review, and warm-up. Athletes who demonstrate competence with the muscle clean can then work on their power clean. Otherwise, they keep working on their muscle clean.

2. Explain the catch position of the power clean. Ask your group of muscle clean-competent athletes to adopt it. This serves as a movement screen: if an athlete can't hit a decent receiving position, thinking carefully and moving deliberately, he's not ready for the power clean. He should stick with the muscle clean, but he'll add another step: after receiving the bar on his shoulders, he'll sit down into a partial front squat, stretching, self-assessing, self-correcting. Meanwhile, you take those who *are* ready for the power clean through the appropriate Positional Drills.

3. From there, challenge your power clean-competent students by adding a front squat. Those whose front squats are still developing could stick with the power clean, or practice the front squat in this new context, at your discretion. In the background, those constrained to muscle cleans are still doing muscle cleans, and you take care to check in regularly with them.

4. Finally, you introduce the clean. Only a fraction of your group has proven advanced enough to work on the full movement. Has their time been wasted by drilling the positions of the muscle clean, power clean, and power clean + front squat variations? No way! Practicing perfect fundamentals always, *always* makes for improved performance of complex movements. It's the willingness to practice and perfect the basics that distinguishes the excellent from the mediocre.

The whole process takes about ten minutes. Small, correctible mistakes are okay. Large mistakes of positioning or sequencing are not—they're an indication fundamentals have not been mastered. By the end, all of your athletes will have found the variation that challenges, but doesn't exceed, their ability. From here it's very important that you make time and space for them to practice and internalize what they've just learned—we'll discuss Practice Mode in Chapter Three.

Movement Hierarchies Applied Prescriptively

In a class setting, it's appropriate to use a technical review of a Movement Hierarchy to determine appropriate level of challenge. For instance, earlier we described a WOD involving power cleans, dips, and toes-to-bar. If you were going to run a group of five athletes through that workout, how would you use the Movement Hierarchy concept to figure out what version of the toes-to-bar each athlete should use?

According to By the Numbers, toes-to-bar is under the category Hip and Trunk Flexion (straight leg, hanging). Even though everyone in your group claims to know how to do toes-to-bar, you start at the bottom of the hierarchy anyway: "Okay, crew, we'll begin with supine straight leg raises." You describe and demo the movement. The supine straight leg raise is a toes-to-bar reduced to its essence: lying on the floor, gripping the post of a pull-up bar for an anchor, you bring your extended legs from parallel with the floor to perpendicular. You then contract your abdominal muscles to curl your trunk, bringing your toes up to tap the post behind you.

Then you have your group try it. Everybody gets five reps of the supine leg raise. Great! You up the ante. "If that was easy, next try a hanging straight leg raise." Again, describe and demo. Although the range of motion of the hip is a little shorter than in the supine version (just a bit over 90 degrees), the hanging leg raise (hLR) is much more difficult, as a) you are suspending your full weight by your hands, and b) the rising feet move away from the line of gravity and acquire moment, increasing the load on the hip.

Aha! When the group tries out the hLR, only three of the athletes can do a set of at least five high-quality reps. You instruct the two who failed to get 5 reps to stick with the supine leg raise in today's workout. Meanwhile, they can keep practicing their hLRs while you go over the strict toes-to-bar bar with the remaining three athletes.

In gymnastics, the toes-to-bar is a slow, controlled movement. Hanging from a bar, with feet together and legs straight, the athlete flexes the hip, then curls the trunk and extends the shoulder until the toes meet the bar. The feet describe a semi-circle in the air. This exercise requires a great deal of hip, trunk, back, and grip strength, as well as flexibility in the hamstrings and lower back.

One athlete can do eight in a row, the next gets four, the last, only three. The latter two will be instructed to begin the workout doing strict toes-to-bar. However, when intensity degrades their performance past a certain threshold, a simpler movement, one that preserves the intended stimulus, should be substituted. At that point, they'll default back through the hierarchy to the next movement down—hanging leg raises. For now, though, they can work on increasing their strict toes-to-bar numbers while you teach your eight-reps athlete the kipping T2B.

Only a trainee who can do at least five strict toes-to-bar should be allowed to do the "kipping" variation so popular today.* Why? Because's she earned it. The kipping toes-to-bar should be reserved for those who meet a baseline of strength and body control. This athlete has met that standard, so now she can increase the intensity by upping the tempo.

But shouldn't the others learn to kip the movement too, if it means they do more work in less time? Isn't that the whole point? No. Teaching new athletes the toes-to-bar as a swing-up-and-kick does them a grave disservice. It will never help them achieve a strict toes-to-bar, thus missing an opportunity to develop their strength, flexibility, and coordination. Often, their attempts to implement the "coaching" they've been given will put them in danger, as they lack basic grip strength and shoulder stability to buffer against the force created by globally extending and flexing the torso while hanging from the pull-up bar. And finally, at some point, their progress will be halted by their lack of a fundamental skill. Then they'll really be in trouble; having done the movement incorrectly for so long, it'll be

---

* Please note that "five strict reps" is not a law carved in stone; I think it's a reasonable requirement, but feel free to set the bar wherever you think is appropriate.

very difficult to break bad habits. In the long run, going slow and getting it right in the first place is the superior approach.

Will you hear some grumbling from those athletes who feel "demoted" from doing their usual swing-up-and-kick toes-to-bar? Yeah, probably. Pay it no mind. Cutting corners to do half-baked versions of legitimately challenging exercises subverts MMGPP training's potential to be a vehicle for self-actualization. So don't let your athletes get away with it. Be a hardass and insist your athletes master each element of a progression. Build them a solid foundation of strength and skill before allowing them to advance through the Movement Hierarchy to attempt competition-derived techniques. And if they try to push too hard too soon, insist that they perform WODs only with exercises they've mastered.

Do this, and your gym will be full of awesome. Guaranteed.

Chapter Three
ARE YOU MR. GARRISON, OR MR. CHIPS?

I often tell prospective clients that a MMGPP facility has more in common with a martial arts school than a regular gym. A beginner doesn't take a couple weeks of lessons in muay thai or Brazilian jiu jitsu and then begin cage fighting with only a referee to keep him from getting killed. It takes months and years of rigorous training under the watchful eye of an experienced instructor before a novice fighter is ready to go full power against an opponent.

So it is with MMGPP. Learning how to implement MMGPP training is a non-trivial task. Each of the training modalities we draw on is a discipline in its own right that can take years to master. So you as an instructor have to understand that your responsibility for the edification and guidance of your clients does not end when they've finished their Elements or Fundamentals classes. It also doesn't end after you've finished reading the WOD off the white board or demoing movement standards. For as long as they are paying you, from the moment class begins to the moment it ends, you have an obligation to engage with your clients. *You have to help them learn.*

This engagement is qualitatively different depending on the job at hand. Rather than try to list all the different training tasks that might comprise a class, BtN postulates general modes of activity for instructors and athletes.

Instructors have two modes: **teaching** and **coaching**. Athletes have three: **learning**, **practicing**, and **performing**. These modes are both descriptions of general pedagogic goals, and prescriptions for how trainer and athlete should interact during class time.

ATHLETE MODES

LEARNING

When your athletes are striving to understand new concepts and committing information to memory, they are in **Learning Mode**. Athletes in Learning Mode may be static, standing still while listening to you expound and explain, or they may be dynamic, trying out the positions of an exercise at your direction.

Learning Mode begins within the first five minutes of Day 1. It recurs every time an athlete is introduced to the next element in a given movement hierarchy.

PRACTICE

In **Practice Mode,** athletes are trying to apply what they have learned. They are not working against the clock, and so can relax and concentrate as they experiment, make mistakes, and receive correction. In BtN, Practice Mode activities are usually scheduled for the first part of class, as part of the warm-up. But they could also be used as a reset/technique review session just before a metcon finisher, or at the end of class as cool down work.

Practice Mode has two goals:

1. Turning knowledge into ability.
2. Turning ability into mastery.

Forms of Practice

Skill-based warm-ups, coaching pairs, and strength training sessions all forms of practice.

Skills-based Warm-ups

Skills-based warm-ups include deliberate practice sessions, calisthenics circuits, baby benchmarks, and EMOM/EOMOMs.

Deliberate practice is critical to success in By the Numbers. Too often if you hand someone a barbell and tell them "Go practice your clean" they'll robotically repeat the same motor pattern again and again, and finish the practice period having made no improvement. Deliberate practice, on the other hand, "refers to a form of training that consists of focused, gruelling, repetitive practice" of small and very specific sections of a skill "in which the subject continuously monitors his or her performance, and subsequently corrects, experiments, and reacts to immediate and constant feedback, with the aim of steady and consistent improvement." (quantum3.co.za, 2013)

Deliberate practice is the path to mastery.

BtN advocates setting aside time in every class for your athletes to engage in deliberate practice of the movement(s) they'll be using in that day's workout. Here are some examples of BtN deliberate practice sessions (more can be found in Appendix II):

1. For ten minutes: your choice of Pull Object (ground to shoulder) exercise: muscle clean, power clean, power clean + front squat, clean. Do at least one iteration of each exercise in the hierarchy as you work your way up to the appropriate level of complexity. Once there, work slowly and carefully, pausing to self-assess and correct after assuming each new position.

2. Choose one Push Away from Object (Vertical, inverted, dynamic) exercise and practice its positions for five minutes: down dog pike push-up, pike push-up from box, handstand push-up, deficit handstand push-up.

3. Pick one barbell squat exercise—back squat, front squat, overhead squat—and work on it for seven minutes. Drill its three positions one-at-a-time, spending 5 seconds hanging out in "the hole." If you have mobility issues affecting your front or overhead squats, address them between sets.

The iterative process of assessment and correction can be self-directed, managed by the instructor (you), or performed in coaching pairs.

Calisthenic circuits are effective dynamic warm-ups and offer a chance to get in some additional exercise volume, practiced mindfully, they are a fantastic opportunity to acquire and refine skills. Here are a few examples:

1. Two rounds of Samson stretch x 20 sec., air squats x 10 reps, butterfly sit-ups x 10, PVC good mornings x 10, ring rows x 10, push-ups x 10. As the athlete gains experience and strength, more volume can be added, and more complex exercises substituted (.e.g., overhead squat, GHD sit-ups, back extensions, kipping pull-ups, ring dips, etc.).

2. Two rounds of reverse lunges x 5/side, 10 strict toes-to-bar, single-leg Romanian deadlifts x 5/side, kick up to handstand x 5, 10 kip swings. A more advanced version of the same warm-up would be two rounds of pistols x 5/side, kipping toes-to-bar x 10, contralateral dumbbell single-leg Romanian deadlifts x 5/side, 10 handstand push-ups, 10 chest-to-bar pull-ups

3. Three rounds of the parallette complex (push-up, shoot through, dip, swing back) x 5, plus 10 kip swings. Then accrue one minute of L-sit in three 20 second efforts.

Don't allow your athletes to mindlessly, mechanically bang through these circuits! If there's a time to turn off their brains and just go for it, it's certainly not now. Make sure they understand that technical improvement only comes through attention to detail. And if they don't care about technique, well...change their minds. It's your gym, and ultimately you are the biggest influence on its culture.

Baby benchmarks use minimal loads and are not for time. Couplets with more complex exercises have reduced volume, to allow the trainees time to work on their technique.

1. 21-15-9 reps not for time of calorie row (1-2-3-4-3-2-1*) and GHD sit-ups (3-1-2-3)

2. 15-10-5 of muscle snatches (1-2-3-4-5-6-7) w/ empty barbell and strict chin-ups (1-2-1)

---

* Numbers in parentheses refer to numbered positions that make up the movement.

3. 15-10-5 of hang cleans (4-3-4-5-6-7-8) w/ empty barbell and ring dips (1-2-1)

You don't have to limit yourself to couplets. Just make sure to keep the volume relatively low and keep the focus on technique development. Each exercise should be performed as a series of positions, rather than a complete motor pattern. Emphasize that the goal is skill-development, *not* racing to be the first done.

EMOMs (every minute on the minute) and **EOMOMs** (every *other* minute on the minute) take the couplet concept and turn it into a group activity, e.g., every other minute on the minute for ten minutes (EOMOM 10), on even minutes, everybody does this, on odd minutes, everybody does that. EOMOM warm-ups are usually written so each minute's work takes about 30 seconds.

1. EOMOM 10. Even minutes: wall walks x 2. Odd minutes: L-sit knee extensions x 10.

2. EOMOM 10. Even minutes: chin-ups x 8. Odd minutes: pistols (alternating sides) x 4.

3. EOMOM 10. Even minutes: Turkish get-up x 1. Odd minutes: American swings x 8. Take your time, work good positions.

Coaching Pairs

Coaching pairs put two athletes together to work through BtN positional drills. One of the pair works as athlete, while the other assumes role of coach. The coach calls out positions to the practicing athlete, reviews his performance, and allows him to move on only when his positions meet the standard.

This arrangement benefits you, the instructor, and both of your clients. The "coach" is developing an eye for good movement, the "athlete" is moving under close supervision, and you don't have to try to have eyes on everyone at once. After a couple of supervised drills, the athletes reverse roles, and continue switching back and forth for the duration of the practice period.

Strength Training

Strength training is not done against the clock, and there's plenty of time for feedback and correction, so it's considered practice. Increasing load over time improves the athlete's capacity for force production, stress tests the athlete's technique, and, programmed correctly, can help determine proper loading for the day's WOD.

The movement hierarchy ensures that everyone strength training is working at the correct level of challenge. Not everyone needs to train the same movement. For instance, an athlete who lacks (and will lack for some time) the mobility to set up correctly for the deadlift can still use his practice time to get stronger by increasing loads on the Romanian deadlift, even as training the rDL helps improve his flexibility until he is eventually able to do a full deadlift from the floor.

Programming Skills-based Warm-ups

Skills-based warm-ups should be part of every single class. Keep their format constantly varied, as you might the elements in the WOD; over a seven day microcycle, try to make sure at least four days include deliberate practice sessions. And there's nothing wrong with doubling up, combining, say, a calisthenic WU and deliberate practice, or deliberate practice, and then an EOMOM. Five minutes of dynamic warm-up, twenty minutes of dedicated skill work, fifteen minutes of strength work, a ten minute ass-whupping finisher, ten minutes of cooldown mobility work—now that's a class!

PERFORMANCE

MMGPP training is rightfully famous for its wild metabolic conditioning ("metcon") workouts, which are done for points or for time, with the goal of maximizing power output. Friendly competition among peers to get the highest score or fastest time to completion drives athletes to push harder than they might on their own. There are benefits and drawbacks to this model, but ultimately, metcons are the *sine qua non* of MMGPP.

In the By the Numbers system, during metcons, athletes are in **Performance Mode**. An athlete in Performance Mode has two goals:

1. To display mastery of the assigned movements under conditions of stress.
2. To develop work capacity by striving to increase power output.

With these goals in mind, it should be obvious that the exercise written on the white board is not necessarily the correct choice for every athlete in the group! In choosing the optimal movement for an athlete in a given WOD, BtN always prefers a simple exercise well-performed to a more complex movement executed poorly. So an athlete in Performance Mode who exhibits a breakdown in form needs to either a) respond to corrective cues from the instructor (who is in his own complementary mode, Coaching for Performance), or b) default to an exercise lower in the hierarchy, one that preserves the desired training stimulus.

The instructor may also choose to pull the athlete having trouble out of Performance Mode into Practice Mode for remedial instruction; more about switching modes during the WOD in a bit.

INSTRUCTOR MODES

When you halt group activity so that you can convey information without distraction, you are in **Teaching Mode**. When your group is working, either practicing or performing, and you're observing and giving feedback, you are in **Coaching Mode.**

TEACHING

In **Teaching Mode**, you are imparting new information or conducting a remedial review. You move, and the athletes watch. You have the space and time not to just explain a movement in detail, but talk about its underlying principles and how it's related to other exercises.

It would be nice if you only had to show your athletes something once, and then they had it forever. But more often you'll find yourself teaching people the difference between, say, the muscle and power clean a half dozen times before it finally sticks. Think of their knowledge as a delicate orchid. You only have to plant the seed once, but you have to cultivate it carefully if you want it to survive. So be prepared to teach every day. And if the thought of teaching every day makes you groan, you'd probably be better off in another line of work.

BtN puts a variety of tools at your disposal to ensure you are able to communicate the necessary information to your athletes as clearly as possible. Those tools are...

1. Classroom arrangement
2. Presence
3. Teaching scripts
4. Positional breakdowns
5. Positional drills
6. Defining cues

Most of these will still be available when you switch over to coaching.

Classroom Arrangement

Teaching can be directed to an individual or a group. When teaching a group By the Numbers, you have a couple of options as far as how to arrange your pupils on the floor. Traditionally, trainees set up in a circle. The instructor does her initial explanation and movement demo at the center of the circle. This can be awkward, because at any given time, no matter which way the instructor turns, a third of the group is looking at the back of her head. She then drills the athletes while walking the perimeter, making adjustments on individuals as necessary while keeping an eye on the group as a whole.

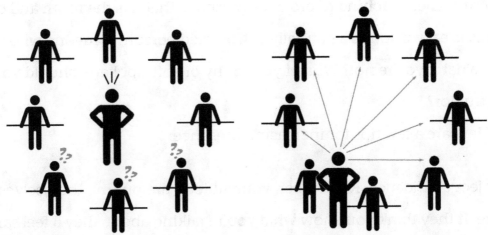

Traditional teaching in a circle   *Traditional coaching in a circle*

BtN suggests you have the athletes set up in staggered ranks facing you. This has two advantages: when teaching, you can see all of your athletes at once (and they can see [and hear] you), and while coaching, by alternating front and side views, you can see at a glance if anyone is making basic positional errors, which usually occur in the frontal and sagittal planes.

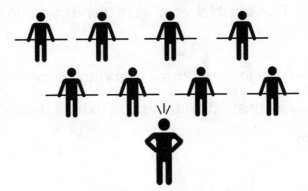

BtN teaching in ranks

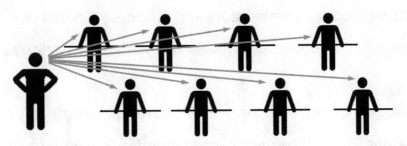

BtN coaching in ranks

Presence

It's important when teaching to project a presence that fills the room and commands attention. This is easy if you're a naturally extroverted person, someone who enjoys performing, but what if you're not? What if you're shy or soft-spoken—should you give up on being an instructor?

No way! Here are a few tips for increasing presence:

1. Project confidence. Remember, your athletes are putting themselves in your care. If they think you know what you're talking about, they'll feel safe enough to leave their comfort zone. And even if you don't feel confident, you can "fake it 'til you make it" if you...

2. Use your "outside" voice. Talk to the person in the back of the group. Also,

3. Be funny. It puts people at ease. And if you can't do that,

4. Be warm. Teaching is a privilege your clients have bestowed on you. Let them know you appreciate it, and that you're glad to see them. Look people in the eye, one at a time. Don't just let your gaze travel over them—make them feel seen. Finally,

5. Be humble. You're not going to know everything, and you don't need to. If someone asks you a question and you don't know the answer, promise to find it. And then do so.

Teaching Scripts

Good teaching is an art. Not only must you master the material, you must be able to impart it with clarity, authority, compassion, and kindness. To that end, it helps to have a script to follow, so you don't have to think about *what* you're saying as much as *how* you're saying it.

There's a great sequence on Mark Rippetoe's "Starting Strength" DVD in which he teaches the back squat. The video editor spliced together Rip working with at least a half dozen athletes, cutting back and forth between them without any disruption of the continuity of his rap. Obviously, Mark had delivered this speech so many times over the years that it was completely automatic, and his mind was free to attend to the situation at hand.

When I first started out, I often quoted Rip almost word-for-word. Now that I've taught these exercises thousands of times, I have my own teaching scripts. I offer these here in *By the Numbers* not in hopes you memorize them, necessarily, but that you'll use them as a scaffolding upon which to begin building your own style. Practice, practice, practice! Rehearse your lines as if you were going to get up and recite them on stage. In a sense, you are.

Positional Breakdowns

Positional Breakdowns are how exercises are taught in BtN. A positional breakdown is created by analyzing an exercise and reducing it to a series of discrete positions, each of which is assigned a movement code and a number. If your athletes learn to accurately model each position of an exercise in correct sequence, when they execute at speed, they will demonstrate outstanding, if not perfect, form.

Positional Drills

Positional Drills are how we transition athletes from segmented, mechanical positional work to full, smoothly executed movement. Positional drills are also the best way to address organizational or sequencing issues.

In a *static positional drill*, when a pose number is called, the athletes adopt the position, then hold while the instructor makes her corrections. We encourage our instructors, through study and experience, to construct a mental model of what perfect form looks like for a given exercise—one that they can see so clearly that they can draw it correctly with simple stick figures (see Appendix II, "Positional Diagrams", pg 544).

In actual practice, the instructor imagines this idealized position superimposed on what he or she is observing, and adjusts the athlete until the abstract and the concrete match—sculpting, essentially. The process continues until the instructor is satisfied with the result. We encourage our instructors to take their time and get it right. This is art, after all (please read that as [semi] ironic).

As noted earlier, this approach makes teaching large groups a snap. By putting an example athlete at the head of the class and forming your trainees into ranks and columns, rather than the traditional circle, you can scan a couple dozen athletes at a glance, easily picking out those whose position does not conform to the ideal standard you've established and making corrections as necessary.

Obviously, many people aren't initially capable of a beautiful squat (for example). Experience and mercy will govern how much of a stickler you should be. Just remember, there is an aesthetic ideal for every movement, and although no two athletes' squats will look exactly alike, both athletes' squats should be a real-world instantiation of that Platonic form, filtered through and expressed by the athlete's unique anthropometry. Insist on beautiful movement from your athletes, and eventually you'll get it, even if it takes months or years.

Once the athlete can, on command, hit all poses of an exercise to standard, then it's time to introduce *dynamic positional drills*. In a dynamic positional drill, athletes execute part or all of a movement at speed. For instance, the "1! 2! 3! Go!" drill for the air squat has athletes moving through the 3 positions of the squat one at a time. They wait in the bottom position for the command "Go!", at which point they stand up through position 2 before coming to rest in position 1.

Using this step-by-step method is a lot more effective than having the athletes execute a movement and then trying to fix mistakes of position or load sequencing after the fact. Instead of "You broke at the knees too soon, so at the bottom of the squat your weight went to the balls of your feet. Next time, hinge back first," it will be, "Show me Air Squat 2. Okay, in Air Squat 2 your hips are back, but your shins should be almost vertical, like this (*adjusts athlete's position*). Now go back to Air Squat 1. Air Squat 2. Better. Again, 1. Two. One. On my 'go', show me the full movement. Ready, go! Okay, good." Now the athlete has a clearer understanding of what went wrong, and thus much improved chances of doing it right the next time.

Defining Cues

As you correct flaws using positional drills, you are also defining for your athletes the cues you'll use while coaching. **Cues** are short, positive reminders of basic points of performance. It's important to have an arsenal of different cues, because people learn in different ways; some are verbal learners, some visual, some tactile. If one cue doesn't work, try another that says the same thing in a different way.

For instance, suppose you have a new trainee who is having difficulty hip hingeing into the second position of the air squat. You show her what you want, establishing a visual cue, while simultaneously describing/explaining what it is she is supposed to be seeing and imitating, thus defining a verbal cue. "Alice, to move from Air Squat Position 1 to Air Squat Position 2, I want you to push your *butt back, like this." Butt back* is now a verbal cue. The action indicated by *like this* is now a visual cue.

COACHING

As you lead your trainees along their path of development, you'll be their taskmaster, baby sitter, drill sergeant, cheerleader. There's one word that sums up all those roles: coach. The goal of coaching is to help athletes progress through the four stages of skills acquisition:

1. Unconscious incompetence. The athlete doesn't know how to do a movement, and maybe doesn't care. You demonstrate what you wish him to learn and he gives you a look like, "Really, guy?" He may go through the motions, but he'll never really begin learning until he makes up his mind to do so.

2. Conscious incompetence. The athlete wants to perform the movement correctly, but has no idea how. This is where frustration can build for trainees, and part of your job will be keeping them from getting so frustrated they want to give up.

3. Conscious competence. Breakthrough! The athlete retains the instruction he's received, and can perform the movement fairly well, as long as he carefully

works through it step-by-step.

4. Unconscious competence. Once the athlete has rehearsed a given movement one or two thousand times (kidding, but not really), it becomes second nature and he can execute flawlessly, even under the stress of increased load and/or time constraint.

In By the Numbers, coaching begins when the initial transfer of necessary information is complete. It is directed to one athlete at a time, and has two sub-modes: Coaching for Practice, and Coaching for Performance.

COACHING FOR PRACTICE

Once you've presented your athletes with enough information to get started, you shift from Teaching Mode to **Coaching for Practice Mode**, just as your athletes shift from Learning to Practice. Coaching for Practice may be directed toward an athlete at any of the four stages of skill acquisition, although by the time unconscious competence has been achieved you will not be coach so much as collaborator, as the athlete begins developing his own style.

During Coaching for Practice, you may halt the athlete at any time—in the middle of a set, if necessary—to offer detailed critique and recommendations for improvement. Your goal is to correct flaws before they become habits.

When Coaching for Practice, you'll have the following weapons in your arsenal. Keep them sharp.

1. Seeing and distinguishing
2. Prioritization
3. Using cues
4. Positional Drills
5. Prescribing orthoses

Seeing and Distinguishing

Before you can start offering help, you first must be able to tell good movement from bad. Seeing and distinguishing is about visual perspicacity and pattern matching. Once you understand a movement well enough to have a clear image of its ideal positional breakdowns, you'll be able to watch an athlete, compare his execution against your mental model, and identify flaws. It's not about checking off a list of points of performance (although thorough familiarity with the points of performance of each exercise is critical for effective cueing), it's about noticing that something is off, and instantly knowing what's wrong, and why.

When seeing and distinguishing,

1. Learn to spot movement errors up close, peripherally, and at a distance. Develop a "spider-sense" that tingles when someone is moving badly, whether it's across the room, in the corner of your eye, or right in your face.

2. Once you've identified an athlete committing an error, keep a global view of the situation, and attempt to identify the cause of the problem, rather than just trying to correct the symptom. For example, an athlete may be rolling onto the balls of his feet at the bottom of his squat, but if it's because he's initiating the squat with his knees, telling him "Weight back!" or "Heels!" isn't going to fix it.

If you're lucky, the athlete will only display one fault. Often, though, poor movement is due to a constellation of problems. In that case, you have to prioritize.

Prioritization

It's easy to overwhelm an athlete with information. "So, your weight is shifting forward onto the balls of your feet, which is probably because your stance is too narrow, and your knees are caving in, and I think you've got some butt wink happening, and…" It's too much. Pick one thing and fix it. But how do you decide which one? Prioritize faults as follows:

1. Safety. Does the fault predispose the athlete to injury?

2. Efficiency. Does the fault make the exercise more difficult than it has to be?

3. Aesthetics. Is the fault minor enough to not pose an immediate threat, but inhibits long-term progress?

For example, you have an athlete who is doing front squats. He cranks his head back to look at the ceiling throughout the movement, his grip is too narrow, his elbows are pointing at the ground, and his back rounds in the bottom position.

Four faults. Which one seems most unsafe? The rounded back, right? For loaded exercises, a straight spine is paramount. Well, that was easy! But what about the other problems? I'd say that his elbow position would be next in priority, because it limits what he can comfortably support, and then the grip. Those two you could probably work on at the same time. Save his head position for last. It puts an unnecessary strain on his cervical vertebrae, but unless he has previous neck problems, it's more of a matter of "it just doesn't look good"—in other words, aesthetics.

Once you've figured out which error to fix first, your next step will be to try to resolve the problem with a cue.

Using Cues

Before we get into cueing, let me point out that you can't teach with a cue. If an athlete never learned that the rack position for a push press is different than for a press, all the various cues you can employ won't be as effective as simply stopping him so you can explain what you want.

Cueing is a matter of personal style, but when you're first getting started as a coach, try ordering your cues like this:

1. Verbal. "Knees out!" Start by assuming your athlete has achieved conscious

competence—he only needs a reminder to tune up his performance.

2. Visual. Indicate what you want with a gesture (tapping your knees and pushing them out, for example), or by demonstrating the correct version of a position for the athlete to imitate. If that still doesn't work, then go...

3. Tactile. Use your hands or feet to provide a target for the athlete's movement, or physically adjust athlete into desired position. Something to keep in mind: coaching exercise is necessarily a hands-on job. When you have to adjust an athlete's position, try to use your hands in a manner that can't be misconstrued (e.g., use a closed fist, or the back of your hand), and if you do have to directly touch your athlete, try to be as uninvasive as possible, making contact at the shoulder, the outside of the hip, and the outside of the knee. Be clinically brisk. Attitude is everything.

As you work with an athlete, you'll grow familiar with his learning style, and can tailor your cues appropriately. For instance, from a verbal cue, you may elect to skip straight to tactile, if you think that's what will be most effective for that athlete.

Here are a few rules of thumb for cueing:

1. Always begin a correction by using the athlete's name. This will focus their attention on you, even if you're across the room. "James! Drive elbows up!"

2. Verbal cues depend on prior communication of meaning. In other words, during instruction and practice it should be well established that the phrase "Knees out!" means "Contract your glutes and quads to externally rotate the legs as you squat, translating the knees laterally." Verbal cues are shorthand, not explanation.

3. Effective verbal cues often have the structure body part / direction. For instance, for an athlete breaking neutral midline by gazing straight ahead while setting up for a deadlift, you might try, "Jane! Chin toward floor!" An athlete squatting his kettlebell swing might be told, "Jeb! Knees stay back!"

4. Visual cues usually need a verbal component: *Do it like this!* For example, for someone initiating a squat with his knees, you might say, "Bill! Like this!", pointing to your hip as you mime hinging back into Air Squat Position 2.

5. Tactile cues often have a verbal component, as well. For example: "Don't touch my hand!" as you crouch to block the knee of an athlete squatting his kettlebell swing.

The cues provided in the "Common Faults and Fixes" section of each movement are not meant to be a definitive list. They're my go-to's, that's all. Every coach will have her own go-to cues, and this is an area where constant creativity is completely encouraged. The more ways you have of putting an idea across, the better chance you have of being understood.

Positional Drills

The positional drills you used to help teach a movement can be an effective corrective technique if an athlete starts making mistakes. To correct errors, simply have them execute the positions of the movement one at a time. As they hold, make the necessary corrections. For example, a client with exhibiting a valgus error (knees caving) in his squat would be told, "Show me Air Squat Position 1. Position Two. Three. Okay, down here in Air Squat 3, push your knees out. Good. Up to Two. Hips forward into One."

If cues are ineffective, and Positional Drills didn't help, either, it's time to employ your last line of defense: an orthosis.

Prescribing Orthoses

Learning new exercises will expose myriad problems with a trainee's strength, balance, flexibility, and coordination. These issues can and should be corrected using mobilizations outside of class. But during class, you just need to get your athlete moving competently so they can stay with the group without getting hurt. To that end we've come up with a variety of ways of using standard gym equipment (boxes, Abmats, PVC pipe, bands, etc.)

as proprioceptive feedback devices to help our trainees get into the right poses. In BtN, we refer to these as **orthoses**. Think of them like corrective braces—they are a temporary solution, one your client should strive to outgrow. One day you should able to shout at them, "SQUAT, FORREST, SQUAT!" as their orthoses fly away in pieces.

In most cases, if you keep putting your athletes in ideal positions, over time their issues will tend to resolve. That said, if an athlete complains of persistent or acute pain, or if his positions remain stubbornly unimproved, insist he sees a medical professional.

COACHING FOR PERFORMANCE

Excuse me while I climb up on my soapbox for a moment. I feel a rant coming on.

BtN's **Coaching for Performance** mode involves giving verbal, visual, or tactile cues while an athlete is in the midst of a metabolic conditioning workout. Sometimes it might also involve prescribing an orthosis. The goal is to make corrections without hindering the athlete's activity. That's the goal—*not* an ironclad law, as we'll see. But as long as that goal remains situationally appropriate, Coaching for Performance is congruent with a concept known as "threshold training".

Threshold training takes place during metabolic conditioning workouts when intensity has risen to the point mechanics begin to break down. This is the zone where stress elicits the greatest adaptations. Therefore, if an athlete is to get the most out of his workout, a certain amount of form degradation is acceptable, if not desirable. (This used to be referred to as "20% slop", although the term has gone out of style.) Essentially, perfect form means you're not working hard enough.

Because the emphasis is always on doing more work in less time, trainers supervising threshold training workouts are told to correct an athlete's poor movement with cues, but to avoid interrupting his workout. And this can work: a cue will work for an athlete who is already competent with a movement and, in his metcon daze, just needs a reminder to fix his execution.

But the form breakdowns we see happening in many MMGPP gyms these days have less to do with experienced athletes pushing the envelope of their ability, and more to do with the fact that most people training MMGPP are too new to know what the hell they're doing. Whether an athlete is just out of Foundations or has been training for a year is immaterial. If he doesn't actually actually understand what the movement is supposed to look like, you'll never fix him with a pithy phrase.

And all too often, these relatively inexperienced athletes aren't even *getting* cues! Their trainers simply stand to the side and watch. They'll step in if someone appears to be in danger, but otherwise, they won't interfere. I've seen this in enough of the gyms I've visited to believe the issue is systemic. What in the world is going on?

I've come to believe this pattern of neglect—I can't put it any other way—is the result not of incompetence*, but of a misunderstanding or misapplication of the threshold training concept. Trainers aren't correcting shoddy technique because they think the fact their athletes are moving badly is a sign of adequate intensity. At one gym I dropped in on, the head trainer told his staff, in my hearing, "Once the clock starts, that's the clients' time to get their conditioning in. Don't interrupt them." At another, a trainer told me, "If you insist on good form, nobody would get a workout."

In a word—bullshit. **If athletes WODing under your supervision are not moving well and you're not trying to do something about it, you are not doing your job.** If you think it's okay that they're not squatting to below parallel when doing wallballs, or that they catch power cleans as if trying to do the limbo, or that their chins don't quite get over the bar on the pull-up, because, hey, it's "20% slop", *I'm calling you out*. YOU MUST GET OUT THERE AND FIX THEM. Mountain Athlete, Gym Jones, Orange Theory, whatever: if your athletes are not moving to standard, cue and correct them, but if those cues don't work, *stop them* to explain what they're doing wrong, and what you want to see.

Of course, one other reason a trainer might avoid making corrections is a lack of confidence, either in his knowledge, or in his ability to win a contest of wills with a stubborn athlete. As a remedy to the former, there are known, objective standards for the movements we teach; they are clearly described in this book, so if you're ever unsure of what's acceptable and what's not, just check out the photo references. As for the latter, you just have to make up your mind that what happens on the gym floor when you're in charge is a reflection on you, and that you'd rather lose a client than lower your standards and tarnish your reputation.

The threshold concept is fine for the athletically accomplished. But in the real world, where the soccer moms and overweight firemen and skinny teenagers in your classes are just learning how to train, athletes hacking their way through metcons are just building bad habits. If you don't intervene, if you wait until end of the workout before making corrections, well, that just means that they've had that much more practice with doing things wrong. And as weightlifting legend Tommy Kono says, *Practice makes permanent.* Letting people people work out with bad form so they can stay at "threshold" trades a short-term gain in work capacity for a long-term retardation of progress. It's a devil's bargain—don't take it!

When coaching athletes in Performance mode, prioritize movement integrity over exercise intensity. I'm begging you. I promise, the intensity will still be there! And it will increase with time as skill increases. There's no need to rush that development. Even if your athletes are only going at 85% instead of 95%, they are still getting fitter, I promise.

While Coaching for Performance, your tools are as follows:

1. Sharking
2. 60 Second Correction Clock
3. Cueing for Performance
4. Switching Athlete Modes
5. Assigning Defaults

Sharking

Remember that very, um...*motivating* speech that Alec Baldwin delivers in the movie *GlenGaryGlennRoss*? When he writes "ABC" on the blackboard and pounds it for emphasis: "ALWAYS. BE. CLOSING." If I had a blackboard I'd hammer my fist on it and say, "ALWAYS. BE. COACHING."

When Coaching for Performance, By the Numbers requires you to never stop moving, never stop interacting with your athletes. We call this "**sharking**" (for the way that sharks [supposedly] never stop swimming, even when they sleep).

To "shark", make circuits of the room. Constantly shift your focus from macro—the class as a whole—to micro—the athlete proximate to you. As you pass an athlete, assess his performance. If you are satisfied with his efforts, tell him, "Good job, So-and-so," and move on. (As Dale Carnegie says, there's not a sweeter sound in all the world to anyone than their own name.) And if you're not satisfied, halt your perambulation to make a fix. As soon as you stop, the Sixty Second Correction Clock begins.

In addition to constantly scanning for movement error, you should be also be acting in your role as safety monitor, making sure people aren't in danger of dropping equipment on each other or falling off the pull-up bar, as well as looking out for anyone displaying signs of emotional breakdown. When running a class, there's no room for standing still, or god forbid, being on your phone. You are personally responsible for every person in your class. Act that way.

Sixty Second Correction Clock

Once you engage with an athlete for purposes of correction, you have roughly one minute to effect the desired change. Any longer, and you are neglecting the rest of your class, who have just as much of a right to your attention. The Sixty Second Clock starts as soon as you give your first cue. Then you check for improvement. If your cue worked, you are on your way after about 10 seconds. If not, give a second cue, catering to a different learning style, and see if that makes a difference. If it does, again, move on.

But if that second cue didn't work, order the athlete to stop (see "Switching Athlete Modes", below). You're now about 20 seconds in. Run a Positional Drill. (If an implement is being used, it'll be too heavy for static holds, so have you trainee execute the drill with an imaginary barbell, kettlebell, etc.) Make corrections, then have the athlete do a test rep. If things are looking better, awesome! If not, you make a choice: go back to sharking, and give the athlete a chance to practice a bit and get better before being evaluated again, prescribe an orthosis, or Assign a Default (see below). Either way, the Sixty Second Clock is running out, and you need to get moving.

The point is, *Don't get stuck.* There are a lot of other people in class depending on you.

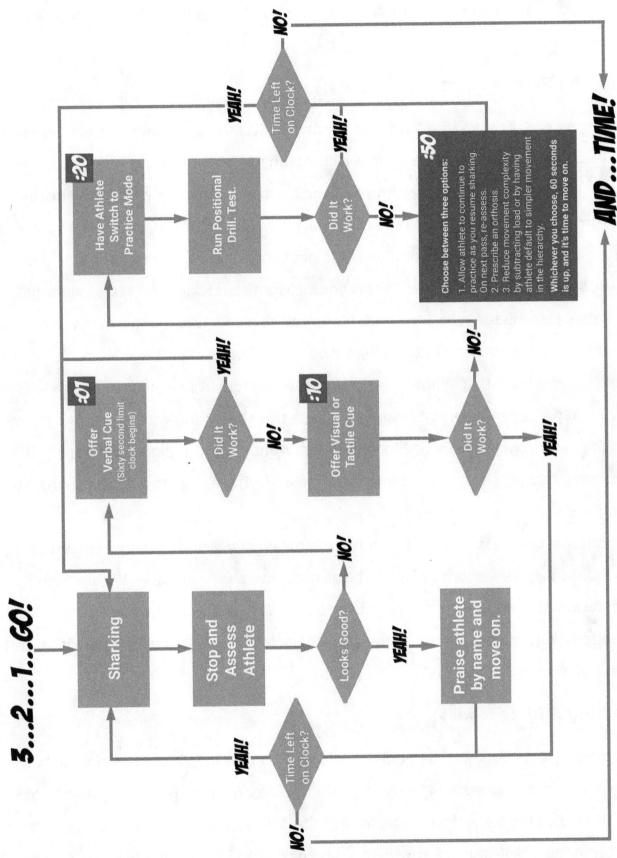

BtN Coaching for Performance Work Flow

Each athlete can have up to a minute of your attention at a time, but no more. Luckily, if you are disciplined about following the sixty second clock, you'll be back around soon to offer more help.

Cueing for Performance

Have you ever heard of the "criticism sandwich"? It's the idea that when it's necessary to make a correction, first you're to offer a compliment, then a critique, then another compliment. That's fine if you're Coaching for Practice, but when athletes are in Performance Mode, time is of the essence, so you have to be pithy, almost brusque. With a whole roomful of athletes to look after, you don't want to get bogged down. Get right to the point.

Next, some tactile cues offered in this book's "Common Faults and Fixes" sections are appropriate for athletes in Performance Mode, but some require the instructor to take athlete out of Performance and into Practice Mode. See "Switching Athlete Modes."

Finally, remember that by the time you see the problem, it's already too late to fix that particular rep. For example, if you spot an athlete front squatting with his elbows pointing at the ground, yelling, "Dave! Elbows up!" or "Wendy, tight upper back!" won't achieve anything on that rep. It's a reminder to the athlete of what he has to do to make the next rep better.

If your first cue doesn't work, try another. Whatever cues you employ, remember the goal in Coaching for Performance is to be as non-invasive as possible. We are trying to guide the athlete's efforts, not slow or impede him. That said, if your cues are not effecting the desired change, don't be shy. Order you athlete to stop what they're doing. It's time to switch modes.

Switching Athlete Modes

In BtN, metcon workouts are performance—an opportunity to demonstrate movement skill, while developing work capacity. If, during a metcon, an athlete is not moving to standard, and Coaching for Performance doesn't effect the desired change, you may temporarily bring the athlete out of Performance and back into Practice mode—that is, make him pause to receive more detailed instruction and/or perform Positional Drills.

The athlete may object. If she's been brainwashed to believe in "Go hard or go home," she may cry, "BUT MY FITNESS!" Acknowledge her qualms, and try to reassure her: slowing down a little or even stopping so she can get a movement right is only going to help her in the long run. It certainly won't hurt her overall "fitness."

Once the athlete is in Practice Mode, have her run one positional drill, and then have her perform a rep to show that she's understood. If it's good, move on.

If not, well...here's the hard truth: an athlete exhibiting a movement fault that cannot be corrected with two cues and a Positional Drill is functionally incompetent with that movement, and should be doing a simpler variation that preserves the desired training stimulus.

You've come to another decision fork. If the error is not particularly grievous or dangerous, you can allow the athlete to continue in Practice Mode while you get back to sharking, which is to say, she's to keep working slowly and carefully on improving her execution until you return for another assessment.

However, if what you're seeing is just plain bad, and you don't think the athlete will be able to work it out on her own, or if she's just too exhausted to perform the exercise correctly, you can solve the problem by reducing movement complexity with an Assigned Default.

Assigning Defaults

You can reduce the complexity of an assigned movement in two ways: lighten the load, or make the athlete default to a less complex version of the exercise he's doing (sometimes, that's the same thing). The choice you make depends on context.

For an example of when and how to reduce movement complexity, let me introduce Phil. Phil dropped in to the gym the other day. He's been doing MMGPP-style training for about two years. He's definitely a strong guy, a guy who knows his way around a WOD, but I make it plain to him that we have pretty strict standards, and that we're not shy about enforcing them. He seems okay with that.

Today in class we did some barbell pressing, and now, as a finisher, we're doing 20-15-10 reps for time of deadlifts (at 225lbs) and handstand push-ups. Phil assures me that he's done similar workouts before, and that the deadlift weight and HSPU will pose no problem. Just in case, I take him and the rest of the class through the movement hierarchy that contains handstand push-ups, which is called "Push Away from Object (vertical, inverted, dynamic)". The hierarchy goes like this: down dog push-ups, pike push-ups from box, handstand push-ups, kipping HSPU.

Phil demonstrated for me that he can do 5 strict handstand push-ups, so I allow him to do kipping HSPU. His deadlift warm-up sets look okay, too, so he's waiting for the clock to start with the Rx'd weight on the bar.

At "GO!", I begin sharking, keeping one eye on Phil, who's my wildcard today. Good thing, too, because not even halfway through the first set of deadlifts, Phil's back is already starting to round. As soon as I stop to fix him, the Sixty Second Correction Clock starts in my head. I cue him, "Phil! Chest up! Flat back!" His positions improve, and I move on, having spent only 10 seconds.

The next time around I catch him at the tail end of his handstand push-ups. Reps 18, 19, and 20 are done as singles—he's already starting to tire.

As I continue to shark, my attention constantly veers from the micro (the athlete right in front of me) to the macro (the class as a whole). I'm across the room when I notice that Phil's back is now rounding badly on his deadlifts, and that he's pulling only two reps at a time. In between efforts he stands staring at the bar, sucking wind.

The mental correction clock starts. I yell, "Phil! Chest up!", because it worked last time. But now it doesn't. I walk over to him. "Phil!" I say. "Like this!" and I mime picking up and putting down the bar with my spine neutral. That's my visual cue. He nods, but on the next rep, nothing's changed, so now it's time to take temporarily take him out of Performance Mode.

"Stop for a second," I order him. "Using an imaginary barbell, show me a good deadlift." If he were one of my athletes, trained with BtN, I would've had him run a Positional Drill:

DL 1, DL 2, DL 3, DL 2, DL 1. As it is he does okay. I say, "Okay, do another rep. Keep your back flat, just like you showed me."

He tries, but his back rounds like a rainbow. And he's not even halfway finished with the WOD! To keep him safe, and to help him continue to demonstrate mastery, I have to reduce the complexity of his task. The deadlift is a simple exercise, compared to, say, the clean, but a heavy load makes it a real challenge to the athlete's posterior chain strength, his ability to stabilize his midline, his balance and kinesthetic awareness. I have him take weight off the bar.

"Pull a 45lbs plate off each side," I tell him. "Finish the workout at 135lbs."

He doesn't like it, but it's my gym, so he does it. What he doesn't understand is that switching to a lighter weight not only makes the exercise safer, it can actually increase his power output. At the rate he was going, this workout might've taken him 12 minutes or more, as he stood and rested in between single reps. Now he can move continuously.*

Sixty seconds is more than up. I go back to sharking. But Phil's not done with me yet, apparently!

In his last set of handstand push-ups, he totally comes off the rails. His head crashes to the floor, he pulls his knees to his chest, and kicks out wildly. His feet never come near the wall. Working with another athlete, I observe out of the corner of my eye as he does this once, twice, three times.

Phil's already gotten a good share of my coaching attention today, but this situation has now gone critical—he's in real danger of injuring himself. Not to mention the fact that not one of the last three reps "counts", nor the fact that sort of flailing is just embarrassing.

I don't even bother with cues, or Positional Drills. It's obvious to me that Phil is too exhausted to do any more HSPU. So instead I reduce the complexity of his task. This time, I do it by having him default to a simpler version of the movement.

Assuming an even split between time spent on deadlifts and time on HSPU (unrealistic maybe, but play along for a second), the deadlifts in a 12:00 finish on this WOD yields a power output of 56.25 foot pounds/sec (45 reps x 225lbs x 2' travel, divided by 360 seconds), or 76.2 watts. The deadlifts in a 7:00 finish @ 135lbs yield an average power output of 57.85 foot pounds/sec, (45 reps x 135lbs x 2', divided by 210 seconds) or 78.4 watts.

Luckily, he had gone through the Movement Hierarchy for the HSPU with the rest of the class, so he was familiar with the subs I was about to make, and even more fortuitously, I had prepared for this eventuality. "Set up for Pike Push-ups from the box," I tell him, maneuvering a box against the wall. "Let's see it." He manages two, and then stops. He is really, really tired.

"Okay," I say, "finish up with Down Dog Pike Push-ups." This beginner version of the HSPU would be easy for him...*if* he was fresh. But he's not. Phil is tired, and so cranking out seven dPK isn't trivial for him. His shoulders are definitely burning. But just like with the reduced load deadlift, he's able to move continuously until all reps are completed. So although the movement challenge has been drastically reduced, he still gets a good ROI on his training time. Remember, intensity is movement agnostic. By using a lighter load and a simplified version of the HSPU, he has done more in less time, so intensity has been maintained.

Sometimes you'll reduce complexity for other reasons. If an athlete is doing power cleans at a moderate weight, but despite your cues can't seem to receive the bar without jumping her feet out wide enough to do the splits, you'd have her switch to muscle cleans. Why? Because you prefer to see a simple movement well-executed to a more complex movement performed poorly. This isn't so much about preventing injury as bad habits. **In Performance , don't let your clients do a movement incorrectly over and over.** Find the version of the movement they can do well, and then help them develop the more complex version during Practice time.

Setting Up Your Athletes (and Yourself) for a Successful Performance

Many coaching headaches during metcons can be avoided by insisting athletes choose exercise variations appropriate to their current abilities. Happily, athletes trained up under BtN will be thoroughly familiar with Movement Hierarchies, and will know which version of a prescribed exercise they should perform, because of frequent opportunities to practice and develop.

That's not to say your BtN-trained athletes won't pose constant challenges. As they start trying to apply new skills in metcons, to "level up", as it were, there's always a chance (a likelihood, really) that fatigue will force a breakdown in technique. No worries! Having started at the bottom of the Movement Hierarchies and worked through the progressions, if they need to default back a notch, they'll know just what to do.

As long as your athletes are performing well an exercise that preserves the desired training stimulus, it's all good. And next time, they'll be able to push the envelope of their ability a little further. *It's all about progression.*

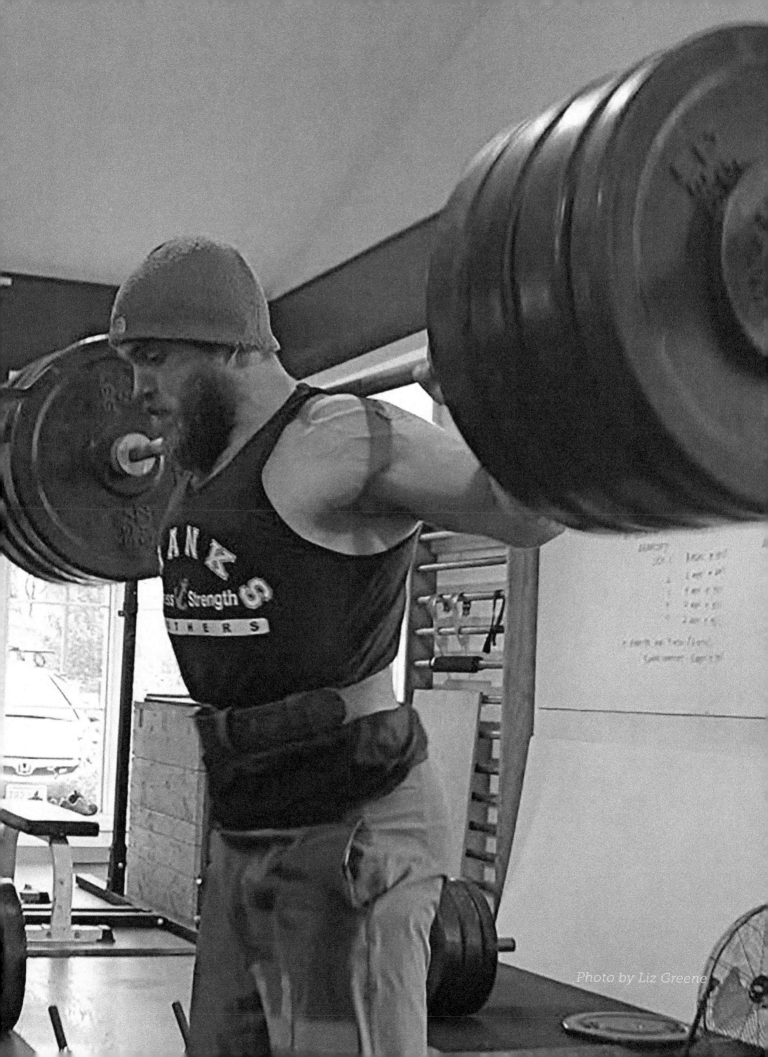

PART TWO:
BY THE
NUMBERS
Teaching and Coaching

Chapter Four
TEACHING AND COACHING OVERVIEW

In Part II, I hope to make more clear how the concepts detailed in the last few chapters—movement hierarchies, classroom modes, teaching scripts, positional breakdowns and drills, etc.—are actually applied in a small group setting.

Three Archetypal Athletes

At the beginning of each section, we'll discuss whether the movement to be taught is appropriate for each of the members of a hypothetical group of MMGPP athletes:

- Harry is a twenty-three-year-old former Marine. He's a great natural athlete, and he and his buddies used to do MMGPP workouts together when he was stationed overseas.

- Amy played multiple sports in high school and went to college on a lacrosse scholarship. Out of school now for 10 years, she's stayed fit through a combination of running, hot yoga, and bootcamp-style workouts. However, she's never done any barbell-based strength work.

- Tim is a professor at the local university. He's in his early fifties, and has never worked out a day in his life. But he's determined to get in better shape, and that's good enough for me.

As the weeks progress, there will be more and more movements that are not appropriate for all our trainees; I'll explain why, and what do to about it.

Movement Instruction

Each movement is presented the same way. First, there is a brief overview, describing the exercise, any necessary prerequisites, and where it might be found in "classical" MMGPP programming.

The prerequisites and recommended movement screens are integral to the concept of Movement Hierarchies. After the first "week", when we'll cover foundational movements accessible to almost anyone, the exercises will grow increasingly challenging. Athletes must meet certain requirements before they'll be able to perform these more advanced exercises correctly. Sometimes the requirement might be having already learned a simpler version of the movement. Sometimes it will be passing a certain test of flexibility. Sometimes it will be a base level of performance. There's little point, for example, in teaching someone ring push-ups if they can't do at least five standard push-ups in good form.

After the overview, our "virtual class" begins as you enter Teaching Mode. Teaching Mode sections are divided into Teaching Scripts, which have gray a background, and Positional Drills, which do not.

Positional Breakdowns

As explained earlier, in BtN each exercise is broken down into a series of positions. These positions are identified with a two letter code and a number, e.g., Air Squat Positions 1, 2, and 3 are designated AS 1, AS 2, AS 3. Movement variants have a lower case letter modifier; e.g., the first position of the Pull-up is PL 1, and the first position of the kipping pull-up is kPL 1.

Each position is represented with photographs shot from the front and from the side. For some movements it was necessary to use a 3/4 view; either way, I tried to make sure the points of performance were always clear.

Teaching Scripts

Each set of photographs is accompanied by a teaching script. Teaching scripts are in quotes, and accurately reflect the way in which I instruct these movements. (In fact, the first drafts of these sections were dictated into my phone as I stood in front of a white board pretending to teach a group.) The teaching scripts describe the actions necessary to get into each position ("Sit back, knees out," etc.), and also offer additional insight into the role the position plays in the context of the full movement.

Are these scripts the only way to explain these movements? Of course not! But each script has been honed by hundreds of repetitions. The information is doled out in a logically progressing manner. Getting thoroughly familiar with these scripts is a good way for a new coach to feel a little bit less "at sea" as he begins teaching. Once you've got a handle on the material, feel free to alter, embellish, and improve as you see fit.

Although not included in these sections, in Appendix III there are Positional Diagrams that can be drawn on the whiteboard as part of your movement explanations.

Positional Drills

After each teaching script, there are Positional Drills. Positional Drills are still considered part of Teaching Mode; the attention of the athletes is fixed on you, as you call out

 There will also be occasional important notes about performance or safety. These will be marked with a large exclamation point, like this one.

sequences of positions, assess their performance, and make corrections. For simple movements, there may be only one Positional Drill. For more complex exercises, there may be a half dozen or more, followed by more teaching scripts.

Common Faults and Fixes

Upon completion of the final Positional Drill for the section, the athletes enter Practice Mode, which means you, the coach, are in Coaching for Practice Mode. After teaching a new movement, you should allow athletes at least ten minutes to internalize and apply all the new information you've just imparted.

Athletes new to a movement will at first make many, many mistakes in execution. These are catalogued in the Common Faults and Fixes sections. As your athletes practice and you identify and address their errors, you'll be collaborating to find the corrective cues most effective for them. Remember, people learn in different ways, so be prepared with an

Verbal cues. Verbal cues will always be your weapon of first choice. Remember, use the athlete's name to get his attention, make the cue short and direct, and when possible specify a direction ("Shoulder blades in your back pockets!").

Visual cues. Visual cues work best when accompanied by a verbal command: "Like this!"

Tactile cues. Some tactile cues are useful when an athlete is in Performance mode, but most will require you take the athlete back into Practice Mode. For instance, it's probably not advisable to kneel in front of athlete and order "Push your knees out into my hands!" while she's banging out 50 air squats as fast as she can! Bring her to a halt, fix her position, and then turn her loose.

Orthosis. You can use a wide variety of objects commonly found in the gym to provide proprioceptive feedback to an athlete and improve his performance without you having to stand there monitoring every rep.

arsenal of commands and work-arounds.

After identifying commonly seen errors of execution, the Common Faults and Fixes section offers remedies, which are categorized like this:

Benchmark WODs

At the conclusion of each "week" a benchmark WOD is analyzed, and we'll figure out how best to adapt it to the needs of Harry, Amy, and Tim at their current level of development. Issues of exercise selection, assigning correct loads, and determining proper volume will all be discussed. Finally, I offer hypothetical workout scenarios to help illustrate the kinds of issues you'll come up against coaching these athletes of very different ability levels while they are in Performance Mode.

THE (VERY) BASICS

When teaching movement, it's important that you and your trainees use a common language to describe positions and actions. This language could be as technical as a scholarly article in the *International Journal of Kinesiology and Sport Science,* or simple enough for a second grader to understand—that's up to you.

The first part of this section, "Just So We're on the Same Page", is the teaching script I use with brand new trainees. The desired result of telling someone "Move your feet in" might seem perfectly obvious to you, but often it's not to the person getting the instruction. Take a minute before you start showing them how to perform exercises to make sure they know what your terminology means.

The second part, "(Very) Basic Anatomy and Kinesiology", is not a teaching script. It defines body parts referred to in this book, and explains and illustrates some terms borrowed from the science of body mechanics. While it can be very helpful for your athletes to know this information, too, it's not necessary for them to begin training. They'll pick it up in context.

I. "Just So We're on the Same Page..."

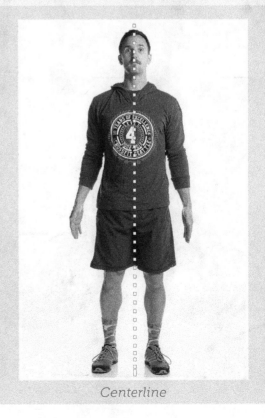

"Stand up tall. Imagine a line running down the middle of your body, dividing right from left. The correct term for that imaginary line is 'sagittal plane' but we're going to refer to it as our **centerline.**

Centerline

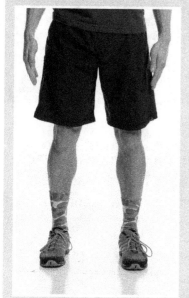
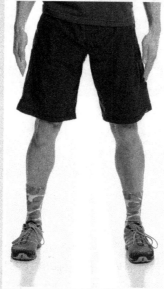

Hip-width stance *Shoulder-width stance*

"The distance between your feet is your **'stance.'** There are two basic stances to be familiar with: **hip-width**, which for most people means heels set 6-9" apart, and **shoulder-width**, anywhere from 12-18".

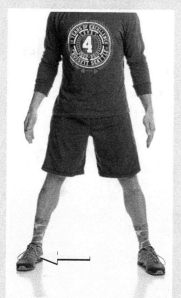
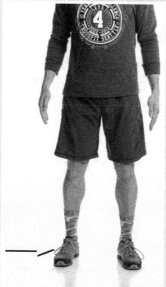

Right foot out *Right foot in*

"When I say '**Out**', that means 'sideways away from my centerline' (the technical term is 'laterally.') When I say '**In**', that means 'move sideways toward my centerline' (the technical term is 'medially'). So here's me moving my right foot out, and my right foot in.

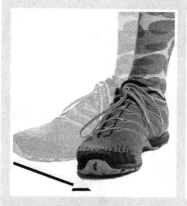
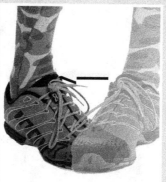

Right toe in *Right heel out*

"For convenience, we'll divide your foot into two parts: toe and heel. If I ask your to move one part of your foot, the other should stay in place. For instance, if I say, 'Right toe in,' that means, 'Plant your right heel and slightly pivot your right forefoot in toward your centerline.' 'Right heel out' means 'With your toe remaining in place, move your heel away from your centerline.'

"When I say '**Forward**', I mean, 'in the direction before me' (or 'anteriorly'.) When I say '**Back**,' I mean 'in the direction behind me' ('posteriorly'). Here's my right foot going forward, and my right foot coming back.

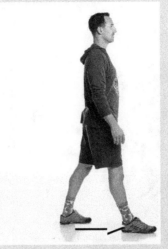 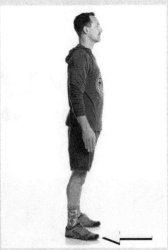

Right foot forward *Right foot back*

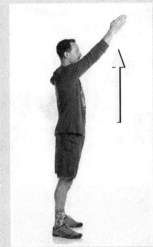 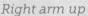

"'**Up**' ('superior') is toward the ceiling, '**Down**' (inferior) is toward the floor."

Right arm up *Right arm down*

II. (Very) Basic Anatomy and Kinesiology

1. The **ankle** is the joint between the foot and the lower leg.

2. The lower leg has two bones: the shinbone, or **tibia**, and the **fibia.**

3. The **knee** is the joint between the lower leg and the upper leg. It is a modified hinge that opens, closes, and rotates slightly.

4. The **femur** is the bone of the thigh.

5. The **hip** is the ball-and-socket joint where the proximal head of the femur attaches to the pelvis. It has multiple axes of movement.

6. The **pelvis** connects the legs to the skeleton of the torso.

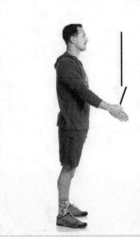 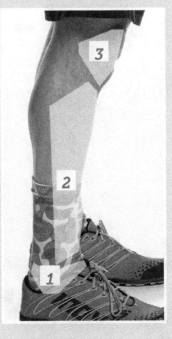 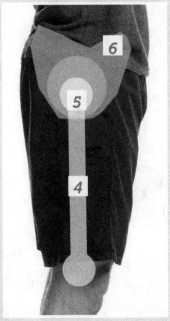

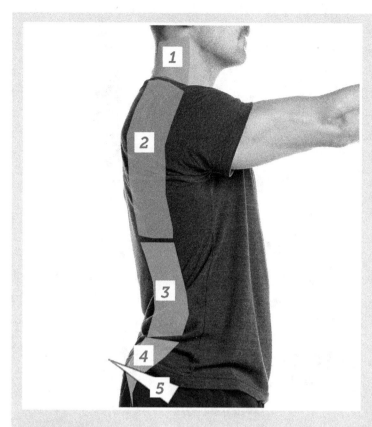

The **spine** is a series of small bones ("vertebrae") separated by discs of cartilege. We'll refer to these regions of the spine:

1. **Cervical,**

2. **Thoracic,** and

3. **Lumbar.** The lumbar vertebrae are set upon the

4. **Sacrum.** The sacrum connects to the pelvis at the

5. **Sacroilliac (SI) joint,** an area often involved in lower back pain.

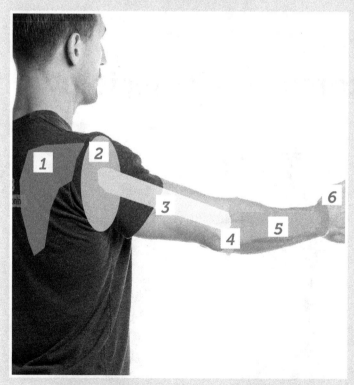

1. The **shoulder blades** (scapulae) are the attachment point for the muscles that connect the upper arm bone (or "humerus") to the collar bone ("clavicle").

2. The **shoulder** is the ball and socket joint where the upper arm attaches to the trunk. It has multiple axes of movement.

3. The **humerus** is the bone of the upper arm.

4. The **elbow** is the joint between the upper arm and the forearm. It is a hinge joint.

5. The **forearm** has two bones, the radius and the ulna.

6. The **wrist** is the joint between the forearm and the hand.

Here are some of the muscles to which we'll be referring:

1. **Quadriceps**. A muscular group on the front of the thigh, they work to extend the knee, as well as flex the hip.

2. The **hip flexors,** or iliopsoas, close the hip.

3. **Abdominals**. The abs flex the spine and, as utilized in the Valsalva maneuver, perform a vital role in stabilizing the midline.

4. **Pectorals**, or chest muscles, adduct and flex the arm.

5. **Deltoids**, or shoulder muscles, abduct, flex, and extend the arm.

6. The **biceps** is the muscle of the upper arm that flexes the elbow.

These muscles, with the exception of the biceps, comprise the **Anterior Chain.**

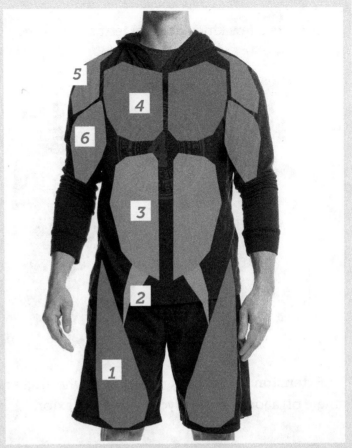

1. The **triceps** is the muscle on the back of the upper arm that extends the elbow.

2. The **rotator cuff** is a group of muscles and tendons whose primary function is to stabilize the glenohumeral joint.

3. The **trapezius** moves the scapula and supports the arm.

4. The "**lats**," or latissimus dorsi, are the large muscles of the back that extend and adduct the arm.

5. **Spinal erectors** are a bundle of muscles and tendons that extend the spine.

6. The **gluteal** muscles extend the hip.

7. The **hamstrings** flex the knee and help extend the hip.

These muscles, with the exception of the triceps, comprise the **Posterior Chain.**

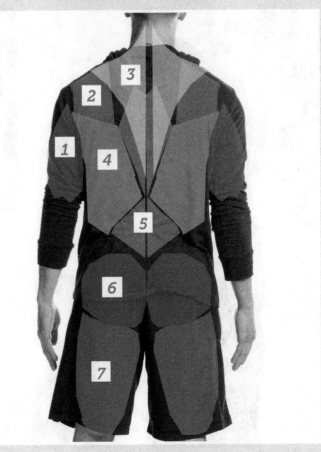

Here are a few kinesiological terms with which it'll be helpful to be familiar.

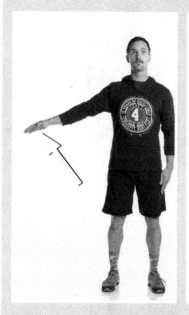
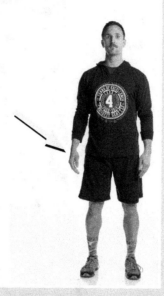

Abduction means to move a limb away laterally from the body.

Adduction is to move a limb in toward (medially) the body.

Extension closes (that is, decreases the angle of) a joint. **Flexion** opens (that is, increases the angle of) a joint. Here is your spine in flexion (1), neutral (2), and in extension (3).

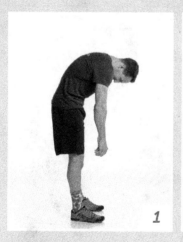
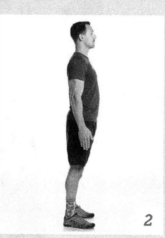
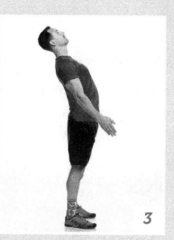

1

2

3

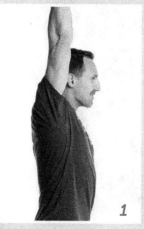
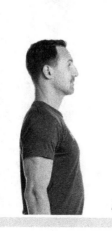

1

2

Shoulder in flexion (1) and extension (2).

Elbow in flexion (1) and extension (2).

Hips in flexion (1) and extension (2).

Knee in flexion (1) and extension (2).

Your ankles flex in two direction. Photo (1) depicts "dorsiflexion". Photo (2) depicts "plantar flexion".

Some joints not only flex and extend, but rotate as well. Turning in toward the centerline is called **internal rotation.** Turning away from the centerline is called **external rotation.**

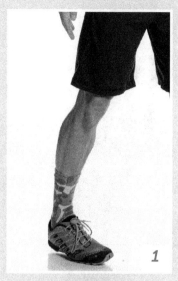
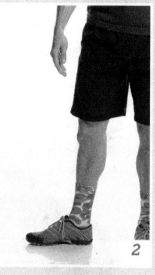

Internal rotation: toe in/ heel out

External rotation: toe out/ heel in

Here is the leg in internal rotation (at the hip) (1).

Here is the leg in external rotation (2).

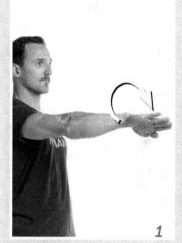
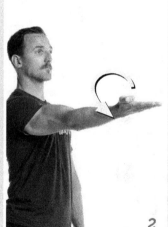

Internal rotation: turn thumb in

External rotation: turn thumb out

Here is the upper arm in internal rotation (1).

Here is the upper arm in external rotation (2).

In many movements, proper set-up will require externally rotating a limb against a fixed point. For example, when learning the squat, we'll talk about "screwing your feet into the floor," and when learning to bench press, "trying to snap the bar in half." This action winds the head of the femur or humerus tight in its capsule, creating torque, which promotes stability and the efficient transfer of power.

The scapulae (shoulder blades) play a critical role in helping to keep the shoulder joint stable under load, as in a bench press or pull-up. Conscious positioning of the shoulder blades is an important part of setting up the front rack position, as well. Here's how we'll refer to movement of the scapulae.

Retraction means the shoulder blades are drawn toward each other across the spine.

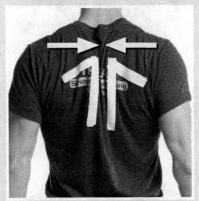

Scapular retraction pulls the shoulders back

Protraction means the shoulder blades are pulled apart, away from the spine.

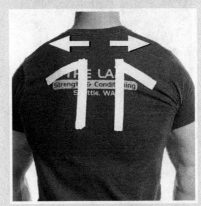

Scapular protraction dumps the shoulder forward

Here is the shoulder with scapulae pro-tracted (1) and retracted (2). The position of the shoulder is usually, but not always, dictated by the action of the shoulder blades.

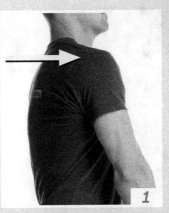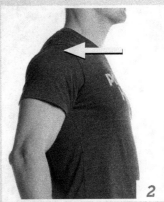

Protraction moves shoulder forward   *Retraction moves shoulder back*

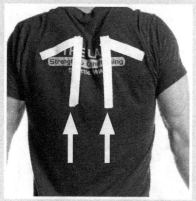

Scapular elevation shrugs the shoulders up

Elevation means the shoulder blades are raised up toward the ears.

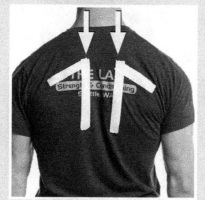

Scapular depression packs the shoulder down

Depression means the shoulder blades are pulled down toward the feet.

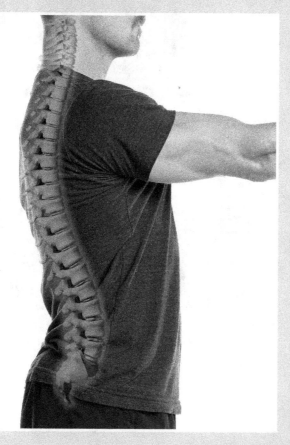

Midline stability is a term you're going to use quite a bit. Efficient transfer of power from the hips in core-to-extremity movements and the safety of the spine under load both depend greatly on midline stability.

The term refers to the neutral spine and to its relationship with the pelvis. The neutral spine has a gentle 'S' shape: from the pelvis, it turns concave through the lumbar spine, then convex through the thoracic spine before terminating at the base of the skull. From the front, it is straight and congruent with our imaginary centerline.

For optimal midline stability, the pelvis must remain in line with the spine. If it tilts forward or backward, it puts the lower spine in a mechanically disadvantageous position.

In every exercise we perform, we'll be careful to use the muscles of the trunk to preserve midline stability. Here's how you set up to preserve midline stability. This is important, so I'm putting it in giant type:

To stabilize your midline, squeeze your butt cheeks, pull your rib cage toward your pelvis and lock in your abs like you're making a "six-pack" in front of the mirror, then finally set your shoulders back and down, "packing" them toward your back pockets.

This will apply to virtually every exercise we'll be examining in this book, so start getting your athletes in the habit of stabilizing their midlines. Don't forget to do it yourself!

 Remember! The neck is part of the spine, so try to keep them in line—what's referred to as a neutral head position. If your hips travel back and your torso tilts forward, your nose should point at the floor. When the hips extend and your spine returns to vertical, your nose should point forward.

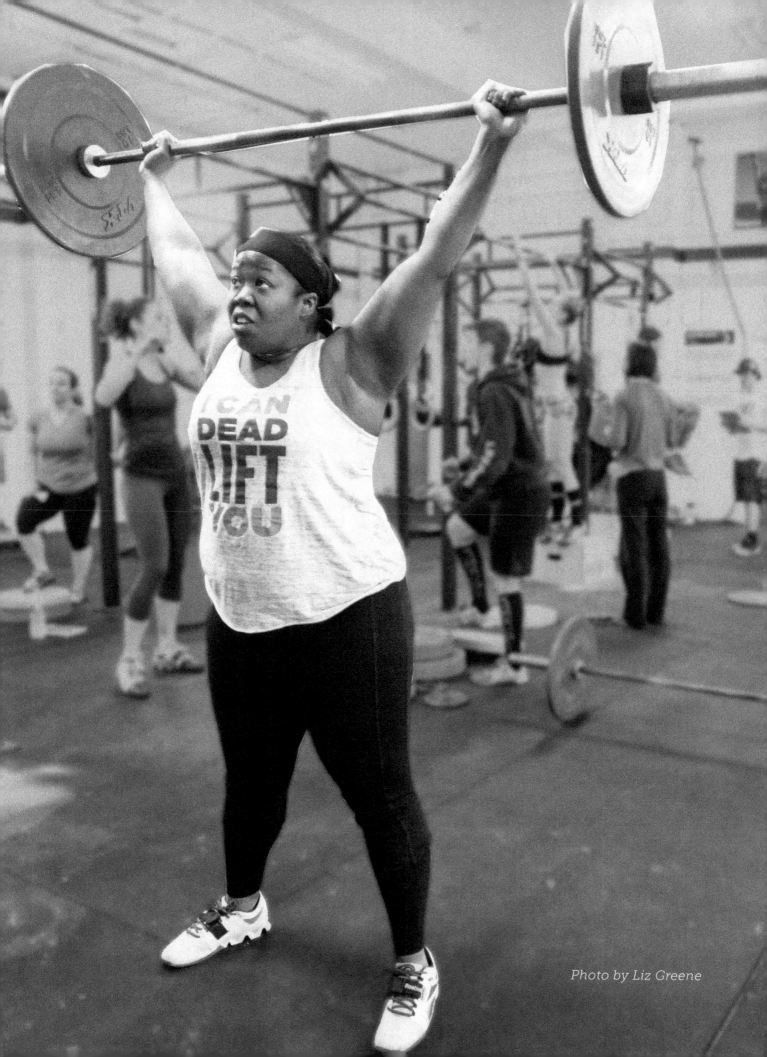

THE SAMSON STRETCH

Category: N/a

Movement screen: N/a

Ability screen: N/a

While generally speaking it is advisable to avoid static stretching before working out, many of us have very tight hip flexors and shoulder extensors, so it's helpful to elongate these tissues so don't impede our efforts as we squat and press.

We'll learn a lot about Harry, Amy, and Tim from how they fare with the Samson stretch. If a new athlete has difficulty stepping into a lunge, holding a pose, and the stepping back up, you'll know to keep an extra careful eye on him as you introduce the squat. If she overarches her back, spinal hypermobility might make correct squat and deadlift positions a challenge. If he is unable to raise his arms in line with his vertical torso, all manner of overhead movements (press, push press, push jerk, American kettlebell swing, overhead squat) will be unavailable to him, at least for awhile. For you as an instructor, knowing that an athlete will have issues even before you start teaching is a distinct advantage. Forewarned is forearmed.

Samson Stretch Teaching Script

"Stand up tall, with your feet hip-width. Without moving your feet, try to screw them into the ground, right foot clockwise, left counterclockwise. Squeeze your butt tight, lock your abs down, set your shoulders back and down. This is **Samson Stretch Position 1 (SS 1).**

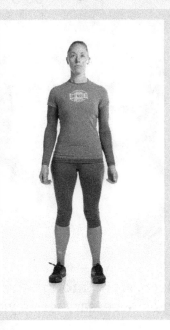
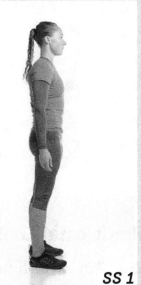

SS 1

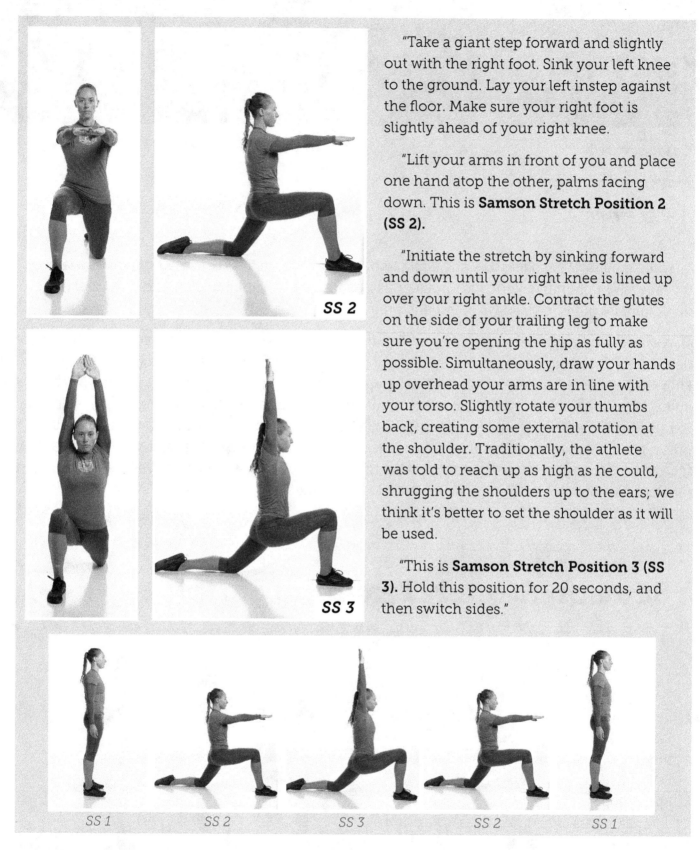

SS 2

SS 3

SS 1   SS 2   SS 3   SS 2   SS 1

"Take a giant step forward and slightly out with the right foot. Sink your left knee to the ground. Lay your left instep against the floor. Make sure your right foot is slightly ahead of your right knee.

"Lift your arms in front of you and place one hand atop the other, palms facing down. This is **Samson Stretch Position 2 (SS 2).**

"Initiate the stretch by sinking forward and down until your right knee is lined up over your right ankle. Contract the glutes on the side of your trailing leg to make sure you're opening the hip as fully as possible. Simultaneously, draw your hands up overhead your arms are in line with your torso. Slightly rotate your thumbs back, creating some external rotation at the shoulder. Traditionally, the athlete was told to reach up as high as he could, shrugging the shoulders up to the ears; we think it's better to set the shoulder as it will be used.

"This is **Samson Stretch Position 3 (SS 3).** Hold this position for 20 seconds, and then switch sides."

Positional Drills

"1! 2! 3! 1!" Have your athletes work through the positions of the Samson stretch, holding each position as long as necessary while you make corrections.

Samson Stretch Common Faults and Fixes

1. Knee jammed forward over foot.

Samson Stretch Position 3 fault. As the athlete settles to the floor into Samson Stretch 2, care must be taken that the foot of the leading leg is in front of the knee. That way, when she sinks forward and down into SS 3, her knee will line up over the ankle.

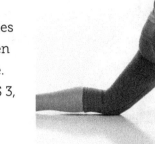

Fault

 "Bigger step!"

 Demonstrate a correct SS 3.

 Tap the heel of the leading foot to get the athlete to move it forward.

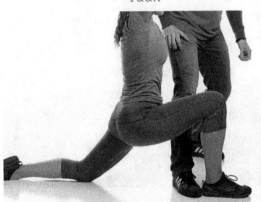

Tactile

2. Not stretching enough.

Samson Stretch Position 3 violation. Sometimes an athlete doesn't understand that although this is a static hold, it's still supposed to feel like hard work! She shouldn't feel comfortable or relaxed. Encourage her to squeeze her glutes to force the hip to open, and to engage the muscles of the upper back to open up the shoulder.

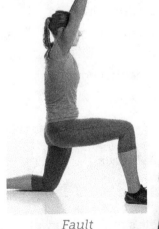

Fault

 "Sink forward and down!"

 Demonstrate a correct SS 3.

 A hand or knee gently pushing at the small of the back will encourage the athlete to move her hips into position, while pressure on the wrist will increase the angle of the arm relative to the body.

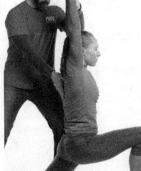

Tactile

Samson Stretch Common Faults and Fixes, cont.

3. Arms out front.

Samson Stretch 3 violation. In the Samson Stretch, the shoulders must be in full flexion, with the arms perpendicular to the ground.

 "Pull hands back!"

 Demonstrate a correct SS 3.

 Gently guide the arms to the proper position. Don't allow the trainee to compromise midline stability.

 Attach a resistance band to a pull-up bar and have the trainee grasp it in both hands as she steps into the stretch. If she concentrates on keeping her ribs locked down and her midline neutral, the band will help stretch her shoulders.

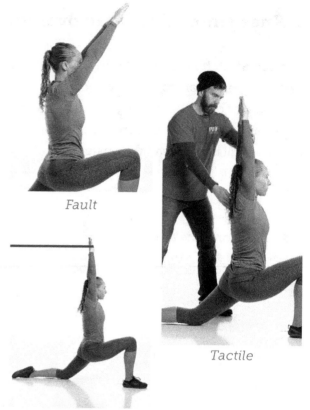

Fault

Tactile

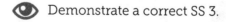

Orthosis

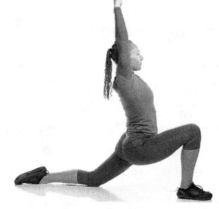

Fault

4. Hyperextended spine.

Samson Stretch Position 3 violation. Often an athlete lacking shoulder flexibility will overarch her spine in an attempt to get her hands to the right place. When you return her spine to a neutral position, you may reveal an issue with her shoulder flexion.

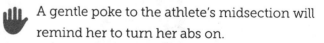 "Pull your ribs down!" or "Six pack!"

Demonstrate a correct SS 3.

A gentle poke to the athlete's midsection will remind her to turn her abs on.

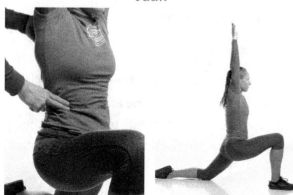

Tactile   *Correct SS 3*

94

GOOD MORNINGS

Category: Hip and Trunk Extension

Movement screen: N/a

Ability screen: N/a

The good morning exercise develops the ability to hinge at the hip while maintaining a neutral spine. The athlete holds a piece of PVC pipe across the traps, and then, with knees unlocked, pushes his hips back, inclining the torso toward the floor. When the athlete has gone as far as he can while maintaining his lumbar curve, he then brings his hips forward to stand. Performed with PVC, the good morning is a very effective warm-up for the hamstrings, glutes, and spinal erectors. Performed with a loaded barbell, the good morning is a staple posterior chain strengthener.

If your athlete has trouble with the positions of the good morning, he'll likely have problems with the squat and the deadlift. Remedial mobilization should begin immediately.

Having taught Harry, Amy, and Tim the Samson stretch, what can we expect with the good morning? Well, Amy is flexible and easily hit the positions of the SS, so the GM should prove no problem. Harry's lunge was good, but he couldn't get his shoulders into full flexion. That will affect his overhead work, but not the GM. Tim, on the other hand, was very stiff in the hips and back. I'm anticipating a correct good morning might prove a challenge for him.

Good Morning Teaching Script

"Grasp a 5' length of PVC pipe in both hands, then lift it over your head. Place it on your traps just below the nape of your neck. Set your feet hip-width. Create some torque at the hip by screwing your feet into the ground (right foot clockwise, left foot counter clockwise). Contract your glutes, lock down your abs, set your shoulders back and down. This is **Good Morning Position 1 (GM 1).**

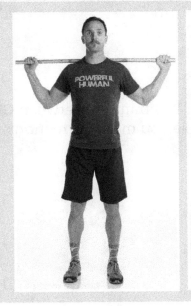 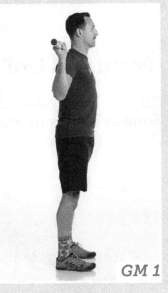

GM 1

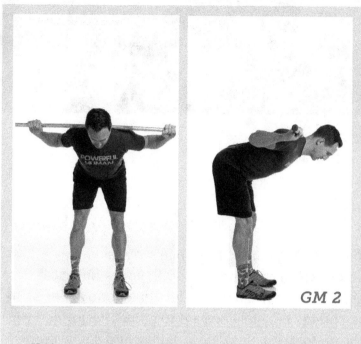

"Unlock your knees. Now, keeping your chest up and without allowing your knees to come forward, pull your hips back until you feel a strong stretch in your hamstrings. Torso parallel to the floor is preferred, but only go as far as you can without your spine going into flexion. This is **Good Morning Position 2 (GM 2)**."

GM 2

"Lift your shoulders and squeeze your glutes to bring your hips forward to return to **GM 1**.

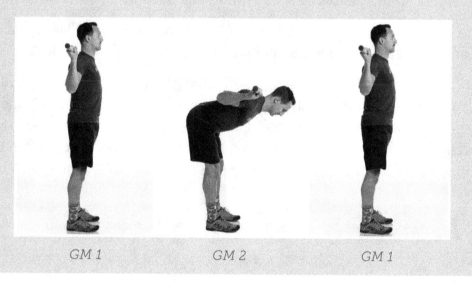

GM 1   *GM 2*   *GM 1*

Positional Drills

"1! 2! 1!" Have your athletes translate between **GM 1** and **GM 2**, holding each position as long as necessary while you make corrections.

All Hinges, Great and Small

"Rhyming positions" are poses different exercises have in common. Sometimes the positions are identical; other times, merely similar. Start looking for them now, so you'll be able to point them out to your athletes later. When athletes can relate a new movement to a pattern they already know well, it greatly accelerates the learning process. (More rhyming positions can be found in Appendix IV, "Rhyming Positions", on page 552.)

While there are only two poses for the good morning, if you break down the transition between GM 1 and GM 2 into two additional phases, you'll find there are strong positional transferabilities to other, more complex movements.

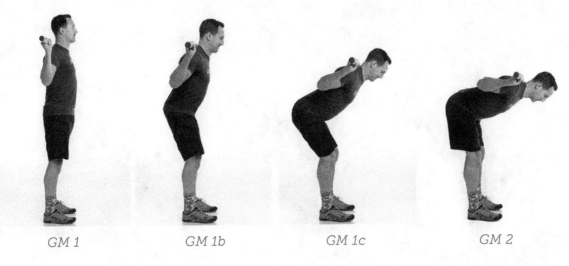

| GM 1 | GM 1b | GM 1c | GM 2 |

Except for the width of the stance, GM 1b is virtually identical to Back Squat Position 2. In both cases, the hips have moved back just enough to load the posterior chain, while the barbell borne on the back shifts slightly forward, placing it in the "line of gravity", where best leverage is obtained. (More about the line of gravity in Week One, Day Three's Deadlift section.) Meanwhile, the knees bend, but shins remain vertical.

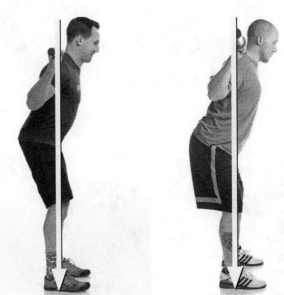

GM 1b and BS 2 both shift the load directly into the line of gravity .

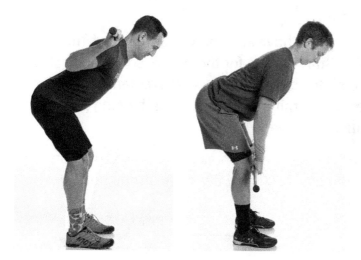

As we'll soon see, the torso and knee angle of GM 1c are very similar to Deadlift Position 2.

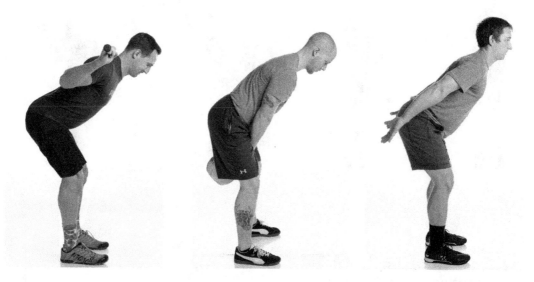

GM 1c also matches Russian Swing Position 1 and Jump Position 2.

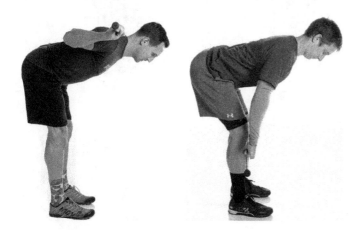

Finally, except for the fact the bar is held by the hands against the leg, and is not sitting on the back, Romanian Deadlift Position 2 is the same as GM 2.

Good Morning Common Faults and Fixes

1. Back rounds

Good Morning Position 2 fault. Some athletes, due to inflexibility, motor control issues, or both, will have a difficult time maintaining a neutral spine as they hinge back at the hip.

 "Chest up!" or "Flat back!" or "Tight lumbar!"

 Demonstrate proper GM 2 positioning.

As the athlete hinges slowly, manually adjust his back position, switching between a light pull at the hip (to keep the hips moving in the correct direction), a lift at the shoulders (to encourage thoracic extension), and a tap between the shoulder blades (to remind the athlete to keep his shoulders back).

Have the trainee hold a 5'length of PVC pipe behind his back, one hand high, the other hand low. The pipe should make contact at the back of trainee's head, between the shoulder blades, and at the tailbone. Point out that he feels no contact of the pipe with the lower back because of the natural concavity of the lumbar spine. If he loses contact with his sacral spine, he has lost a neutral spine.

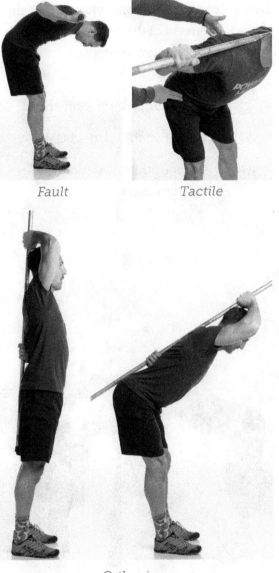

Fault   *Tactile*

Orthosis

Good Morning Common Faults and Fixes, cont.

2. Knees locked back

Good Morning Position 2 violation. Maintaining locked extension of the knees puts an unnecessary strain on the athlete's lower back.

 "Knees unlock!" or "Soft knees!"

 Demonstrate a correct GM2.

 Tap the athlete behind the knees to encourage him to unlock.

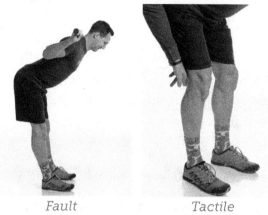

Fault   *Tactile*

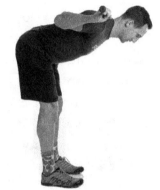

Correct GM 2

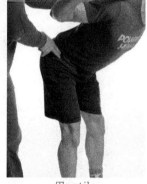

Fault   *Tactile*

3. Pitching forward

Good Morning Position 2 violation. Rather than pushing his hips back, the athlete leans forward until the weight is distributed to the front of his foot and he's almost tipping over. Ask the trainee to imagine he is a bow, as in bow and arrow. The string attaches at the shoulder and the knee. The hips are the point where the fingers grasp the string to draw it back. It's easiest to use a tactile cue here: put one hand on his shoulder, two fingers at his hip, and draw his hips back.

 "Hips back first!" or "Heels!"

 Demonstrate proper transition from GM1 to GM 2.

 Two fingers at the athlete's hip can encourage proper hip draw.

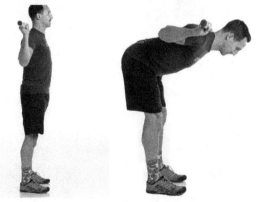

Correct Transition from GM 1 to GM 2

AIR SQUATS

Category: Squat

Movement screen: N/a

Ability screen: Good morning x 5 (box squat), 12" box squat x 5 (air squat)

The squat has been referred to as a "universal motor pattern"—it seems as if it was coded in our DNA. Toddlers need no coaching to rest in a well-organized squat, and it's the seated position of choice for people all over the world. Only in the industrialized nations have we lost the ability to squat, and it's been to our detriment.

As a calisthenic exercise, the squat can be a wickedly effective conditioning tool. And when loaded with a barbell, the squat becomes the foundation for any effective strength and conditioning program. The barbell back squat, front squat, and overhead squat are all based on the air squat, as are the clean, the snatch, and MMGPP staples like burpees, thrusters, and wallballs.

Just as you can know a lot about someone by the way they shake hands, you can tell how carefully (or not) an athlete has been trained by the quality of their squat. All too often the humble air squat hasn't received the attention it deserves. Don't skimp, or somewhere down the line, your athletes will pay the price. As Kelly Starrett says, "The bottom line is that if you want to optimize performance and escape pain and injury, it's imperative that you learn how to squat correctly."

In By the Numbers, instruction of the air squat begins with the reduced range-of-motion box squat. Many trainees joining your program simply won't have the strength, flexibility, coordination, or balance to squat on Day One. So rather than embarrass them in the first five minutes of their first class (and no matter how nice you try to be, if someone can't do a simple movement seemingly everyone else can perform without difficulty, he is going to be embarrassed), by starting with the box squat, you'll ensure their first experience of learning MMGPP is a positive one.

How will our three new athletes fare with the air squat? (They need a catchy name. How about "Team Space Monkey"?) Based on the Samson stretch and the good morning, I predict Amy will have an excellent squat right out of the box. Harry's will be pretty good, too. As likely as not, though, Tim won't be air squatting today; I think he'll be sticking with the box squat. Let's find out.

Box Squat Teaching Script

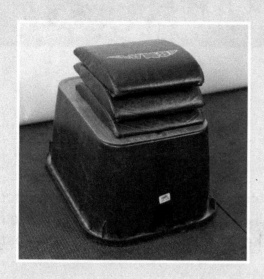

"If you can sit down on a chair, you can box squat. The box squat teaches how to hinge at the hip, lower yourself under control to a seated position, and then stand, without imposing the strength and flexibility demands of a full range-of-motion squat.

"Start by stacking three Abmats on top of a 12" box.

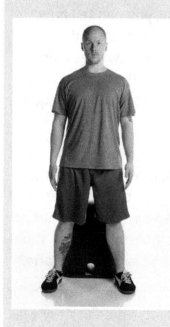
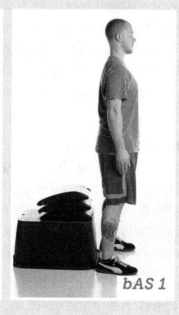

bAS 1

"Stand with the box about 1" behind your heels. Set your feet shoulder-width apart. The squat is essentially sitting down between your feet, so if your stance is too narrow, at the bottom there won't be room between your heels for your hips. Your feet should be only slightly turned out—5-10 degrees. With your weight centered over a point between your heel and the arch of your foot, screw your feet into the floor, right foot clockwise, left foot counterclockwise. Try to grip the floor with your toes.

"Stand as tall as you can. Brace your midline by squeezing your glutes and contracting your abs. Then pack your shoulders.

"You are now in **Box Squat Position 1 (bAS 1)**—the start and finish of every repetition.

"Unlock your knees and sit your hips back. Your ribs remain locked down. Push your knees out. You should feel tension in your hamstrings. Flex your elbows to lift your hands. This is **Box Squat Position 2 (bAS 2).**

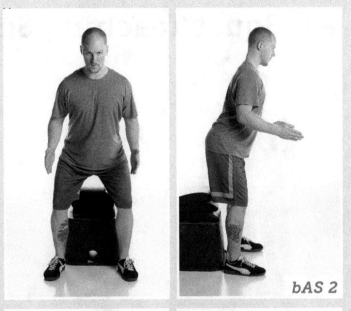

bAS 2

"Keeping your knees out, sit straight down until your butt touches the Abmat. Do not come to rest! Maintain tension in your hips and hamstrings. Keep your weight just in front of your heel and your back straight. Lift your hands up high for balance. This is **Box Squat Position 3 (bAS 3).**

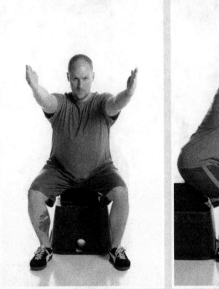
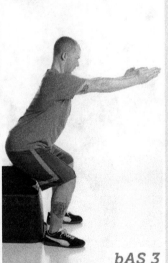

bAS 3

"Stand back up to **bAS 2.**

"Squeeze your glutes to bring your hips forward into **bAS 1.**

"If you sat and stood with good form, take a mat away. Repeat the process until you're sitting to the box only."

Positional Drills

"1! 2! 1! 2!" Practice the stand and hinge positions one at a time, with your trainees holding the pose as necessary while you make corrections.

"1! 2! 3! 2! 1!" Practice all three Box Squat positions one at a time, making corrections as necessary.

Air Squat Teaching Script

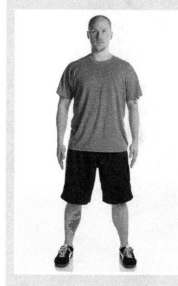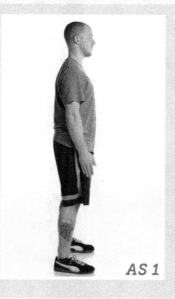

AS 1

"When you've got a handle on the box squat, it's time to air squat.

"Air Squat Position 1 (AS 1) is the same as Box Squat Position 1: standing tall as possible, heels shoulder-width, slight turnout of the toes, feet screwed into the ground by contracting your quads and glutes, toes gripping the ground, abs locked down, shoulders packed.

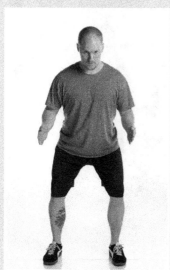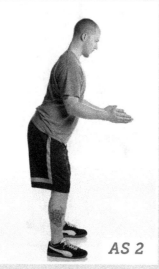

AS 2

"Unlock your knees and sit your hips back. Push your knees out. Flex your elbows to lift your hands for counterbalance. This is **Air Squat Position 2 (AS 2).**

"This is a critical step. When people complain that squats hurt their knees, it's often because they squat with the knees first, allowing the weight to roll forward onto the balls of the feet. This puts unnecessary shear force on the knees. Hinging back puts the stress in the hips, where it's easily borne.

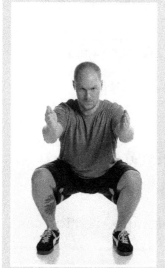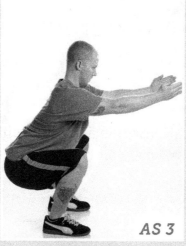

AS 3

"Keeping your knees tracking over your feet, sit straight down. 'Pull' yourself into this position by engaging your hip flexors. Your spine remains neutral.

"As you descend, raise your arms to help maintain balance, taking care to keep your shoulders back. Stop when the crease of your hip is below the top of your knee. Weight remains at center of foot, with a slight emphasis on the heels. This is **Air Squat Position 3 (AS 3).**

"Drive up until you've returned to **AS 2.**

"Squeeze your glutes to bring your hips forward into **AS 1.**

"Let's take a closer look at the definition of legal depth. Imagine a plane parallel to the floor placed just at the top of the knee (1). In **AS 3**, the crease of hip (2) must be below that invisible plane for the squat to count. This applies in metcon workouts as well as 1RM strength training efforts.

"If you wish, you may squat lower, as long as the lumbar curve is preserved. But for the general fitness trainee, this is deep enough."

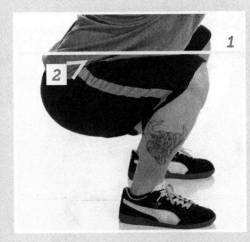

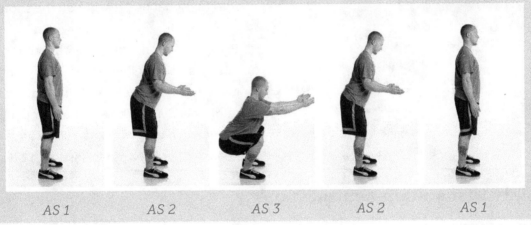

| AS 1 | AS 2 | AS 3 | AS 2 | AS 1 |

Positional Drills

"1! 2! 1!" Practice the stand and hinge positions one at a time, with your trainees holding the pose while you make necessary corrections. Make sure knees are unlocked and shins remain vertical as trainees push hips back into **AS 2**.

"1! 2! 3! 2! 1!" Take athletes through the positions of the air squat one at a time, with trainees holding the poses as necessary while you make corrections.

"1! 2! 3! Go!" Take athletes from stand through hinge to squat, with trainees holding the poses as necessary while you make corrections, and then have them rise on their own through the hinge to stand.

"1! 2! Go!" Take athletes from stand through hinge, then have them sit and stand through **AS 3, AS 2, AS 1** on their own.

"1! Go!" Full air squat.

Air Squat Common Faults and Fixes

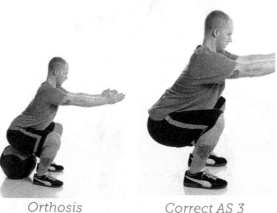

Fault

Tactile

Orthosis

Correct AS 3

1. Insufficient depth.

Air Squat Position 3 violation. Legal depth for the squat is defined as "crease of the hip below the top of the knee."

 "Sit lower!" or just "Lower!"

 Demonstrate correct depth, or, after making eye contact, just point forcefully at the ground.

 As athlete holds in AS 3, gently push him deeper into the squat by pressing on the shoulders and

 Place a box or medicine ball about 1" behind the athlete's heels Tell him to sit down until his butt just lightly taps the box, then stand. Tall athletes might need a medball atop a bumper plate or an Abmat on a box, whereas a short athlete might need a stack of bumpers less than 12" high.

2. Inability to maintain neutral spine.

Air Squat Position 2 and Position 3 violation. Sometimes an athlete will have a hard time maintaining a flat back as he squats. Assuming his spine is not kyphotic, this is a motor control issue.

1. IN POSITION AIR SQUAT POSITION 2:

 "Chest up!" or "Shoulders back!"

 Demonstrate hinging from Air Squat 1 to Air Squat 2 with a flat back.

With the athlete holding in AS 2, tap him between the shoulder blades to get him to pull his shoulders back, which will lift the chest and return him to a neutral position. Failing that, put one hand at his hip to serve as fulcrum, and then put the other on his shoulder to lift his chest.

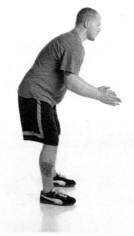

Fault in AS 2

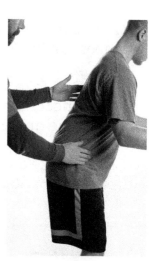

Tactile

Air Squat Common Faults and Fixes, cont.

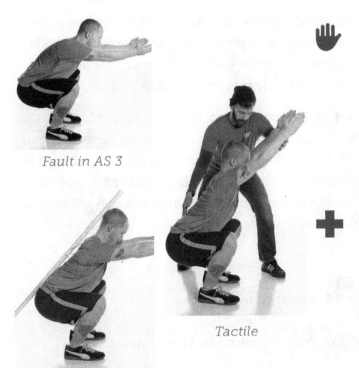

Fault in AS 3

Tactile

Orthosis

2. IN AIR SQUAT POSITION 3:

Lift athlete's arms to raise his chest. Keep your other hand on his hip, effectively making that the fixed fulcrum point.

Use "The Tail"! The Tail is a 5' length of PVC pipe with a hole drilled through it. Thread twine, a broken jump rope, shoelaces, or what have you through the hole to create two shoulder loops. Have the athlete slip his arms through the loops so that when he stands tall, The Tail is in contact with his tailbone, thoracic spine, and the back of his head. As the athlete practices the positions of the air squat, he should strive to maintain these points of contact with the Tail. Loss of contact at the tailbone means the athlete failed to maintain a neutral spine position.

3. Spinal overextension.

Air Squat Position 2 violation. If an athlete fails to keep his abdominal muscles engaged as he hinges back into Position 2, he may arch his spine in an exaggerated fashion. Not particularly dangerous in the air squat, but will cause problems later when the squat is loaded.

 "Abs on!" or "Ribs down!" or "Six pack!"

 Demonstrate pulling your ribcage toward your pelvis by contracting your abs.

 A light tap with the back of the hand will encourage ab engagement. Use with discretion.

 THE TAIL! If the PVC loses contact with the t-spine, the athlete is hyperextending his back.

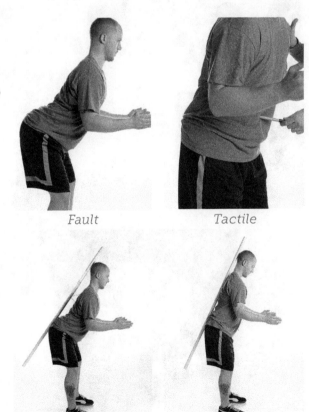

Fault

Tactile

Orthosis

Air Squat Common Faults and Fixes, cont.

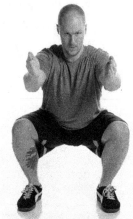

Fault

Correct

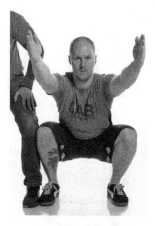

Tactile

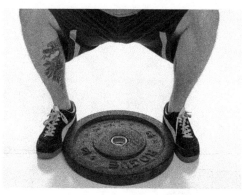

Orthosis

4. Excessive toe turn-out.

Air Squat Position 3 violation. Sometimes an athlete's feet externally rotate (turn out) as he descends, while his knees continue traveling forward, twisting a joint that's really only meant to hinge open and closed.

Is it a motor control problem? Tight hips? Tight adductors? You can make a diagnosis later. The specific etiology of the symptom isn't that important—you need to get him moving well now. And most of the time, continually working toward the ideal position will resolve the issue, whatever it is.

 "Screw your feet in!"

 Demonstrate correct toe turnout in AS 1.

 Block one of your athlete's feet with your foot. Have him squat. He'll feel additional tightness in his hips, but also what a correct foot position feels like.

Grab a 10lbs bumper plate (for people 5'10" and and above) or an Abmat (for people under 5' 10"). Place it on the ground, and tell the athlete to fix his feet to the sides of the object. Make sure sides of heels and sides of balls of his feet are in contact. Explain that as he squats, he is to keep the sides of his feet fixed against the object. Cue him through the positions of the squat. It might be difficult, but he'll quickly get the idea. The orthosis provides immediate proprioceptive feedback, as well as a point against which the leg adductors can work to help prevent unwanted rotation.

Air Squat Common Faults and Fixes, cont.

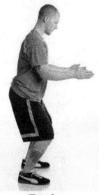

Fault

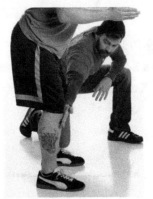

Tactile

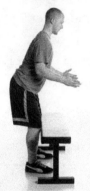

Orthosis

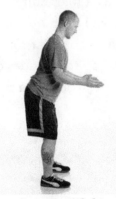

Correct AS 2

5. Weight on balls of feet.

Air Squat Position 3 violation. The athlete's weight is distributed toward the balls of his feet, putting shear on the knee, and reducing posterior chain's contribution to the squat. This can have any of several causes.

1. BREAKING AT KNEES TOO SOON. The athlete initiates his squat by sending his knees forward while his torso remains vertical. The result is his weight shifts onto the balls of his feet, and his legs and hips compress straight down like the folds of an accordion.

🗣 "Sit back!" or "Butt back!" or "Hips first!"

👁 Demonstrate the hip hinge in a correct AS 2.

✋ Block the athlete's knee with the back of your hand as he initiates the squat.

➕ Have athlete stand with his knees touching the side of a utility bench. Run "1-2-1" Positional Drill. The bench will block the forward translation of his knees—he'll quickly get the idea.

2. TECHNICAL ERROR. The most common cause, and the easiest to fix, is a simple misunderstanding of how the body's weight should be distributed across the foot. Explain to the athlete that for best leverage, he must keep the load in the line of gravity (more about this in the Deadlift section). Tell him to try to be aware of the greatest concentration of pressure on the soles of his feet, and to keep that point between the arch of the foot and the heel.

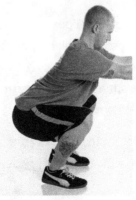

Fault

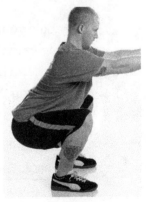

Correct AS 3

🗣 "Heels!" or "Weight back!"

👁 Demonstrate weight distribution in AS 1. AS 2, ad AS 3.

Air Squat Common Faults and Fixes, cont.

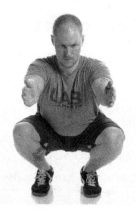

Fault (caused by narrow stance)

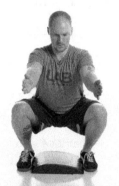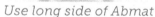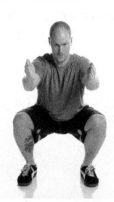

Use long side of Abmat   *Correct AS 3*

3. NARROW STANCE. If the feet are too close and there's no room for the hips in the bottom of the squat, in AS 3 the athlete will tend to pitch forward.

 "Wider stance" or "Move your feet out!"

 Demonstrate AS 3 with proper width stance.

 Grab a 10lbs bumper plate (for people 5'10" and above) or an Abmat (for people under 5' 10"). Place it on the ground, and tell the athlete to fix his feet to the sides of the object. This serves as a rough guide for proper stance width.

4. LOSS OF BALANCE ON DESCENT. Motor sequencing is correct but athlete rocks forward in bottom of squat. May also be caused by tight ankles (see Air Squat Fault 9).

 "Wriggle your toes" or "Toes up". Curling the toes toward the ceiling will help your athlete understand proper distribution of weight on the foot during the squat, but make sure he understands this isn't a permanent fix.

 Demonstrate AS 3 with weight in toes, then rock back onto heels to show proper weight distribution.

 As the athlete holds in AS 3, shift your athlete into the desired position by gently pushing him back at the knee. It's helpful if you place a knee behind him at the tailbone, so he feels supported.

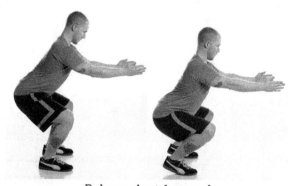

Balance lost forward

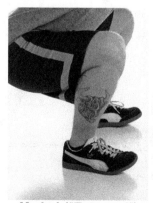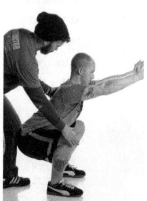

Verbal ("Toes up!")   *Tactile*

Air Squat Common Faults and Fixes, cont.

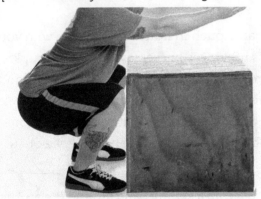

Squat initiated by knees sends weight forward

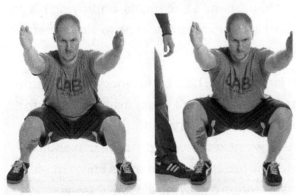

Orthosis

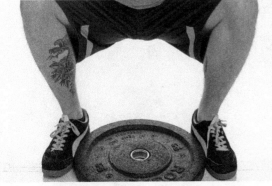

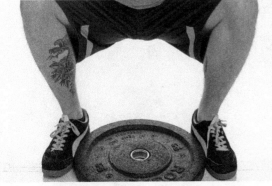

Fault   *Tactile*

Orthosis

Weight on balls of feet, cont.

5. JAMS KNEES FORWARD IN BOTTOM POSITION. Often but not necessarily the result of initiating the squat with the knees. Sometimes caused by hyper-flexible ankles and a lack of clarity about proper bottom positions. A third cause: inability to sit back due to tight hamstrings. Not to be confused with the knees-past-the-toes A2G squat of a competent weightlifter.

 Have the athlete stand with his toes touching the side of a box. Not close, actually in contact. Then ask him to squat. If he tries to drive his knees to far forward, the box will block him, sending him sprawling back. After a little practice he'll break the bad habit. If this fault is accompanied by a pronounced lean athlete may need a counterbalance.

6. Knees cave in.

Air Squat Position 3 violation. This is called a "Valgus fault". When the knees cave in, it puts twisting rotational force on a joint that functions mainly as a simple, opening-and-closing hinge. This can have any of several causes.

1. TOO-WIDE STANCE. A wide stance will tend to make the knees bend in (the exception is powerlifters consciously using a wide stance).

 "Move your feet in!"

 Demonstrate a proper width stance in AS 1.

 Tap athlete's foot with your own to get him to move his foot in to a proper stance width.

 Grab a 10lbs bumper plate (for people 5'10" and and above) or an Abmat (for people under 5' 10"). Place it on the ground, and tell the athlete to fix his feet to the sides of the object. Explain that as he squats, he is to keep the sides of his feet fixed against the bumper and push his knees out.

Air Squat Common Faults and Fixes, cont.

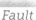
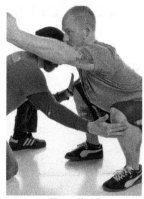

Fault

Tactile I

Knees cave in, cont.

2. LACK OF EXTERNAL ROTATION OF HIP. If athlete does not consciouly engage the quads and glutes, knees may cave in.

🗣 "Knees out!" or "Spread the floor!" or "Screw in your feet!"

👁 Demonstrate proper knee position in AS 3.

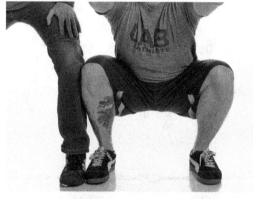

Tactile II

✋ You can crouch in front of the athlete with your hands beside his knees, saying, "Push your knees into my hands!" If that's too awkward, try standing beside the athlete, bracing his foot with your own, and crouching so that your knee becomes the objective. Tell him, "Push your knee out to mine, and match it on the other side."

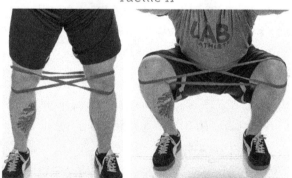
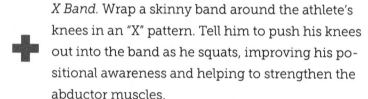

X Band

✚ *X Band.* Wrap a skinny band around the athlete's knees in an "X" pattern. Tell him to push his knees out into the band as he squats, improving his positional awareness and helping to strengthen the abductor muscles.

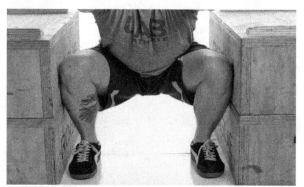

Barrier Method

✚ *Barrier method.* The X band works, but it's cumbersome, and difficult to get in and out of during a workout. Instead, try putting the athlete between two boxes, set at a distance that approximates the ideal placement of his knees in Air Squat Position 3. Having a goal—*Push your knees out to the boxes*—seems to help expedite learning the correct motor pattern.

Air Squat Common Faults and Fixes, cont.

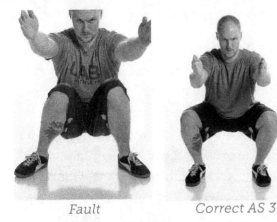

Fault   *Correct AS 3*

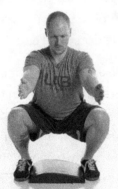

Orthosis

Knees cave in, cont.

3. EXCESS EXTERNAL ROTATION OF FOOT. Turning out the feet too far nearly always leads to a cave-in of the knees. If this is part of the basic set-up, it's an **Air Squat Position 1** violation. If it happens as the athlete descends into the bottom of the squat, it's an **Air Squat Position 3 violation.**

 "Toes in!"

 Demonstrate proper foot position in AS 1 or AS 3 as appropriate.

 Grab a 10lbs bumper plate (for people 5'10" and and above) or an Abmat (for people under 5' 10"). Place it on the ground, and tell the athlete to fix his feet to the sides of the object. Pressing his feet against the bumpers fires the adductors, which can act in a synergistic fashion as external rotators and push out the knees!

7. Loss of Lumbar Curve.

Air Squat Position 3 violation. Athlete rounds his lower back in the bottom position of the squat. Not particularly dangerous in the air squat, but if not corrected will be very problematic when the athlete attempts weighted squats.

1. DUMPING. If an athlete loses hamstring tension and collapses at the bottom of the squat to sit on his haunches, his pelvis will rotate posteriorly, causing loss of lumbar curve. Often caused by squatting too deep.

 "Chest up!" or "Too low!", as appropriate.

 Demonstrate a correct AS 3.

 With athlete holding in AS 3, lift his hips to correct height, and then raise his arms to lift his chest.

 Use a box or medball to set correct height.

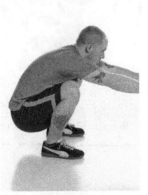

Fault

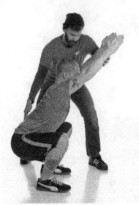

Tactile

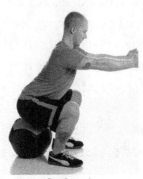

Orthosis

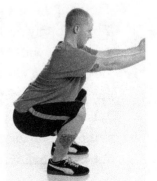

Correct AS 3

Air Squat Common Faults and Fixes, cont.

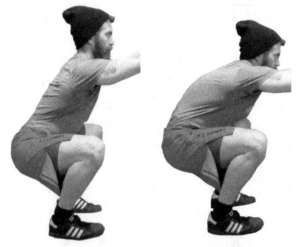

Extension to neutral: ok, not great

Extension to flexion: ugh, no way

Loss of lumbar curve, cont.

2. BUTT WINK. Ideally, as the athlete squats, the pelvis stays perfectly in line with the spine. However, several factors—hamstring inflexibility, tight hip flexors, and even the shape of the acetabulum (hip socket) itself—can limit the pelvis's ability to follow the spine as the hips drop low in the squat. If the pelvis is immobilized so it can't tilt to follow the spine, the back will round in compensation. This rapid shift of pelvis angle is referred to as "butt wink". A little bit of butt wink is not the end of the world, as long as the spine stays neutral. But if the lumbar spine goes into flexion, it's a cause for concern.

Pry squats, detailed at the end of this section, will do wonders for butt wink if the problem is in the hamstrings. If the problem is short hip flexors (which pull the head of the femur forward in the acetabulum, causing impingement and preventing pelvic tilt), one of Kelly Starrett's mobilizations would be appropriate.

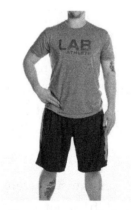

Two fingers placed

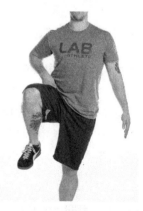

Captain Morgan

3. LACK OF HIP FLEXOR RECRUITMENT. Sometimes loss of lumbar can be ameliorated by teaching the athlete to strongly fire his hip flexors in the bottom position.

➕ Have your athlete put two fingers at the crook of his hip. Then tell him, "Pretend you're Captain Morgan!" As he raises his leg, ask his to notice how strongly his hip flexor is firing. Next, have him squat with fingers placed at both hips, and as he descends, ask him to "pinch" his fingers with his hip flexors. If tight hamstrings are the issue, this contraction will resist the hamstrings' attempt to pull the pelvis into a posterior tilt, keep the pelvis in line, and preserve the lumbar curve.

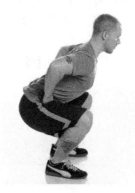

Pinching

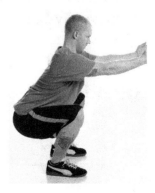

Correct AS 3

Air Squat Common Faults and Fixes, cont.

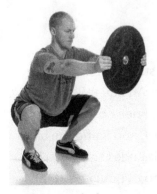

Fault

8. Immature squat/excessive lean

Air Squat Position 3 violation. A squat can be technically correct—feet shoulder-width, weight back toward heels, hip crease below the knees, spine neutral—but still suboptimal because of a pronounced forward lean (remember, the weighted squats require a more and more vertical torso). This can have any of several causes.

1. BORN THAT WAY. Some athletes, due to unusually long femurs and a short torso, will always squat with a lean. Later, those athletes will be good candidates for the lowbar back squat.

2. TIGHT ANKLES. Here's a simply test to determine if an athlete lacks ankle flexibility: with his feet together, have him sit down on his haunches without falling over. If the shins cannot reduce their angle relative to the ground as the athlete descends in the squat, he'll be forced to lean forward to keep his balance.

If the athlete is unable to pass this test, no amount of cueing will fix anything. Extracurricular mobility work is required. Orthoses, however, can help the athlete improve the quality of his squat.

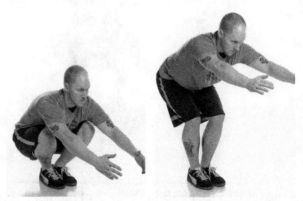

Ankle Test pass   *Ankle Test fail*

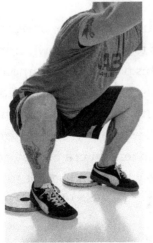

Counterbalance

Heel lift

Counterbalance. Hand the athlete a light (5-10lbs) plate, kettlebell, or dumbbell and instruct him to hold it at arm's length as he squats. Often this small load, counterbalancing the resistance of the ankles, will allow him to keep a more vertical torso. Over time the weight can be reduced until the athlete is "weaned".

Heel lift. Another alternative is to put 5 or 10lbs plates or bumpers under each of the athlete's heels. This elevated heel will often make it easier for him to maintain an upright torso in the squat. A good pair of squat shoes will also do much to alleviate this problem.

Air Squat Common Faults and Fixes, cont.

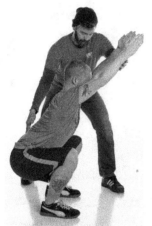

Tactile

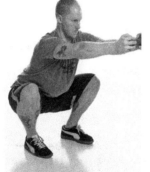

Orthosis

3. LACK OF BALANCE. The body's weight must be kept centered over the foot—if the athlete sits back too far, he'll feel like he's going to tip over backward, and will compensate by leaning forward.

 "Sit straight down!" or "Weight forward!"

 With one hand at the small of the athlete's back to keep it in place, with your other hand, raise his arms up toward the ceiling. Gradually withdraw support until he is balancing on his own.

 Hand the athlete a light (5-10lbs) dumbbell and instruct him to hold it at arm's length as he squats. Often this counterweight will allow him to keep a more vertical torso without feeling like he's going to fall backward. Over time the counterweight can be reduced as the athlete's balance improves.

4. LACK OF HIP MOBILITY. Lack of hip flexibility is extremely common, and can take a long time to fix. Here are two techniques you can teach that will help your athletes improve their ability to maintain a vertical torso at the bottom of the squat.

a. PRY SQUAT

Have your athlete loop an assistance band around a pull-up post or other upright support. Keeping as much tension on the band as necessary for balance, he is to transition slowly from Air Squat Position 1 to AS 2 and down into AS 3. Make sure everything about his position—toe turnout, knee position, depth, etc.—is on point. Then, after advising him to make sure his feet stay flat on the floor, and using the band as leverage, have him pull his hips in over his heels and lift his chest. Make sure his knees stay out. He'll probably feel a tremendous stretch through the hips. Explain to him his ultimate goal should be to hit this position, and then be able to put slack on the band and remain in a perfectly organized, upright torso squat. Have him do a couple of 15 second efforts. Ultimately he should be able to hang out for a full minute or more.

Air Squat Common Faults and Fixes, cont.

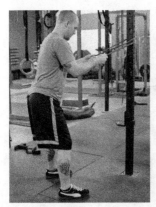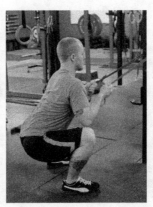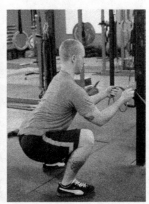

Pry squat: loop a band, use tension on band to pull yourself into good position, release tension to test position

b. HANDS-UP WALL SQUAT

All athletes, no matter how experienced, can benefit from practicing the wall squat. It is the non pareil developer of Air Squat Position 3.

Bring your athlete over to a handy wall ("This is our most expensive piece of equipment") and place him to stand facing it about one foot-length away (that is, the length of the athlete's foot). From there, ask him to take a shoulder-width stance.

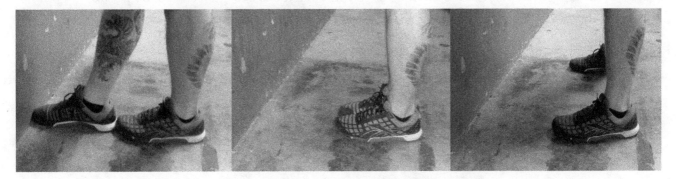

Finding proper distance for Hands-up Wall Squat Test

Talk him through setting up in **Air Squat 1:** bracing sequence, screwing in the feet, etc. Unlike a regular squat, however, have him lift his hands to place his fingertips lightly against the wall. Ask him to sit back into **Air Squat Position 2**, and from there, descend to **Air Squat Position 3**. If he is lacking in hip mobility and/or hamstring flexibility, he will quickly reach a point where he must either stop, or fall backward.

Catch him (if necessary) and then explain you want him to try again, this time by pulling himself back and down. When he hits his sticking point, he's to hold for five seconds before standing. Have him repeat for four more reps. He should do this drill every day.

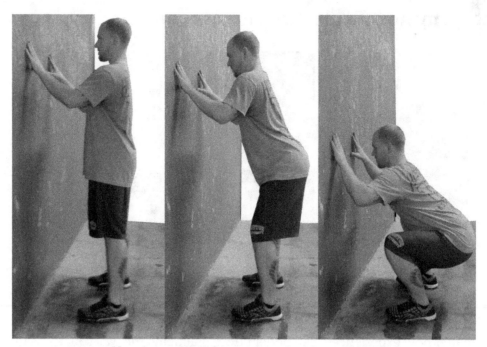

Hands-up Wall Squat start, hold, success!

! The athlete must be disciplined about not allowing his squat form to break down just so he can reach legal depth! If his feet overly externally rotate, if his knees cave in, if he has to splay his arms out for balance, have him stop. Remind him that he is striving for an ideal position. Refresh his memory as to what that looks like, then let him try again.

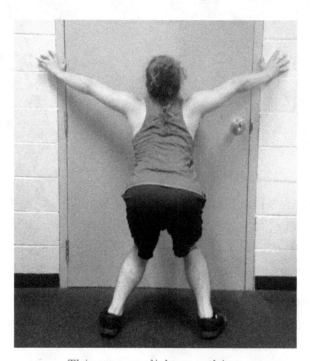

This accomplishes nothing.

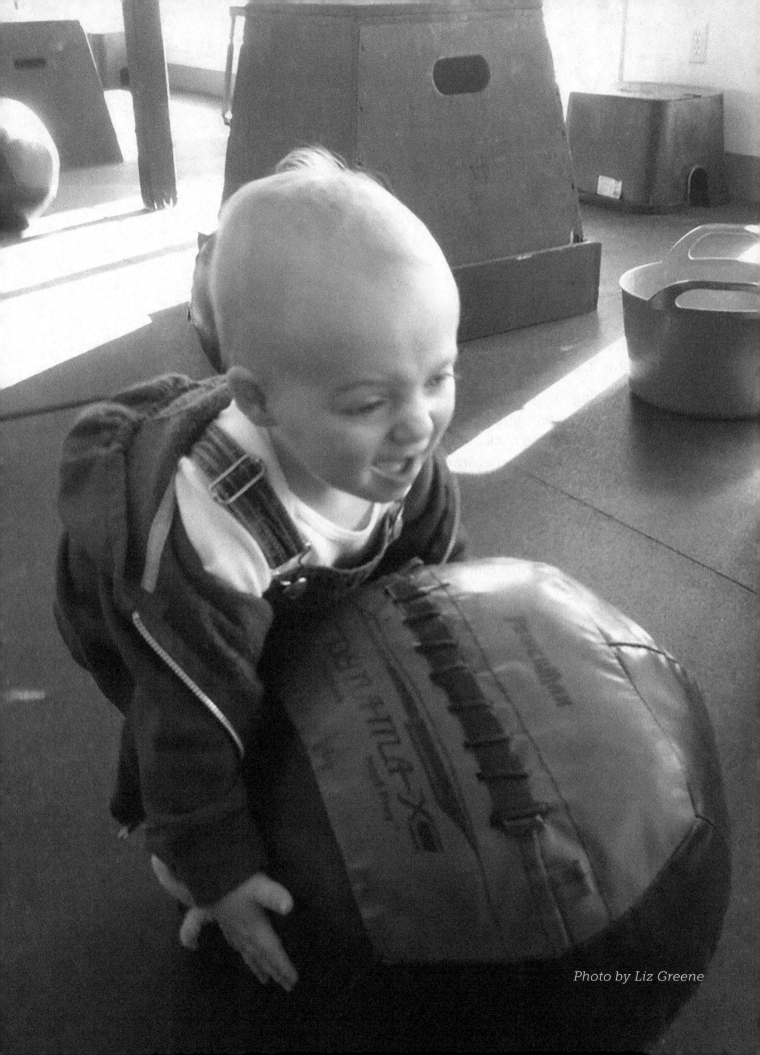

Photo by Liz Greene

RING ROWS

Category: Pull to Object (strict, horizontal)

Movement screen: N/a

Ability screen: N/a

Pull-ups are a big part of MMGPP programming. But only a small percentage of our new members come in able to do strict pull-ups. Most will start with the ring row.

To perform a ring row, the athlete begins by grasping a pair of hanging rings set at about shoulder height. Keeping a straight body line from ankle to shoulder, he leans back until his arms are fully extended. Rocking back on the fulcrum point of his heels, he pulls to bring his chest to the rings. He then straightens his arms to lower himself again, completing the repetition.

By changing the body's angle relative to the ground, the ring row can be made accessible to almost everybody, or made challenging for even the most experienced athletes.

Nobody on Team Space Monkey is elderly or excessively overweight, so I expect they'll all be able to successfully perform a Ring Row.

Ring Row Teaching Script

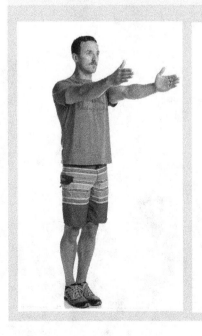
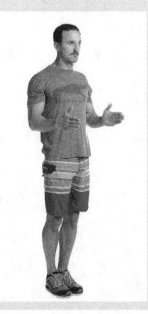

"Start by standing up tall with your feet together. Brace your midline. Elevate your arms until they are parallel to the ground. Pack your shoulders back and down. Rotate your thumbs toward the ceiling. Make a fist.

"From here, pull your elbows back until your fists are beside your ribs. Then, maintaining retraction and depression of your scapulae, punch your fists forward until your arms are straight. This is the action of the ring row.

"Now stand with a pair of rings before you hanging at about shoulder height. Grasp the rings with a thumbs-around grip.

"Maintaining a straight line from ankle to shoulder, lay back until your arms are fully extended. Keep your shoulders packed, and keep your feet together and your toes pointed. This is **Ring Row Position 1 (RR 1).**

"Next, pull until you have reached end ROM. Don't come to a full stand. This is **Ring Row Position 2 (RR 2)."**

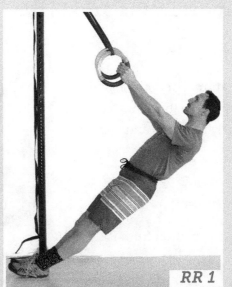
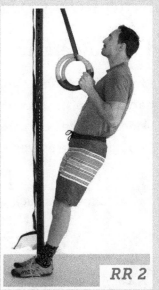

RR 1

RR 2

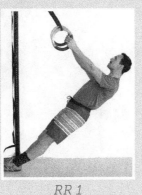
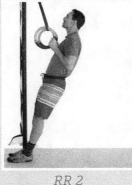
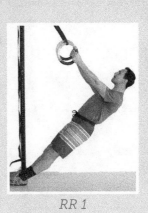

RR 1   RR 2   RR 1

Positional Drills

"1! 2! 1!" Practice the positions of the ring row one at a time, with your trainees holding the pose while you make necessary corrections. Make sure your athletes maintain a straight line from ankle to shoulder as they transition from position to position.

"The Ring Row can be made more challenging by elevating the feet, reducing the body's angle relative to the floor, and increasing the load on the arms and back."

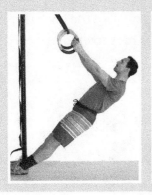
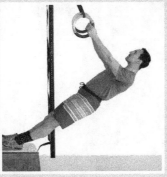
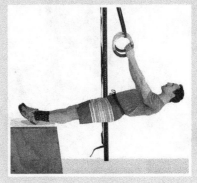

Ring Row Common Faults and Fixes

1. Shoulders dumping in.

Ring Row Position 2 violation. For optimal power transference and shoulder safety, the shoulder blades must be held partially retracted and depressed throughout the movement.

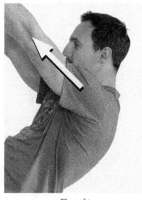 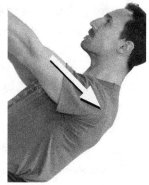

Fault   *Correct RR 1*

 "Shoulders back and down!"

 Demonstrate proper transition from RR 1 to RR 2.

 A tap between the shoulder blades can remind the athlete how to set his shoulders.

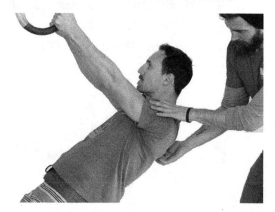

Tactile

2. Sagging at the hips.

Ring Row Position 1 violation. A straight body line must be maintained throughout the movement.

 "Glutes on!" or "Squeeze your butt!"

 Demonstrate proper RR 1 position.

 Press up at the small of the back to get the athlete to bring his hips foward.

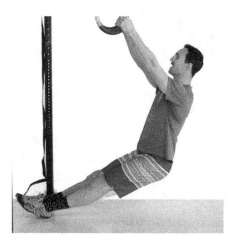

Fault

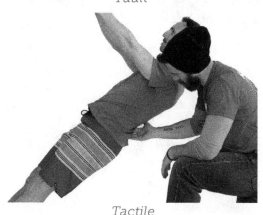

Tactile

Ring Row Common Faults and Fixes, cont.

3. Table top.

Ring Row Position 1 and 2 violation. Sometimes you'll catch an athlete trying to make ring rows easier by bending his knees to shorten the lever. Remember, we're always seeking transferability to more advanced movements, so require your athletes do to ring rows with the body organization they'll ultimate use for pull-ups: feet together, legs straight, midline neutral, shoulders packed.

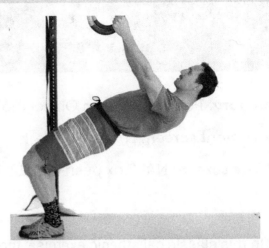

Fault

 "Feet together! Legs straight!"

 Demonstrate a correct RR 2.

 Reduce load by raising the rings or by having the athlete step back to increase the angle of the body relative to the floor.

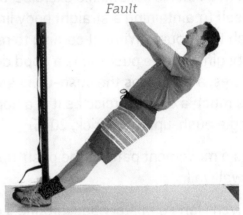

Correct RR 2

4. Kipping the row.

Global positional violation. Athlete throws hips forward to create momentum. The ring row is a strictly upper body exercise. The hips must be static, the body locked in a straight line from ankle to shoulder.

 "Arms only!" or "Lock abs and glutes!"

 Demonstrate proper action of the ring row.

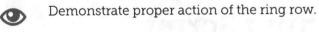 Reduce load by raising the rings or by having the athlete step back to increase the angle of the body relative to the floor.

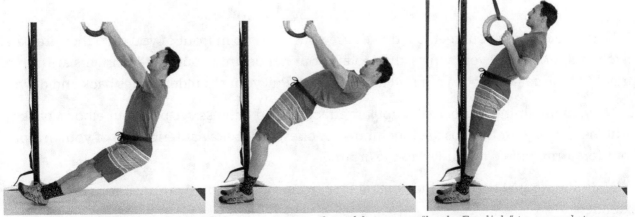

Lacking strength or stamina to ring row correctly, athlete uses "body English" to complete rep

PUSH-UPS

Category: Push Away from Object (horizontal)

Movement screen: N/a

Ability screen: N/a (box push-up), 12" box push-up x 5 (push-up)

In this classic calisthenic exercise, the athlete sets up in a straight-armed plank. He lowers himself (maintaining a straight body line from ankle to shoulder) until his thighs, chest, and chin touch the ground. Without coming to rest, he then pushes until his arms are again fully extended. For beginners, the push-up is a good developer of upper body strength; for more advanced athletes, at high reps the push-up is a valuable conditioning tool. And don't forget: the push-up is as much a core exercise as it is a upper body strengthener. "If the plank is violated, you're not doing a push-up." (Roderick, 2015)

As a movement pattern, the push-up is also fundamental to the bench press, the burpee, and the wallwalk.

Given Harry's military background, I expect the push-up will pose no problems for him—although, beware, a lot of strong guys pick up bad push-up habits in service of their country. Amy says she does push-ups all the time in her bootcamp classes, but we'll see if they meet our standard. As for Tim, given his sedentary condition, I expect he'll be challenged by the easiest push-up variation I can provide.

Push-up Set-up Teaching Script

"Stand up tall with your feet together. Raise your arms up in front of you until they are parallel to the floor. Extend your wrists, then rotate your hands until your middle fingers are pointed straight at the ceiling. Lock your butt and abs tight. Pull your shoulder blades back and down.

"Now, maintaining this partial scapular retraction and depression, pull your elbows back until the tips of your thumbs are touching your chest, just below anterior fold of your armpit. Your forearms should be parallel to the ground.

"Maintaining that scapular and core tension, push your hands away until your arms are fully extended.

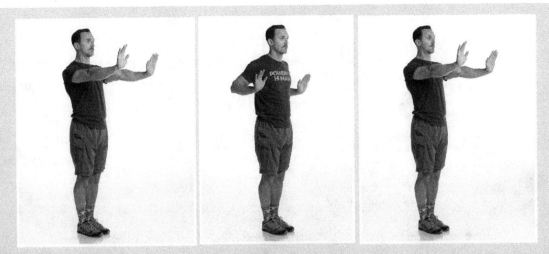

"That's what a push-up should feel like. Although it's mainly practiced to develop upper-body pushing strength, the entire body, especially the core, is involved.

"Many new trainees find executing a full push-up prohibitively difficult. We avoid teaching people knee push-ups because that variation shortens the lever from foot-to-shoulder to knee-to-shoulder, thus reducing the demand (and therefore the training benefit) on the muscles of the core.

"So how do we make the push-up available to people of all ability levels, without compromising a strong plank position? We do it by increasing the angle of the athlete's body relative to the ground."

Box Push-up Set-up Teaching Script

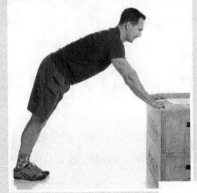

"Start by setting up with the heels of your hands at the edge of a 24" box, just outside shoulder width. Feet are together, with a slight pike in the hips.

"Squeeze your butt and abs to lock your body in a straight line from ankle to shoulder, and to bring yourself forward over your hands. Pull your shoulders back and down. Screw your hands into the box, right hand clockwise, left hand counter-clockwise. This is **Box Push-up Position 1 (bPU 1).**

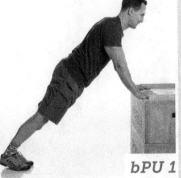

bPU 1

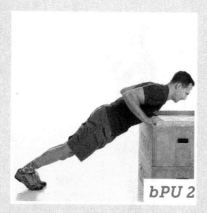

bPU 2

"Continuing to screw in your hands, lower yourself until your chest makes contact with the box, just below the nipple line. This is **Box Push-up Position 2 (bPU 2).**

"Push until your arms are straight again, taking care that you keep you maintain a straight body line from ankle to shoulder.

"When you can do 12-15 reps without stopping, switch to a shorter box, and eventually a short stack of plates. Wean yourself until you can do push-ups on the floor. If, in the course of a workout, you fatigue to the point your form starts to break down, simply increase the angle of your body relative to the floor until you can again perform the exercise correctly."

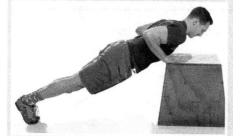 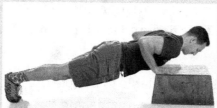 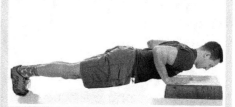

To progress the push-up, nothing changes but the body's angle relative to the floor

This progression can be done using a barbell and a squat rack, if the holes in the posts allow the hooks to be set close to the floor. Also, avoid using bands to provide assistance for push-ups, whether they are hung from pull-up bars or looped around the athlete's elbows. They'll often encourage "snaking", as the trainee lacks the core strength to keep a straight body line in a completely prone position.

Push-up Teaching Script

"To perform a standard push-up, set up with your hands on the floor ahead of you, set about shoulder-width. Feet are together, with a slight pike in the hips.

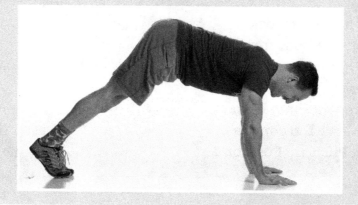

"Squeeze your butt and abs to lock your body in a straight line from ankle to shoulder and bring your shoulders forward over your hands. Pull your shoulders back and down. Screw your hands into the ground, right hand clockwise, left hand counterclockwise. This is **Push-up Position 1 (PU 1).**

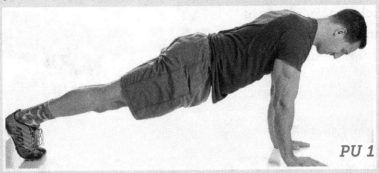

PU 1

"Pull your elbows back until chest, chin, and top of thigh all make brushing contact with the ground. Abs and glutes should be locked in, shoulders packed, forearms vertical. Because you're continually screwing your hands to the floor, the external rotation at the shoulder keeps your elbows from flaring out past 30 degrees or so. This is **Push-up Position 2 (PU 2)."**

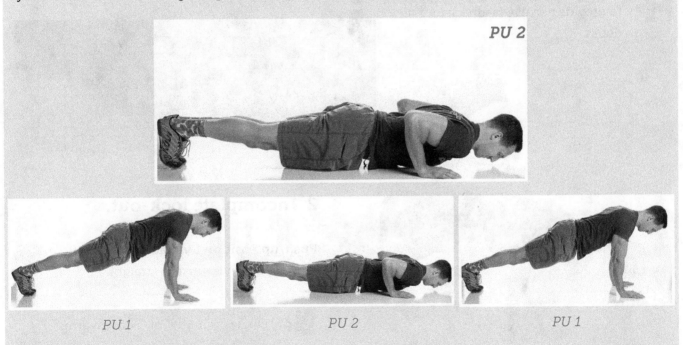

PU 2

PU 1   *PU 2*   *PU 1*

"Hand-release" push-ups are a standard invented for the CrossFit Games and should not be considered good push-up form or a 'scale' for push-ups. Tension should NOT be released in the bottom of the push-up, either through the arms or the core.

Positional Drills

"1! 2! 1!" Practice the positions of the push-up one at a time, with your trainees holding the pose while you make necessary corrections. Make sure your athletes maintain a straight line from ankle to shoulder as they transition from position to position.

Push-up Common Faults and Fixes

1. Insufficient depth.

Push-up Position 2 violation. Full range of motion means chest and chin contact floor in PU 2 (just the chest for Box Push-ups).

 "Chest-to-deck!"

 Get down and demonstrate PU 2.

 Place a hand palm down on deck, and insist athlete's chest make contact with back of your hand. (NOTE: not appropriate for female athletes!)

 Use a squeaky toy under your athlete to provide positive feedback for full depth.

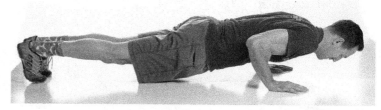

Fault

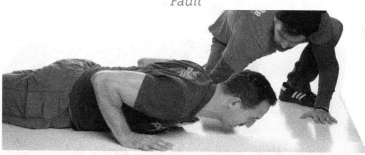

Tactile

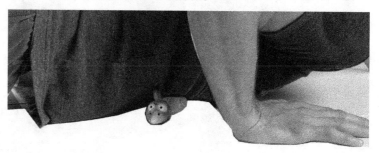

Orthosis

2. Incomplete lock-out.

Push-up Position 1 violation. At top of push-up, elbows must be straight.

 "Elbows straight!" or "Straight arms!"

 Get down and demonstrate proper PU 1.

 Have athlete pause in PU 1 and press his elbows straight.

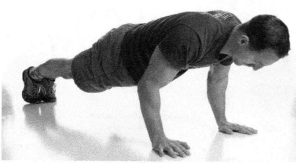

Fault

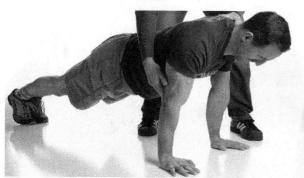

Tactile

Push-up Common Faults and Fixes, cont.

3. Sagging in the middle/snaking/breakdancing

Push-up Position 1 violation. If the athlete does not maintain core tension, his hips will sag, and his lower back hyperextend. If his hips are first down, last up, he'll look like he's doing "the worm." Body line must be straight from ankle to shoulder through ROM.

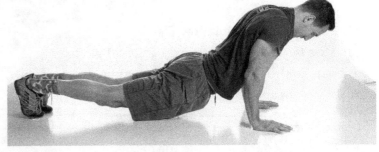
Fault

 "Abs on!" or "Six pack!"

 Demonstrate proper PU 1 positioning.

 Have athlete pause in PU 1, then lift his hips or prod down as necessary.

 Use THE TAIL! If contact is lost with the back of the head, hips have dropped.

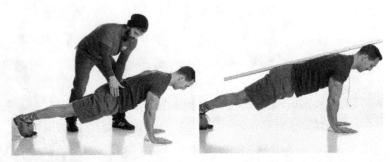
Tactile   *Orthosis*

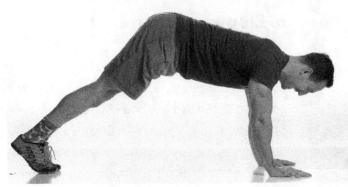
Fault

4. Piked at the hips.

Push-up Position 1 violation. Hips are partially flexed to take load off the arms. Body line must be straight from ankle to shoulder through ROM.

 "Glutes on!" or "Squeeze your butt!"

 Demonstrate proper PU 1 positioning.

 Have athlete pause in PU 1, push down on his tailbone with a closed fist until his feet, hips, and shoulders are in a straight line.

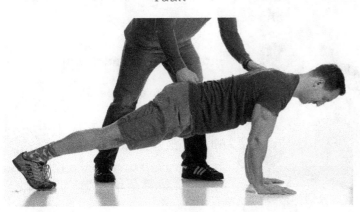
Tactile

Push-up Common Faults and Fixes, cont.

5. Elbows flare out.

Push-up Position 2 violation. Elbows come too far away from the body, internally rotating the shoulder and possibly causing impingement and pain.

 "Screw your hands into the ground!"

 Demonstrate a proper PU 2.

Double-up a skinny (1/4-1/2") band around the trainee's elbows. Have it run across the front of the body if the trainee is weaker, behind the back if the trainee is stronger. A pair of boxes set exactly as wide apart as optimal elbow position works, too.

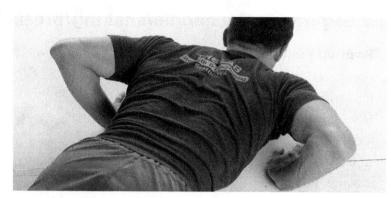

Fault

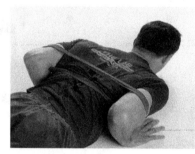

Orthosis

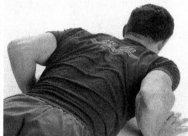

Correct PU 2

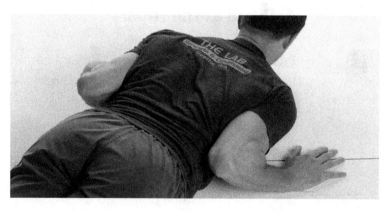

Fault

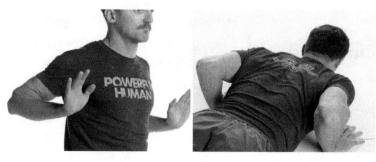

Tactile   *Correct PU 2*

6. Elbows point in.

Push-up Position 2 violation. In PU 2, elbows should be stacked over the wrists. If they collapse in toward the body, it's an indication of insufficient scapular stabilization. Interestingly, it can *also* occur due to too much scapular retraction! The athlete must concentrate on packing the shoulders, that is, back, and down.

 "Shoulders back and down!"

 Demonstrate a proper PU 2.

 Have the athlete stand and review the initial introduction to the push-up set-up. Ascertain he is recruiting the rotator cuff muscles appropriately.

BUTTERFLY SIT-UPS

Category: Hip and Trunk Flexion (seated)

Movement screen: N/a

Ability screen: N/a

By The Numbers introduces anterior core work with the butterfly sit-up. The butterfly sit-up is done in conjunction with an AbMat, which is designed to support the lower back as the upper abdominals contract to initiate the movement. The knees are spread apart to reduce the contribution of the hip flexors. The butterfly sit-up should be performed in a smooth, controlled fashion, not a violent whipping back and forth. Think draw forward, lay back.

I expect Harry, Amy, and Tim will all be able to handle the Butterfly Sit-up without trouble.

Butterfly Sit-up Teaching Script

"The Abmat is designed to conform to the lumbar curve of your spine. Place it on the floor with the logo upside-down relative to you, then have a seat on the floor with your tailbone at the edge of the mat. Do not sit on the mat.

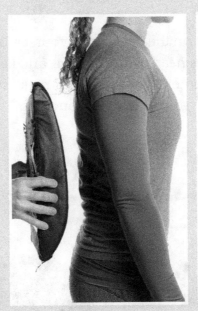
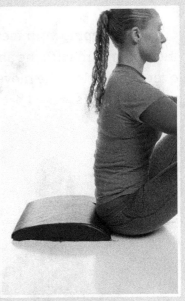

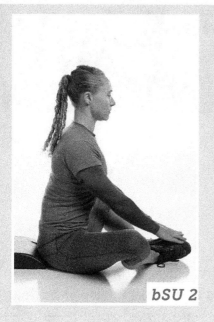

bSU 2

"Put the soles of your feet together and let your knees fall out wide as if you were going to do a butterfly stretch. This reduces the role of the hip flexors in initiating the movement.

"Sit up tall. Pull your shoulders back and down. Straighten your arms and bring your hands together

"Maintaining this tension in the back, hinge forward from the hips until you can touch your toes. This is **Butterfly Sit-up Position 2 (bSU 2)**, the finish position for the butterfly set up.

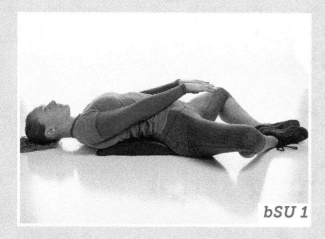

bSU 1

"Keeping your feet on the floor, and your arms low, right over the belly, lay back to bring your head and shoulder blades to the ground. This is **Butterfly Sit-up Position 1 (bSU 1)**, the start of the butterfly sit-up.

"Now, keeping your feet on the floor, draw yourself up to touch your toes. Initiate by pushing down hard with the abs nearest the rib cage, and keep sitting up until your hip flexors take over to complete the movement. Back in **bSU 1**, make sure you keep your arms straight and your shoulders locked back and down. No slouching!"

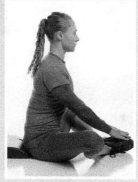
bSU 2

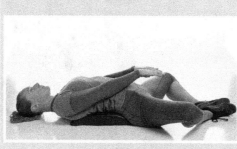
bSU 1

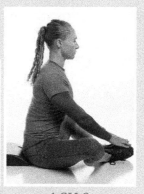
bSU 2

Butterfly Sit-up Common Faults and Fixes

1. Arms overhead/throws arms forward.

Butterfly Sit-up Position 1 violation. Lacking the strength to complete the sit-up, the athlete initiates her sit-up by bringing her arms overhead and then throws them forward to create momentum that carries her through the sticking point.

 "Arms in front, hands low!"

 Demonstrate proper transition from bSU 1 to bSU 2.

If an athlete is unable to sit up on her own, try tying a skinny assistance band to a stable upright post. Set the athlete up so that in bSU 1, with arms extended, there is just a touch of slack in the band. As she sits back, the band will stretch; the tension will give her the assistance necessary to complete the rep.

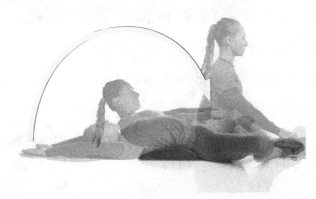

Fault

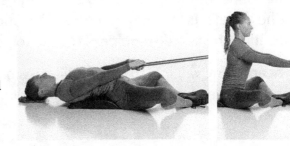

Orthosis

2. Hunchback.

Butterfly Sit-up Position 2 violation. Athlete hunches over at completion of rep. Her back should be straight.

 "Sit up tall!" or "Shoulders back and down!"

 Demonstrate proper bSU 2 positioning.

 Tap athlete between shoulder blades to indicate she needs to pack her shoulders.

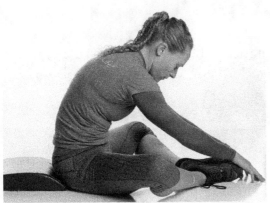

Fault

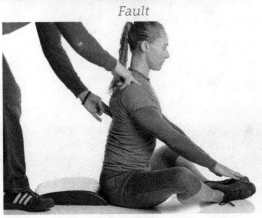

Tactile

133

Category: Pull to Object (strict, vertical)

Movement screen: N/a

Ability screen: N/a

Pull-ups are important part of MMGPP training. But before trainees can begin learning how to pull their body up toward a fixed point, whether rings or a pull-up bar, they have to be strong enough to suspend their weight by their hands. We start them off with the static hang. The static hang teaches correct grip and how to "pack" the shoulders to the keep the shoulder joint stable and safe. Once they can perform a 20 second static hang, athletes work on scapular pull-ups, in which the athlete, from a straight hang, lifts and lowers himself a small amount by depressing and elevating the shoulder blades. This action strengthens the muscles of the rotator cuff.

Harry and Amy will find the scap pull-up a breeze. Tim, I think, may yet lack the coordination to do more than the static hang.

Static Hang Teaching Script

"When you hang from a pull-up bar, the only thing standing between you and a dislocated shoulder is your ability to activate the muscles of your rotator cuff. Well, the situation might not be quite that dire...but almost. Before you hang from the bar, you must understand how to keep your shoulders stable while hanging.

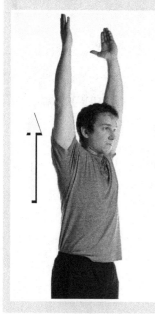 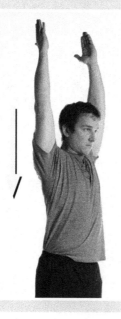

"Reach up straight overhead, as high as you can. Externally rotate your arms to turn your thumbs back. Now, keeping your elbows straight, pull your arms down into their sockets. Again, reach up. Feel your shoulders stretch, and then lock them down one more time. We refer to that locked down position as having 'active shoulders.'

"Now we'll do it on the bar. Climb up on a box and grasp the pull-up bar with a full, thumbs-around grip. ALWAYS thumbs around. This is for safety. Rotate your hand slightly over the bar so that your pinky knuckles point toward the ceiling; this helps create external rotation at the shoulder, which helps keep the joint stable.

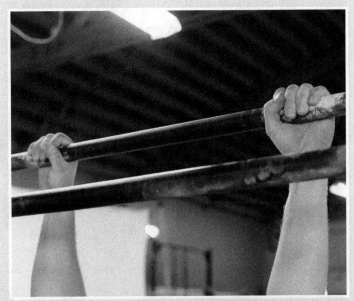

"Contract the muscles of your upper back to pull your shoulder blades down toward your feet.

"When you feel ready, lift one knee just high enough that your foot leaves the box.

"If you feel confident, lift the other knee.

"You are now in a 'static hang.'"

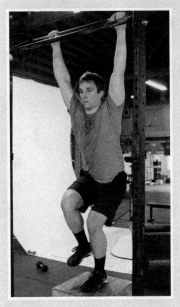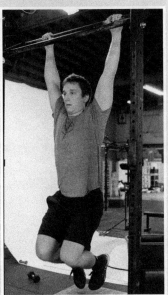

"Hang as long as you can, counting off seconds. If you get to ten, put your feet down. If you feel your grip slipping, immediately put both feet down.

"Work up to a twenty second static hang."

Static Hang Common Faults and Fixes

1. Suicide grip.

Athlete holds pull-up bar with thumbs on the same side as the fingers. It took nature millions of years to give your athletes an opposable thumb for the sole purpose of not falling off your pull-up bar. Make sure they use it!

 "Thumbs around!"

 Demonstrate a correct thumbs-around grip.

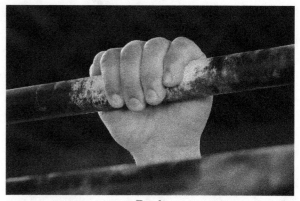

Fault

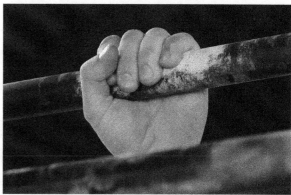

Correct

THE PIKED RING ROW

Category: Pull to Object (strict, vertical)

Movement screen: N/a

Ability screen: Ring row x 10

The piked ring row redirects the direction of the pull in the ring row from horizontal to vertical. This load-reduced vertical pull is a great "training wheels" version of the pull-up.

The only drawback to the piked ring row is that athletes must be disciplined about preserving the verticality of the pull. As they tire they'll automatically lean back or bring their hips forward to change the vector of force and make the pull easier. Let them know that if they want to get the greatest benefit from the exercise, they must continue to sit back and lean forward. If that becomes too difficult, they can default to horizontal ring rows. The convenience of that default is why the piked ring row is presented before the self-assisted and band-assisted pull-up, even though all three are roughly the same level of technical challenge.

I'm going to have Tim continue with standard ring rows. This piked variation will help Amy prepare for strict pull-ups. Harry, who already has pull-ups, goes along with this more rudimentary work good-naturedly.

Piked Ring Row Teaching Script

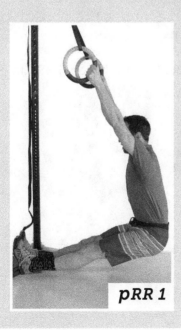

pRR 1

"Standing just behind the rings, grasp them with a thumbs-around grip.

"Maintaining a straight line from ankle to shoulder, lay back until your arms are straight. Keep your feet together and your toes pointed. Then sit back as far as you can, leaning forward so that the arms are in line with the torso. Your shoulders should be actively locked down. This is **Piked Ring Row Position 1 (pRR 1).**

"If you find your feet sliding forward, prop them against a 45lbs plate.

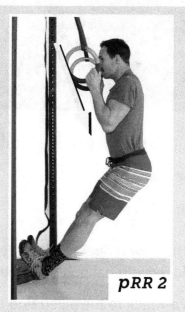

"Continuing to sit as far back as you can, pull the elbows down in a line with the torso until your fists are just above your shoulders and your elbows are tucked into your ribs. This is **Piked Ring Row Position 2 (pRR 2)**. The trick is keeping the hips back as far as possible to maintain a vertical pull."

pRR 2

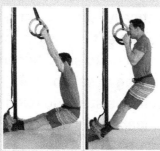
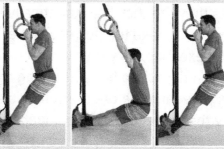

pRR 1   pRR 2   pRR 1   pRR 2

Piked Ring Row Common Faults and Fixes

1. Horizontal pull.

Piked Ring Row Position 2 violation. In order to reap the benefit of the piked ring row, the athlete must pull in line with the torso. As he pulls, he must continue to sit back. Bringing the hips forward reduces the verticality of the pull.

 "Sit back and down!"   Demonstrate proper transition from pRR 1 to pRR 2.

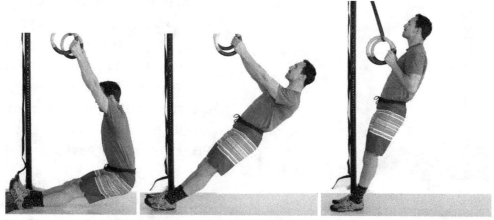

By extending his hips, the athlete turns the pRR into a horizontal pull

Category: Monostructural (row)

Movement screen: N/a

Ability screen: N/a

The C2 rowing ergometer is a terrific developer of aerobic capacity. It also helps teach the principle of 'core to extremity', which underlies much of what we do in MMGPP training.

At my gym, we regularly test our athlete's times for distances of 500m, 2k, and 5k. Teams of two rowing 10k is a fun variation, as well.

Remember, rowing is a sport unto itself; it takes years to master the subtleties of rowing, even on an indoor rower. Our goal, especially at the beginning, is merely to get our athletes moving with basic competence, and to prevent them from forming bad habits.

Amy and Harry will have no problem with this. Given Tim's difficulties with the good morning, however, I expect he'll find it difficult to get in good positions on the rower.

Row Teaching Script

"Have a seat. Set your feet on the platforms and tighten the straps. The straps should cross your shoe just below where your big toe meets your foot; if you need to, loosen the straps and adjust the height of the foot pad.

"Take a wide grip on the rower's handle with both hands palms down and thumbs around. Try to 'snap' the handle in half by rotating your right fist clockwise and your left counterclockwise. Pull your shoulders back and down. I want you to try to maintain this tension throughout the movement.

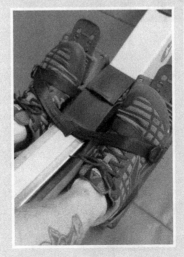 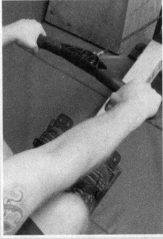

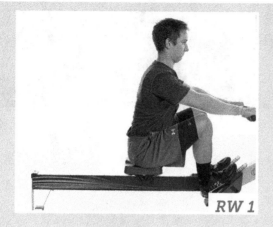

RW 1

"Now slide forward until your shins are perpendicular to the floor. Depending on your ankle flexibility, your heels may lift; that's okay. Don't let your knees knock; push them out slightly, so that they line up under the arms. Keep your arms straight, your shoulders back and down, and lean slightly forward from the hips. This is the 'catch', **Row Position 1 (RW 1).**

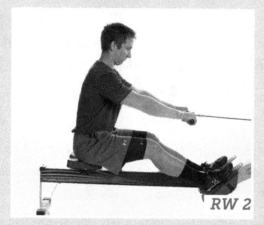

RW 2

"Maintaining a slight forward lean of the torso and strong abdominal bracing, push through the heels until your legs are straight. This is **Row Position 2 (RW 2),** sometimes known as 'legs'.

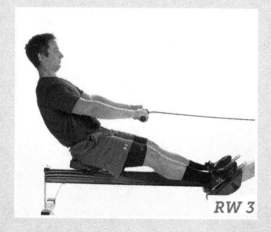

RW 3

"When your legs are straight, sit back to about 10 o'clock (*or 2 o'clock, depending on your vantage point - Ed.*). Keep your gaze directed at the chain to help keep your head in a neutral position. This is **Row Position 3 (RW 3),** sometimes referred to as 'back'.

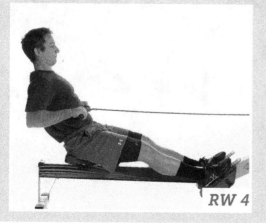

RW 4

"Pull your elbows straight back to bring the handle to your diaphragm, about halfway between your navel and your solar plexus. This is **Row Position 4 (RW 4),** sometimes called 'arms'.

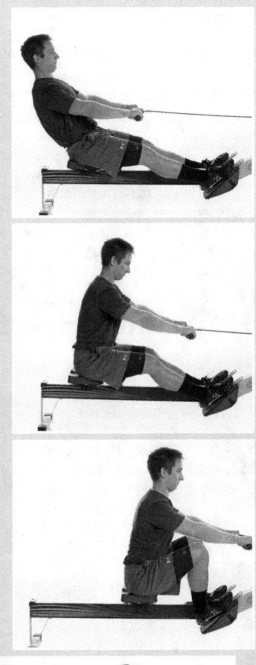

"The same positions in reverse order comprise the return stroke.

"Punch your hands straight ahead. This brings you back to **RW 3**, 'arms'.

"Sit up until you are leaning slightly forward. This is **RW 2**, or 'back'.

"Lastly, engaging your hamstrings, pull yourself forward to return to **RW 1**, or 'legs'. As you pull yourself forward, you are generating tension you can use to help drive the next cycle. Imagine your legs are a pair of compressing springs!"

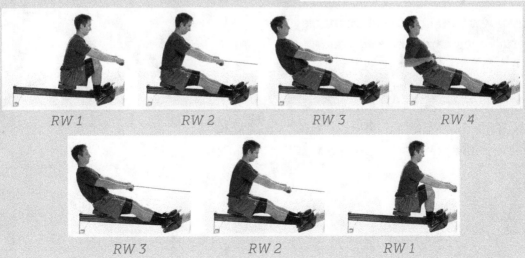

RW 1   RW 2   RW 3   RW 4

RW 3   RW 2   RW 1

Positional Drills

"1! 2! 1! 2!" Practice driving out of the catch while maintaining a light forward lean.

"1! 2! 3! 2! 1!" Practice driving out of the catch and then leaning back only once legs have straightened. Arms remain straight. Then sit up and slide forward.

"1! 2! 3! 4! 3! 2! 1!" Have your athletes row three slow "legs-back-arms-arms-back-legs," then ten more strokes with increasing force. Explain that although they are being taught the movement in a mechanical, segmented manner, ultimately their rows will be smooth and powerful. Once they have a feel for it, explain that the concentric phase of the stroke (legs-back-arms) is twice as fast the the eccentric (arms-back-legs). If you're musically minded, try this analogy: the row stroke is in waltz time, 3/4, with the positive stroke on the 1 and the negative on the 2 and 3.

A (Hopefully) Helpful Analogy

 At this point, you have a group of athletes executing a decent approximation of a correct rowing stroke. Usually, however, some additional explanation of what they're actually supposed to do on the rower can be helpful.

"The C2 rowing ergometer is designed to simulate racing a scull on the water. To that end, the idea is to go fast, and to go fast, one must produce power on the rower. Here's an analogy to help you understand how.

"When I was a kid, I had a toy car. It came with a long thin plastic strip with a serrated edge. You'd feed the strip behind the wheel and pull it to make the car go. Pulling slowly and gently was easy. The problem was, when you put the car down, it wouldn't go anywhere. You hadn't produced any power. Pulling the strap quickly and forcefully was hard—there was significant resistance—but when you put down the car, it would take off. That's how the flywheel in your ergometer works. The harder you pull, the more it will resist, but the further and faster you'll go on every pull.

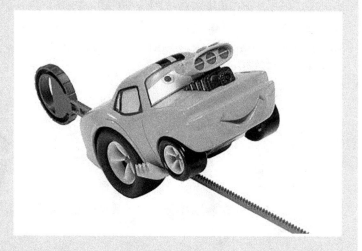

"To get the most out of your pull, get your heels down early, and use the big engine of your legs and hips to drive yourself back. You'll feel a 'catch' as the flywheel resists. Aggressively 'stand up' hard and fast against the platform, then follow through with your back and arms."

Rowing Common Faults and Fixes

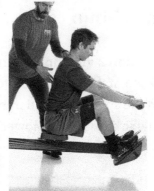

Fault

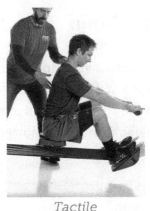

Tactile

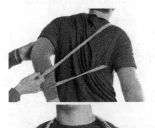

Orthosis

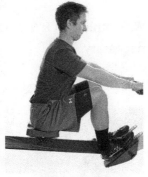

Correct RW 1

1. Loss of neutral spine/shoulder drift.

Row Position 1 violation. Athlete hunches over in the catch position, and/or lets shoulders go slack and drift forward. For safety and efficiency, the spine must remain neutral, with shoulders packed.

 "Pack your shoulders!" or "Chest up!"

 Demonstrate proper transition from RW 1 to RW 2.

 With athlete in RW 1, adjust athlete as necessary.

 Loop a skinny band about your athlete's neck and arms as a "band bra" that will encourage him to keep his shoulders packed.

2. Knees Knock.

Row Position 1 violation. In the catch position, the athlete's legs internally rotate, so the knees come together. The knees should line up under the arms. Explain to your trainee that knees knocking will never be a good athletic position; even with the stance constrained by the footpads, the athlete should push knees out to create some external rotation.

 "Push your knees out!"

 Mime pushing your knees out with a close stance—it'll look like you're doing the Charleston.

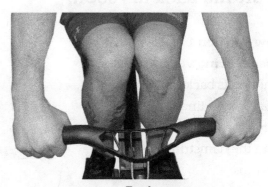

Fault

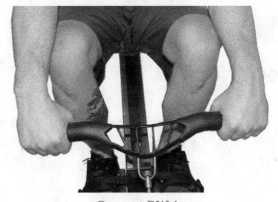

Correct RW 1

Rowing Common Faults and Fixes, cont.

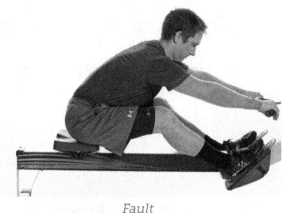

Fault

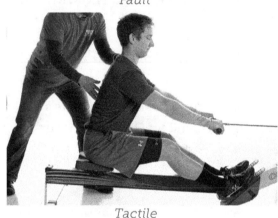

Tactile

3. "Taco"-ing.

Row Position 2 violation. During the initial drive out of RW 1, if the athlete fails to engage the core to support the spine, he'll fold in half like a taco, putting undesirable stress on the lower back.

 "Abs on!" or "Chest up!"

 Demonstrate proper transition from RW 1 to RW 2.

 With athlete in RW 2, adjust athlete as necessary.

4. Sitting back too soon.

Row Position 1 to Row Position 2 sequencing violation. If the athlete sits back too soon, the quads extending the knee become the primary drivers, rather than the hamstrings extending the hips.

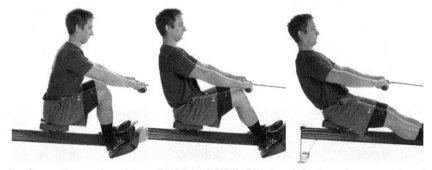

Faulty sequencing from RW 1 to RW 3. Sits back before knees extend.

 "Drive the hips back!"

 Demonstrate proper transition from RW 1 to RW 2.

 Slow the athlete down. Put one hand on his hip and the other on his shoulder, maintaining the desired back angle as he pushes back.

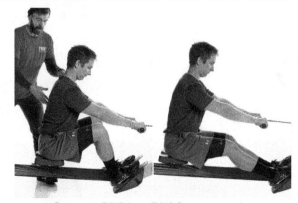

Correct RW 1 to RW 2 sequencing

Rowing Common Faults and Fixes, cont.

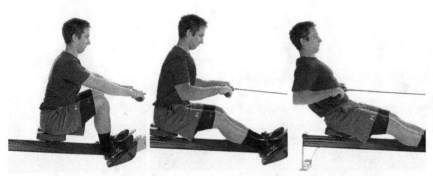

Faulty sequencing from RW 2 to RW 3. Arms pull before hips extend.

5. Pulling too soon.

Row Position 2 and Row Position 3 violation. If the athlete ignores core to extremity, he'll pull early, robbing himself of the power that could be generated by his legs and hips.

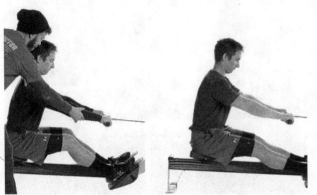

Tactile fix for RW 2, correct RW 3

 "Straight arms!"

 Demonstrate proper transition from RW 1 to RW 2 to RW 3.

 With athlete in RW 2 or RW 3, adjust athlete as necessary.

6. Bending knees too soon on return.

Row Position 3 (return) violation. If the athlete executes the return (arms-back-legs) out of order, he'll end up lifting the handle over the knees, resulting in an inefficient stroke. For an efficient stroke return, the athlete must first extend his arms, then lean forward, then bend the knees.

 "Arms first!" or "Punch in!"

 Demonstrate proper transition from RW 1 to RW 2.

 Block knee with your fist to keep it from bending until arms have straightened and the athlete has sat forward.

(Photos on next page)

Rowing Common Faults and Fixes, cont.

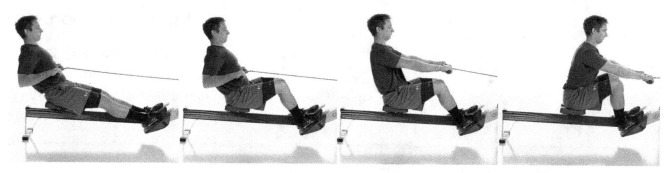

Faulty sequencing from RW 4 to RW 2. Knees bend before arms extend.

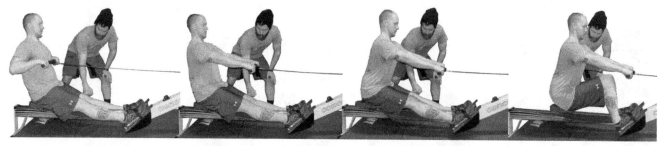

Tactile fix: block knee with your fist during transition from RW 4 to RW 2

7. Head snaps back.

Row Position 2 violation. As athlete drives out of RW 1, he throws his head back, putting unnecessary strain on his cervical vertebrae and violating the neutral midline rule.

 "Head neutral!" or "Look at the chain!"

 Demonstrate proper transition from RW 1 to RW 2 to RW 3.

 With athlete in RW 2, adjust athlete as necessary.

 Have your athlete hold a rolled-up towel between his chest and chin.

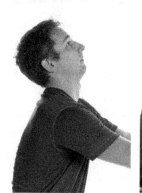
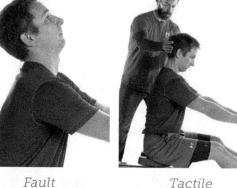

Fault   *Tactile*

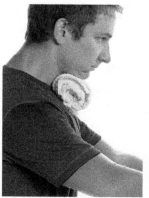
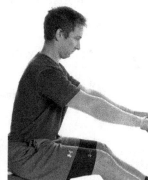

Orthosis   *Correct RW 2*

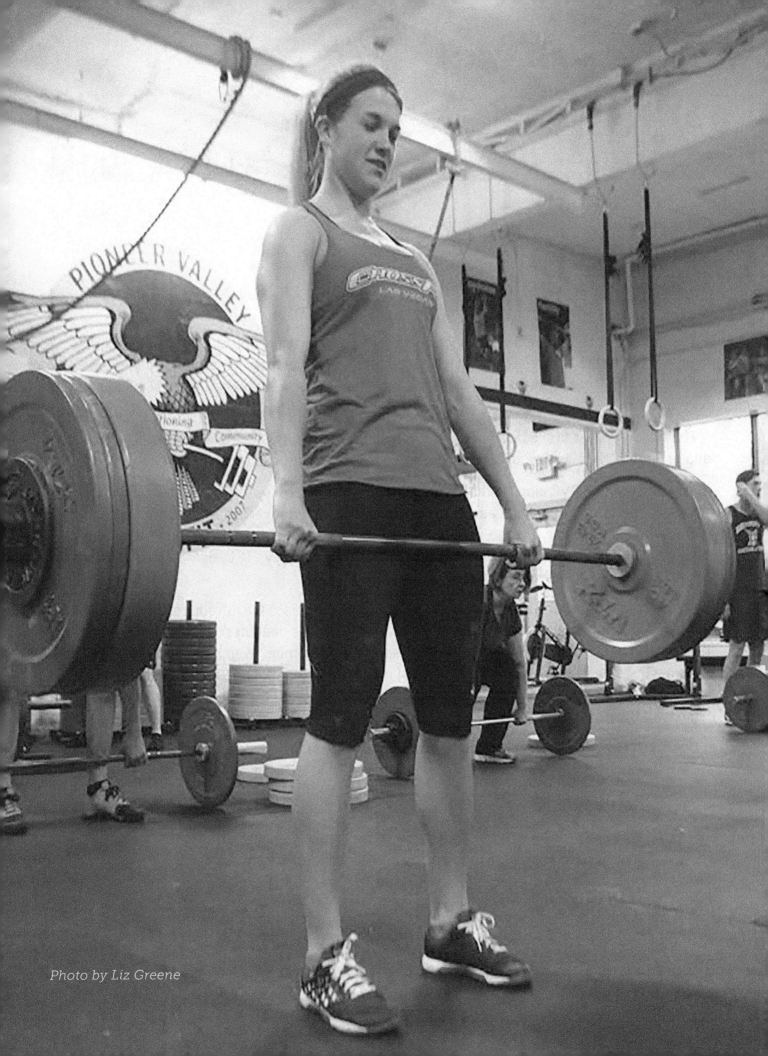

DEADLIFTS

Category: Pull Object (ground to hip)

Movement screen: N/a

Ability screen: PVC Good morning x 5 (Romanian deadlift), RDL x 5 (deadlift)

The deadlift is the biomechanically correct way to pick a heavy object up off the ground. It involves setting the back in a strong, neutral position, then utilizing the posterior chain muscles to drive the hips up and forward, all the while keeping the bar as close to the body's line of gravity as possible.

The deadlift is the first barbell exercise we teach. Even the most wary novice athlete likes the idea of learning how to pick up a heavy object in a safe and efficient manner.

Athletes will use PVC pipe for the initial instruction, and barbells with bumpers to learn the process of setting up. Try to be as explicit as possible with your verbal instructions—pretend your trainees are playing a game, with one rule: if there's any way they can misconstrue something you say, while remaining true to what you literally said, they are to do so. Head them off at the pass by making yourself absolutely clear.

So far, so good for Amy and Harry. Eventually, as the exercises we introduce grow more complex, we'll find something one of them won't be ready for. The deadlift probably isn't it. For Tim, though, who had a difficult time keeping his back straight coming even halfway down in the good morning, the deadlift is almost certainly out of reach at this point. I need to start him off with a stimulus-preserving exercise that will help him progress toward the full lift. Thus, our group will begin with the Romanian deadlift.

But first, I need to explain to them the concepts of efficiency and leverage.

Explaining Leverage and Efficiency

"Generally speaking, when lifting barbells, you want to have the best possible leverage on the load, and you want to move it as efficiently as possible.

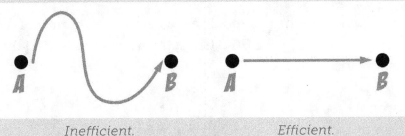

Inefficient.   *Efficient.*

"Efficiency in this context is easy to understand. Everyone knows the fastest way between two points is a straight line. It's also the most efficient, in the sense of achieving maximum effect with minimum effort.

"Leverage is a little trickier.

"Imagine there's a 50lbs bag of dogfood on the ground. You straddle it, bend at the hip, pick it up. No big deal, right? Now imagine that dog food is just a couple of feet in front of you. Bend over, reach out, and try to pick it up—it's nearly impossible. Why? Because leverage is working against you.

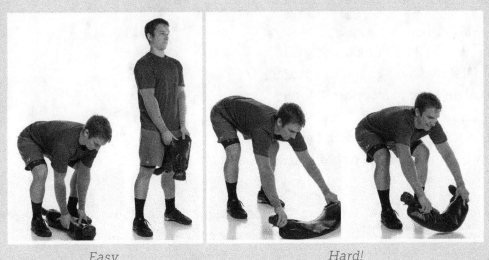

Easy.   *Hard!*

"Leverage is 'the exertion of force by means of a lever.' There are three types of levers; any time you are lifting an object from the ground, effectively a 'third class' lever is created, in which the effort is applied between the fulcrum, or pivot point, and the load.

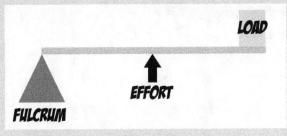

Third class lever in the abstract

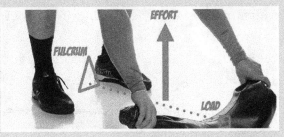

Third class lever in action

"A third class lever is considered a mechanically disadvantaged arrangement, because for the load to be lifted, the effort must be greater than the load. Compounding that, as the lever grows longer, the load acquires 'moment', or a tendency to rotate around its fulcrum toward the ground. The effort required to move the load increases with the load's distance from the fulcrum, because you're contending with both the object's weight, and this extra rotational force. That's why the bag of dog food gets harder and harder to lift the further away it gets.

"The fulcrum of our dog food-lifting lever is on the ground directly below your **center of gravity (COG)**. In an anatomically neutral position, your COG lies at the intersection of **(1) the transverse plane**, which divides the body top from bottom; **(2) the sagittal plane**, which divides left from right, and **(3) the coronal or frontal plane**, which divides the body front to back.

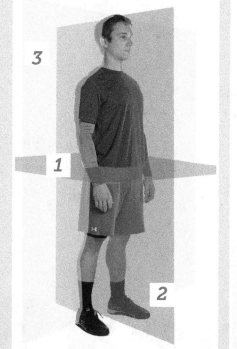
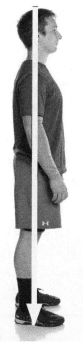

"Passing through your COG is an imaginary **line of gravity**. It describes how gravity is acting on your body: always pulling you straight down toward the center of the earth. It is congruent with the intersection of the frontal and sagittal planes.

"The point at which the line of gravity enters the ground below you is called the **projection of COG within base of support**. (Note that from the side, it's lined up between the arch and heel of your foot, just where I've been encouraging you to place your weight when squatting.)

Transverse, sagittal, frontal planes

Line of gravity

"It's this projection point that serves as the fulcrum for the de facto third-class lever you use to pick up your dog food, and indeed for any object you wish to lift unaided.

"Which brings us back to lifting barbells. To gain the best possible leverage, you must minimize moment by keeping the barbell over the projection of COG within the base of support. The long lever between fulcrum and load in movements like the overhead squat makes this mission critical.

"To summarize: whether squatting, pressing, or deadlifting, move the bar in the straightest path possible, while keeping it as close to the line of gravity as possible. Failure to do so will reduce the amount of weight you can lift, and ultimately cause you to fail, as moment's additional rotational force on the load overcomes the force you can produce.

"To summarize further: when lifting a barbell, do your best to keep it lined up over the front of your heel."

Deadlift Teaching Script

"Hold your PVC pipe in a two-handed grip about thumb's-length outside the thighs. Feet should be between hip and shoulder width. Keep your weight evenly distributed across the foot with a slight emphasis on the heel. Brace your midline by locking your glutes and abs, and pack your shoulders. Continuously try to 'snap' the pipe in half by externally rotating your arms. The pipe should be in contact with your upper thighs. This is **Deadlift Position 3 (DL 3)**.

"Unlock your knees and hinge at the hip. Allowing the bar to slide down your thighs like it's on a ramp, keep pulling the hips back until the bar is in front of your kneecaps, with your shins vertical to the floor. You've reached **Deadlift Position 2 (DL 2)**. During this descent, make sure to keep your lats strongly contracted to keep the bar from drifting away from the LOG."

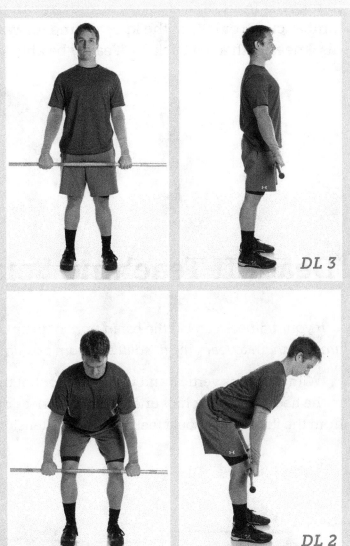

DL 3

DL 2

Positional Drills

"3! 2! 3!" Working from **DL 3** to **DL 2** to **DL 3** reinforces the motor pattern "hip hinge/hip extend" (as opposed to "lean forward/lift from the lower back"). Your trainee is essentially performing a good morning, except the bar is held in the hands, rather than on the back. This is functionally equivalent to performing a deadlift variant called the **Romanian deadlift (rDL)**.

Some trainees, due to flexibility issues, are simply incapable of getting into DL 2 without starting to lose their neutral spine. This means they won't be able to get into a sound set-up from the floor (DL 1). Traditionally, range-of-motion would be reduced for these trainees by resting the bar on bumpers or boxes. However, we believe this does nothing to help improve the inflexible athlete's positional issues. The RDL is a better choice.

Later, when the rest of the group is deadlifting from the floor, inflexible athletes can rDL, taking the bar out of a rack. Load (and hopefully ROM) can be increased over time. In the rDL, Position 2 is as low as the bar can be lowered without the athlete losing his lumbar curve or letting the knees come forward. Once an athlete can get the bar below his knees with a flat back, he'll easily be able to set up and pull from the floor.

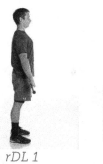 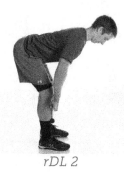 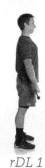

rDL 1　　　　　　　*rDL 2*　　　　　　　*rDL 1*

Deadlift Teaching Script, cont.

If your trainees can get the bar in front of their knees with shins vertical and back straight, it's time for them to learn the deadlift's bottom position.

"With the shins vertical and the bar in front of the knees at **DL 2**, and with the weight firmly in the heels, sink your hips and push your knees out to lower the bar to mid-shin, about 9" from the floor. You should feel tremendous tension in the hamstrings.

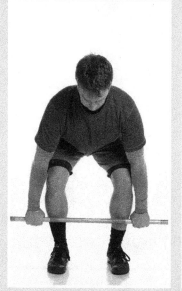 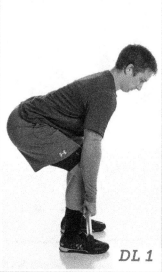

"At this point, the weight is in the heels, with the pipe held against the shin, directly over the knots in your shoelaces. Your hamstrings are in tension. Your back is flat, and your arms are straight. The posterior axillary (armpit) crease is over the barbell, which puts your shoulders slightly in front of the bar. Your gaze directed at the floor a few feet ahead of you, to help keep the neck in line with the spine. This is **Deadlift Position 1 (DL 1)**.

DL 1

DL 1 will look a little different for everybody. If the trainee has a short torso and long femurs, his butt will be higher; a long torso and short femurs, and his butt will be lower. As long as the bar is under the posterior axillary fold and over the knot in his laces (the navicular bones of the feet, for the anatomically-minded), he's good.

"That's the deadlift from the top down—the eccentric portion of the movement. Now let's talk the concentric phase: going from the ground up.

"As we discussed earlier, when lifting weights, you want best leverage and best efficiency. Best leverage meant keeping the load as close to the line of gravity as possible. Best efficiency means moving the bar in a straight line. Now, if this is your finish position (*demonstrate* **DL 3**), and this is your set-up position (*demonstrate* **DL 1**), what's in the way of the bar moving in a straight line?

"That's right, my knees. So when I initiate a deadlift, I push with my legs, rather than pull with my back. My knees straighten just enough so that there is no interference with the bar's vertical travel.

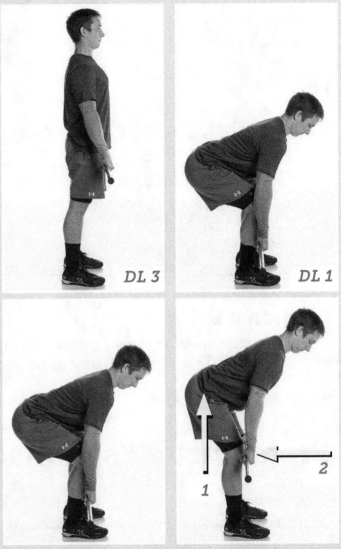

Moving from DL 1 to DL 2, knees squeeze back (2) as hips push up (1). Hips and shoulders rise together.

"To perform a full deadlift from **DL 1**, push through your heels to extend your knees and drive your hips toward the ceiling. The bar should remain in contact with the body as it rises. Notice that the back angle remains constant; the hips and shoulders rise at the same rate. As the bar reaches the knees, you're in **DL 2**.

"Once the bar clears the knees, bring the hips forward to meet the bar.

"When you reach **DL 3**, squeeze your glutes to ensure your hips are fully opened, but keep your abs tight so you don't overextend your lower back.

"Hinge back to return to **DL 2**.

"Keeping your weight back toward your heels, push your knees out to lower into **DL 1**. This resets your hamstrings into tension."

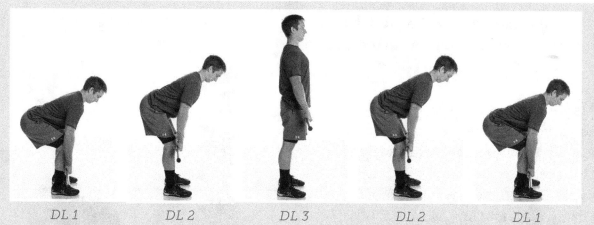

DL 1   *DL 2*   *DL 3*   *DL 2*   *DL 1*

"To call the deadlift a 'pulling' movement is somewhat inaccurate. You are not pulling in the sense of levering from your lower back to move the object. Your trunk is locked and rigid; it's your hips that drive it up, like a crane rising. Once the barbell passes the knees, the crane rotates to vertical...again, not by pulling with the lower back, but by extending the hips. To return the weight to the floor, send the hips back, then down."

Positional Drills

"1! 2! 1!" Practice moving from a correct set-up to squeezing the knees back out of the way. Emphasize resetting the hamstrings into tension as they lower back to DL 1.

"1! 2! 3! 2! 1!" Full sequence.

Frankenstein's Monster Set-up

"When tasked with lifting a heavy barbell from the ground, it's important to learn how to set up correctly.

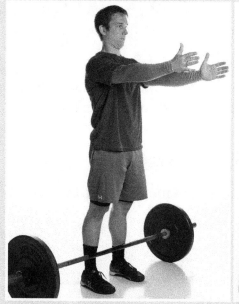
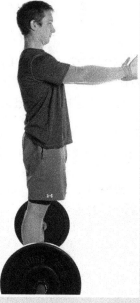

"Stand in your deadlift stance with shins touching the barbell. Lift your arms straight up in front of you. Rotate your thumbs toward the ceiling. Pull your shoulders back and down. Squeeze your glutes and lock your ribcage down.

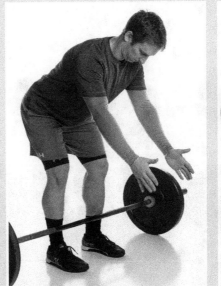
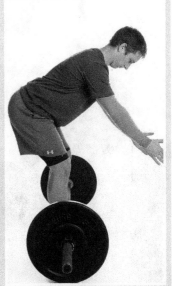

"Hinge back at the hip as far as you can without losing your neutral spine position.

"Then bend at the knees and take a grip of the bar with your right hand. Match it with your left hand.

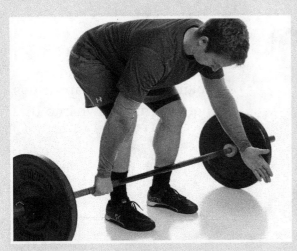
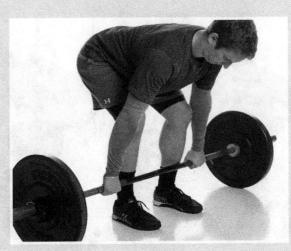

"Lift your chest to pull all the slack out of your arms. The bar should make an audible 'click.'

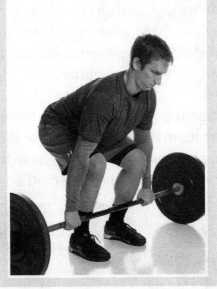
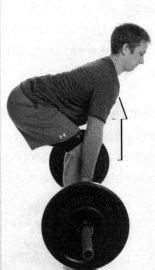

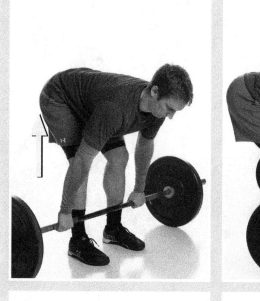

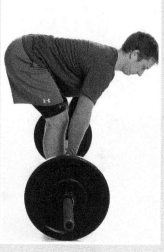

"Still holding the bar against your shins, push your butt toward the ceiling.

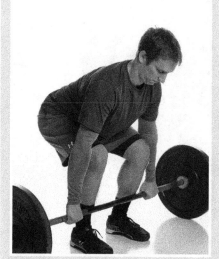

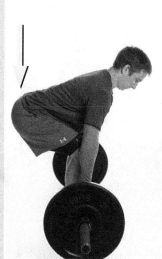

"Pulling with your hamstrings, ratchet your hips down into **DL 1**."

"Attempt to snap the bar in half by externally rotating your arms. With your weight in your heels, bar in contact with the legs, hamstrings in tension, back flat, arms straight, shoulders slightly in front of the bar, and head neutral, you are ready to deadlift. Almost. Before you try to pick that weight up off the ground, we need to discuss the role breath control plays in safe lifting. We need to talk about the Valsalva technique."

But first, a quick word about grip! Trainees have three options: double-overhand, mixed, and hook grip. My advice: have them use double-over for their warm-up sets, and the hook grip for any weight they can imagine cleaning some day. Save the mixed grip for heavy, heavy sets, or for when fatigue or discomfort make the other two methods unworkable.

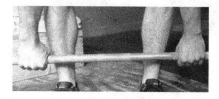

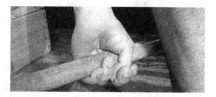

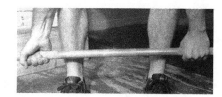

The Valsalva Technique

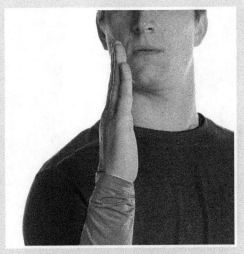

This is your spine, OK?

"Imagine my fingers are your spine. Each knuckle is a vertebra. You can consider the spine as simply a number of joints stacked one on top of the next.

"When you put a heavy load on your spine, that load will try to force your spine into flexion. Going into spinal flexion under load is a bad thing—that's when you can pull muscles, strain ligaments, slip discs...all outcomes we'd rather avoid. So if you're going to load your spine, it's in your best interest to keep it in a neutral position.

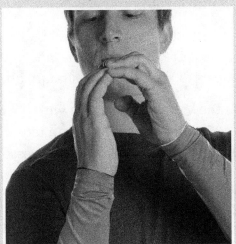

This is your spine going into flexion under load.

"The muscles in your back are not strong enough to accomplish this by themselves. So we're going to utilize a technique that uses all the musculature of the trunk, in conjunction with breath control, to support the spine. It's called the Valsalva maneuver.

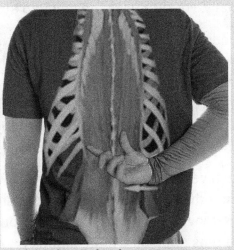

The muscles of your back are not strong enough to keep your spine neutral under heavy load.

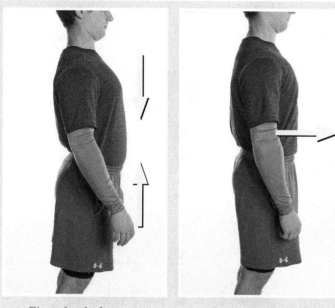

First, lock down...   *...then, pressurize.*

"Here's how you do it: Squeeze your butt, and lock down your abs. To put it indelicately, think about pulling your sphincter toward your belly button. Put a hand on your stomach to make sure that your abs are contracting strongly, like you're preparing to take a punch to the gut.

"Now take a big breath, right from the pelvic floor.

"While holding your breath, try to force your diaphragm out through that wall of unmoving abdominal muscle."

"Did it feel like your head was going to explode? Good, that means you're doing it correctly.

"What you've done is create a bubble of intra-thoracic pressure that stabilizes the spine from the front, like a tire holding up the side of the truck. Now all the muscles of the core are working in concert to keep the back straight and safe.

"To use the Valsalva technique with the deadlift, stabilize your midline as part of the Frankenstein's Monster set-up. Maintain tension as you hinge and get your grip. Just before you initiate the lift, take a big breath and pressurize. Hold your breath as you execute, all the way up and down. When the bar is safely on the floor again, exhale and inhale without surrendering core tension. Repressurize, and go again.

"If you find this makes you light-headed, you may exchange at the top, breathing out and in while holding in DL 3. The rule is, when the bar is in motion, you must be holding your breath and engaging Valsalva."*

Now, finally, your trainees are ready to start lifting!

Remember, there's no rush. Have your trainees start with weights they can easily handle for working through the "1-2-3-2-1" positional drill. 15lbs aluminum bars and 10lbs bumper plates are light enough for all but children and the aged/injured; if you anticipate working with these populations, a pair of 3lbs wooden training bumpers can be handy, or you could simply continue using PVC pipe. Always be conservative when working with new trainees—a 20kg bar might seem feather light to you, but to someone's grandma, it could mean injury risk.

Only when your athletes can consistently hit all three positions correctly should you allow them to smooth the movement into a continuous whole, and only once they can consistently execute the movement correctly should you allow them to begin adding weight. In any event, five sets of five reps should be quite sufficient on their first exposure.

Only provisionally true, as athletes will not be holding their breath when performing lifts in a metcon.

Deadlift Common Faults and Fixes

1. Back rounds/ shoulders go slack.

Athlete loses neutral spine position, with potentially disastrous consequences. In the concentric portion of the lift, we often see an athlete drive his hips up while failing to maintain his lumbar curve. In the eccentric portion, allowing the shoulders to droop forward leads to thoracic flexion and then loss of lumbar curve. It can be helpful to remind the athlete that every time he hits PR 3, he has an opportunity to get re-organized for the next rep.

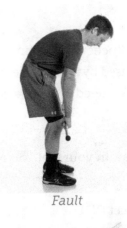
Fault

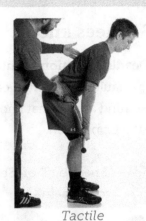
Tactile

 "Chest up!" and "Shoulders back and down!" or "Tight lumbar!"

 Demonstrate a correct DL 1, or lowering from DL 3.

 Tap between the shoulder blades to get athlete to retract and depress scapulae. This will aid thoracic extension.

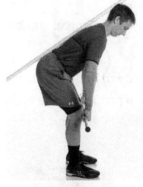
Orthosis

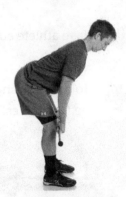
Correct DL 2

 Put The Tail on him! If your athlete can't feel three points of contact—back of head, t-spine, tailbone—at any point during the lift, he's lost neutral spine position.

2. Weight on balls of feet.

Deadlift Position 1 fault. Weight is distributed forward on foot. This can happen either from the ground up, the results of a faulty set-up, or from the top down, as the athlete tilts forward with the descending load.

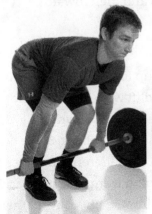
Fault

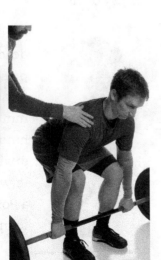
Tactile

 "Heels!"

 Demonstrate DL 1.

 By gently pushing back the knees and pressing down the hips, shift athlete's stance so that the emphasis is on his heels.

Deadlift Common Faults and Fixes, cont.

3. Knees knock.

Deadlift Position 1 fault. Knees are pointing in—Valgus fault. This is often caused by a too-wide stance. Remind athlete that knock-kneed is never a good athletic position.

 "Knees out!" or "Screw in your feet!" or "Move your feet in!"

 Demonstrate a correct DL 1.

 Have athlete adjust to a narrower stance.

 Holding the short side of an Abmat between the feet can establish proper stance width.

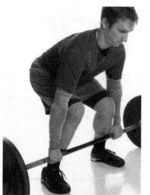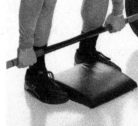

Fault   *Orthosis*

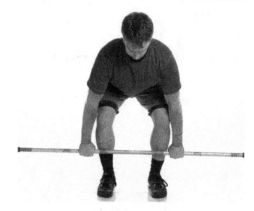

Correct DL 1

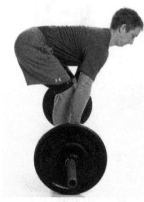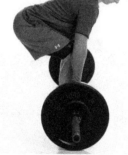

Faulty set-up   *Correct DL 1*

4. Lift from lower back

Deadlift Position 1 fault. If athlete starts with hips too high, he effectively lifts by pulling with the lower back, rather than driving the hips up and then foward.

 "Hips down!"

Set up for an imaginary deadlift while your trainee presses a fist down at the small of your back. Show him the difference between hinging from hips high, and driving the hips up and then forward. Switch places. Run a Positional Drill, telling your trainee to transition from DL 1 to DL 2 by driving his tailbone up against your fist.

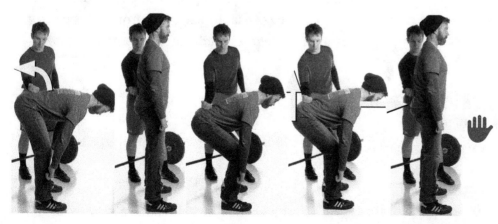

Bad: lifting around fulcrum of hip.   *Good: driving hip up and then forward to meet bar.*

Deadlift Common Faults and Fixes, cont.

5. Hips rise faster than shoulders.

Deadlift Position 1 fault. Remember, as the bar rises from floor to knee height, the hips and shoulders should rise at the same rate. If hips shoot up first, it usually means that during set-up, the hamstrings were not placed in sufficient tension. This fault is difficult to fix with a pithy cue, verbal or otherwise; generally, you'll need to review proper set-up, or how to reset tension as bar is lowered, or go all the way back to 1-2-3-2-1 positional drills.

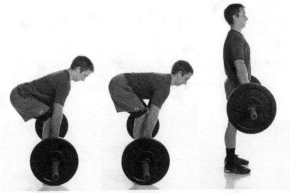

DL 1, hips rise faster than shoulders, DL 3

"Lift with chest!" During eccentric phase of lift: "Heels!" (in hopes athlete will not tip forward, losing tension in hamstrings).

Demonstrate a correct transition from DL 1 to DL 2.

With athlete in D1, place a piece of PVC in line with his spine. As athlete moves from DL1 to DL2, maintain angle of PVC.

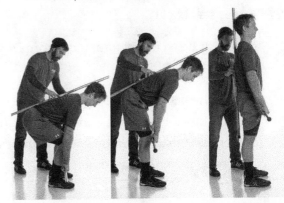

Tactile

6. Pulling bar around knees.

Deadlift Position 2 fault. The athlete failed to squeeze his knees back in the transition to DL 2, or he lifted with his lower back, causing his shoulders to rise more quickly than his hips—either way, the bar is pulled around the knees, rather than traveling straight up.

"Knees squeeze back!" or "Drive hips up!"

Demonstrate proper transition from DL 1 to DL 2.

With athlete in DL 1, place a piece of PVC in line with his spine. As athlete moves slowly from DL 1 to DL 2, maintain angle of PVC.

DL 1, shoulders rise faster than hips, DL 3

Tactile

Deadlift Common Faults and Fixes, cont.

7. Knees come forward during lower.

Deadlift Position 2 violation. If the athlete lowers the bar from DL 3 by allowing the knees to come forward, he creates a "ski jump" that will send the bar way out over his feet. The result? A poor set-up and bad execution of the next rep, or time lost as athlete reorganizes.

 "Knees stay back!"

 Demonstrate a correct transition from DL 3 to DL 2.

 Placing the back of your hand as a barrier in front of the athlete's knee can help him understand when to allow the knees to translate forward as the weight is lowered.

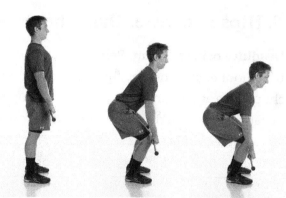

DL 1, shoulders rise faster than hips, DL 3

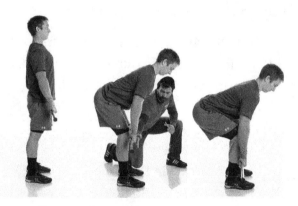

Correct Transition DL 3 to DL 2

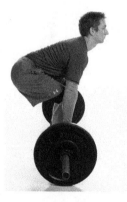
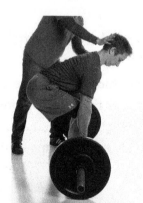

Fault   *Tactile*

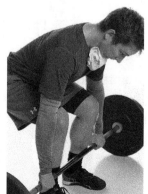
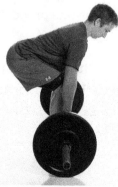

Orthosis   *Correct*

8. Head fault

Deadlift Position 1 fault. Athlete is looking straight ahead in bottom position. Gaze should be directed at floor, keeping neck and spine in a straight line.

 "Chin down!" or "Look down!"

 Demonstrate proper DL 1.

 With athlete holding in DL 1, adjust into desired position.

 Roll up a towel and have trainee hold it between his chin and chest. Alternately, place an object on the floor for them to look at.

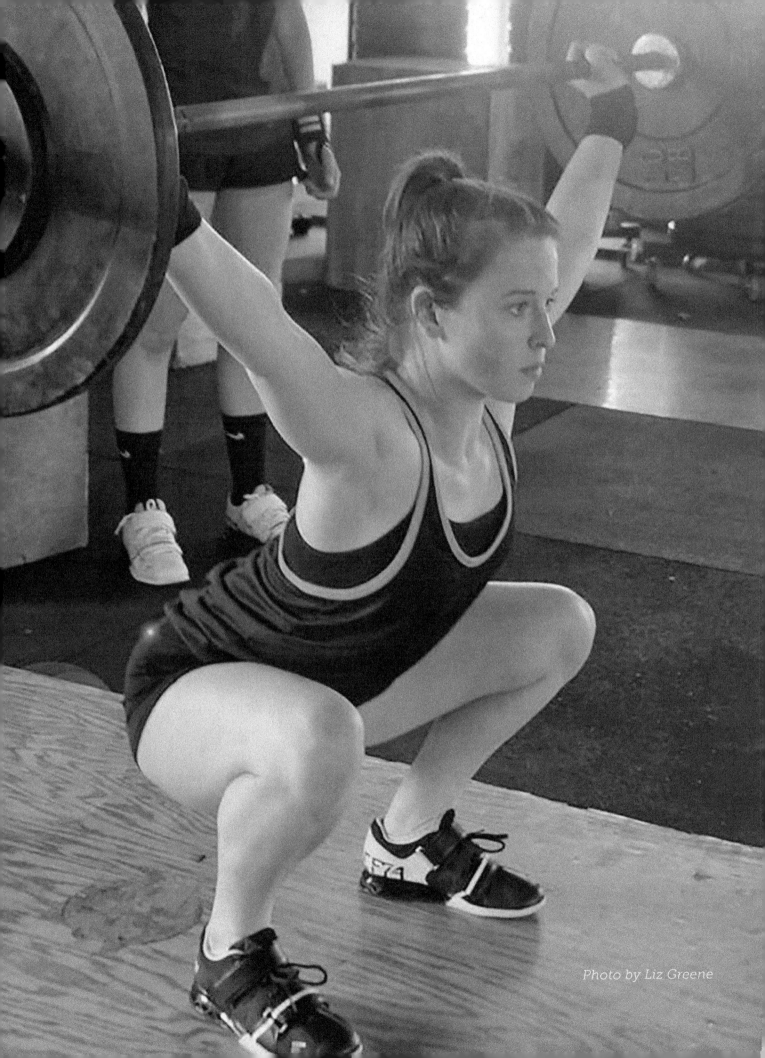

Photo by Liz Greene

THE "CFLA BASELINE"

This week our benchmark workout is adapted from the "CFLA Baseline WOD", written by Andy Petranek. The original version goes like this:

For time:
Row 500m
40 Squats
30 Sit-ups
20 Push-ups
10 Pull-ups

As an introductory benchmark, the CFLA Baseline has a lot to recommend it. For starters, its simple, "chipper" structure is easy to understand— all reps of a given exercise need to be completed before moving on to the next. Next, with the exception of the pull-ups, it draws on movements we've covered in this initial week of instruction. And the volume is relatively low, as it's meant to be administered safely to novices.

But the fact is the CFLA Baseline WOD, as written, isn't necessarily appropriate for all populations. Okay, it can be completed by an experienced athlete in less than five minutes, and your average "in-shape" person averages about seven. But what if that in-shape person brought her ex-jock, gone-to-pot husband? Even scaled, it might take him twelve minutes or more. That might be too much for a deconditioned athlete. And what if she brought her tough, spunky, but undeniably over-60 grandma? How do you make this workout safe for her?

For one possible answer, let's look at how we'll customize this WOD for Harry, Amy, and Tim, the three members of Team Space Monkey.

CUSTOMIZING THE CFLA BASELINE WOD FOR ATHLETES OF VARYING ABILITY LEVELS

Having worked with Harry, Amy, and Tim for three days, what do we know about them?

Harry is very strong, and has had some experience with MMGPP training. Unfortunately, he's never had any formal instruction, so he's acquired some bad habits, like over-rotating his feet in the squat, and he sometimes forgets to squat to correct depth. A more serious problem is the lack of shoulder flexion he demonstrated when trying to do the Samson Stretch. That's not going to make much of a difference today, but later, when we start doing overhead work, it'll be an issue.

Amy's flexibility is very good, as is her physical intelligence--she easily hits any position once it's demonstrated. As noted earlier, she hasn't done any barbell work before, but that's okay, because there's no barbell stuff in this WOD.

A lifetime of sedentary habits and years of working at a desk have left Tim terribly stiff through the hips, back and shoulders. To squat, he needs a 12" box with two Abmats. He also has difficulty translating verbal instruction into bodily movement; he seems to do much better when he has a visual aid. So for today, I'll draw the positions of the row and the squat on the whiteboard for him to reference.

Prescribing Correct Movement

Harry's good to go on the rower. He does have that bad habit of over-rotating his feet in the squat, so I set him up with a bumper plate as an orthosis. He'll cruise through the sit-ups and push-ups. He says he can do kipping pull-ups, but when I ask him to demonstrate, his form is all over the place. His strict pull-ups aren't much better, with much midline-breaking and chin-reaching. There's no time now to instruct and correct him adequately, so I ask him to do piked ring rows instead. Good sport that he is, he agrees.

Amy also looks good on the rower. Her knees cave in on the squats, so I set her between a pair of boxes to serve as orthoses. The sit-ups will be no problem, but it's pretty likely that after 10 reps the push-ups will become too challenging. I keep a 20" box on standby. Standard ring rows are right for her.

For Tim, who is still working to master the various positions of the movements he's been taught, there's no question of going fast. He's simply to practice the four positions of the row, the three positions of the box squat, the two positions of the butterfly sit-ups (perhaps with a band tied to a post for some assistance), the two positions of the push-up on a 24" box, and then the two positions of the ring row. In all cases, he is to concentrate on maintaining a stable midline and keeping his shoulders packed. The period of practice for each exercise is delimited as follows.

Prescribing Correct Volume

Part of the attraction of task-specific WODs, in which a certain amount of work is specified and the time to completion is the variable, is that as you progress through the workout, there is a light at the end of the tunnel. There's comfort in knowing "Only x number of reps left. Only y reps left." But task-specific WODs can be problematic, because the volume of work specified is often beyond what is safe for new or developing athletes.

Traditionally, faced with this fact, you had three options:

A) Let them gut it out 'til they're done. Death before DNF! (Unfortunately, this tends to put people in the hospital.)

B) Time cut-off. You allow your athletes a certain amount of time to complete the workout, and when time's up, they're done, no matter where they are. This is a safer option, but it's often dissatisfying to the client, who feels "cheated" because they "didn't get to finish".

C) Guesstimate appropriate work volume. "You're new, so you do half of what's written on the board. You've been training a few months, you can do 75%." This is inexact, and again can lead to people feeling cheated, because the prescription was too light, and they finished too soon, or because it was still too much, and again they didn't get to finish.

A better way to ensure your athletes are receiving the correct dose of volume for their level of development is to analyze how long it takes an average/good athlete to complete the prescribed work, and then restructure the WOD along those lines. For our group of trainees with varying ability levels, By the Numbers recommends structuring the CFLA Baseline WOD like this:

> AMRAP 2:30 Row. If you get to 500m before time is up, move on to...
> AMRAP :90 Squats. If you get to 40 before time is up, move on to...
> AMRAP :75 Sit-ups. If you get to 30 before time is up, move on to...
> AMRAP :60 Push-ups. If you get to 20 before time is up, move on to...
> AMRAP :45 Ring rows. If you get to 10 before time is up, you're done!

The intervals add up to 7 minutes, which is a good time domain for this WOD. A very fit and experienced athlete like Harry will likely charge right through, easily staying ahead of the clock. His score will be his time to completion.

The athletes concentrate on trying to complete the prescribed work. They don't need to think about the time intervals; that's your job. To make sure you don't get confused, write down (either on the white board or on a note card you carry) the specific times allotted for each interval, e.g., "0:00 - 2:29, row. 2:30 - 3:59, squats. 4:00 - 5:14, sit-ups. 5:15 - 6:14, push-ups. 6:15 - 7:00, pull-ups." Let them know when it's time to transition: "3...2...1... Time for push-ups! Let's go!" Being able to administrate odd intervals *and* cue/correct is no small feat; it won't be easy at first. But when you can do it effortlessly, you'll know you're on your way to coaching virtuosity.

For the less experienced, the time limitations greatly reduce the likelihood that an athlete will be overdosed with volume. For Amy, the correct volume of squats is what she can complete in 90 seconds or less (up to 40). Once those 90 seconds are up, she moves on to the next exercise. If that's only 25 squats, fine; next time, hopefully, that number will be higher. At the end of the workout, she'll have five numbers: total meters rowed in 2:30, total squats in :90, total sit-ups in :75, total push-ups in :60, total ring rows in :45.

This way, everyone gets an appropriate dose of intensity. This approach also provides an easy way to find the deficits in an athlete's capacities (e.g., perhaps an athlete easily finished the squats, push-ups, and ring rows, but not the sit-ups. Guess what needs some extra work?)

I instruct Tim to move deliberately through the positions of each exercise. He need pay attention to the clock only to know when it's time to move on to practicing the next movement.

"3...2...1...GO!"

Harry

Once the clock started, Harry attacked the row. He form was all over the place, but once I reminded him "Legs back arms, arms back legs," he smoothed things out. He hopped off the rower at 1:37, fit his feet around the bumper to help maintain his stance, and then started hammering his squats. In his hard-charging excitement to get 'er done, he wasn't quite getting to legal depth. I used a verbal cue on him ("Lower!"), and when that didn't work, demonstrated what I wanted. When *that* didn't work, I slid a medicine ball under him and told him to be sure his butt hit the ball on every rep. That solved the issue! From there he burned through his sit-ups, push-ups and piked ring-rows, finishing the whole workout in 5:05. He was so excited, and so obviously ready for more, that on the spot I turned the Baseline into a 7 minute AMRAP.* Back on the rower he went. He had finished another 500m row and 15 squats when time was called. Pretty impressive!

Amy

At 2:29, Amy had rowed 460m. Not bad for a new athlete of her height! From there it was on to squats. I think she was a little shocked at how shaky her legs felt after the row, but she still finished 35 squats in 90 seconds. Sit-ups posed no problem. As expected, she hit failure on the push-ups around rep 14, so she finished her last set with box push-ups. Although she was definitely out of breath, she had stamina to spare for the ring rows, and finished at 6:40. Then she turned 'round to cheer on Harry and Tim.

Rather than record her time to completion, I had her write down her time for the 500m piece, and how many squats, sit-ups, push-ups, and pull-ups she got, and at what scale. Here's why: if Amy did the Baseline in 6:40 today, but in three months does it again in 6:55 with strict push-ups and band-assisted pull-ups, does that 15 second difference really mean her fitness regressed? No way! Until athletes are able to do the exact movements prescribed, their time to completion is meaningless. For now, the only data that matters is what specific work she accomplished in the workout, so she has numbers to beat next time.

Tim

Remember, for Tim this is all new. He's never really exercised before, so just performing the five exercises in this workout to even a degree of competence was a big accomplishment. He carefully worked his way through all the positions of the row, practiced his squats, did his sit-ups. Surprising me, Tim did 15 strict push-ups on the floor in the allotted minute! When he stood up from his ring rows shortly before the 7 minutes mark, he was all smiles, and enthusiastically high-fived his humble instructor, saying, "What a great way to end the week!"

I couldn't agree more.

---

* Why did I make a change? When he had finished the workout, Harry was still fired up and ready to go. By letting him show off a bit I kept him "entertrained"—working hard as hell, and having fun doing it.

WEEK 2 / DAY 1
BACK SQUATS

Category: Squat

Movement screen: Hands-up wall squat test

Ability screen: Air squat x 5 (dumbbell squat), dumbbell squat x 5 (back squat)

The barbell back squat is the king of strength exercises. Greater loads are moved with the deadlift, but the back squat, in addition to moving the load a longer distance, places more demand on the athlete's coordination, balance, and flexibility. To barbell back squat safely, an athlete needs a solid air squat, and to pass the Hands-up Wall Squat test described previously.

There are two kinds of back squats: high bar, or Olympic squats, and low bar, or powerlifting squats. High bar means the barbell is sitting on the traps, just below the nape of the neck. Low bar means the barbell is seated a couple inches lower, atop the spine of the scapulae. High bar squatting requires the athlete keep a fairly vertical torso, and evenly loads the anterior and posterior chains. Low bar requires a greater forward lean, and is a very posterior chain dominant movement; in fact, it could be described as deadlifting with a barbell on your back.

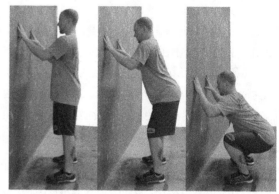
Want to back squat? Pass this test.

In By the Numbers we teach the high bar squat by default. Its more vertical torso position has a better carryover to the front squat, overhead squat, and thruster. However, there are instances—limited ankle mobility, or a trainee with extra long femurs and a short torso—when the low bar is a more practical choice, so I've included instruction for that as well. For the reason stated, however, those low-bar trainees should be transitioned to high bar if and when possible.

I've found it helpful to start everyone with the dumbbell squat. The dumbbell squat is simply an air squat with dumbbells racked on the shoulders. Not only is it accessible to everyone who can at least air squat, it's foundational to dumbbell thrusters and dumbbell clean variations. (The goblet squat is also a workable choice at this point, but it doesn't progress directly to any other exercises.)

Harry and Amy both pass the Hands-up Wall Squat Test, so they will back squat today. (Harry will continue to use a bumper plate held between his feet to correct his over-rotating feet.) Tim will receive instruction about how to set up for the back squat, but when it's time to train, he'll keep working on progressing from Box Squats to Air Squats.

Dumbbell Squat Teaching Script

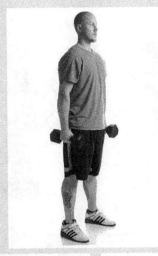

"Grab a pair of dumbbells. Make sure the pinky-side of your hand is closer to the loading plate or dumbbell head than your thumb-side.

"Then set up in Air Squat Position 1: feet shoulder width, weight centered in the foot, feet screwed into the floor, midline braced, shoulders back and down.

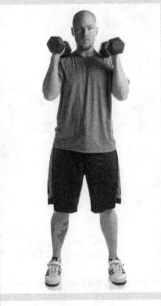
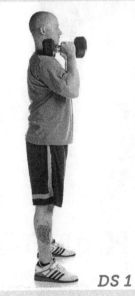

"Seat the head of the dumbbell firmly on your shoulder. Keep the elbows in close to the rib cage. Dumbbells should be parallel to the floor. This is **Dumbbell Squat Position 1 (DS 1)**. The next two positions will be exactly the same as Air Squat Positions 2 and 3, except for the dumbbells you're carrying on your shoulders.

DS 1

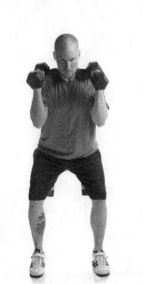
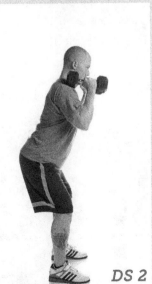

"Unlock your knees. Sit your hips back. Push your knees out. Keep the dumbbells parallel to the floor. This is **Dumbbell Squat Position 2 (DS 2)**.

DS 2

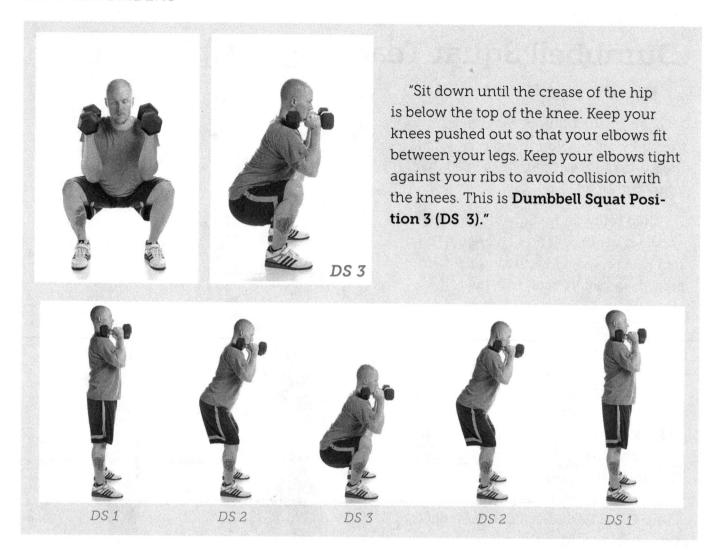

"Sit down until the crease of the hip is below the top of the knee. Keep your knees pushed out so that your elbows fit between your legs. Keep your elbows tight against your ribs to avoid collision with the knees. This is **Dumbbell Squat Position 3 (DS 3)**."

DS 3

DS 1   DS 2   DS 3   DS 2   DS 1

High Bar Back Squat Teaching Script

"As we go through this process of setting up for the back squat, remember, we are trying to create maximal tension in the body. Once tension is set, it remains until the end of the set. No going slack at any point! Here's how to set up for the back squat:

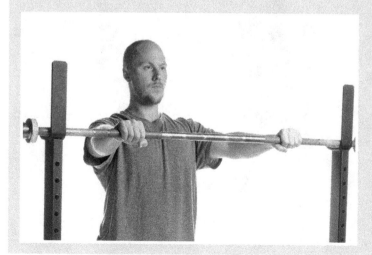

"With the bar in the rack (set about 1" below the top of the shoulders), grip it at arm's length. Try starting with your hands 1" plus thumb's length out from where the gnurling meets the smooth center of the bar, and adjust from there, closer or farther apart as your mobility allows. (A closer grip allows you to bunch the muscles of your upper back, cushioning your spine against the bar.) Finally, wrap your thumbs around the bar.

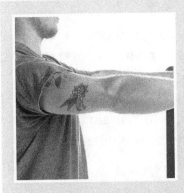 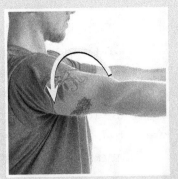

"'Snap' the bar in half by externally rotating your arms.

"Partially retract and depress your shoulder blades.

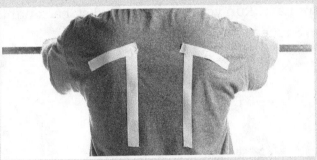 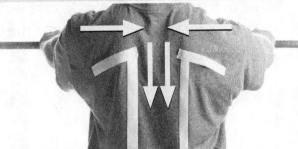

"Plant one foot forward under the bar, and screw it tight to the floor. As you duck under the bar, bring your rear foot forward, arranging your stance so that you are in a partial squat under the bar: feet shoulder-width, a small degree of toe turn-out, knees out, hips back, chest up.

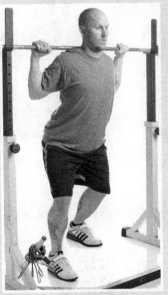 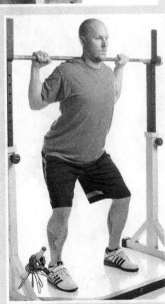

"At this point, your lower back may be over-arched. Squeeze your glutes and lock your abs down to 'hollow out' under the bar.

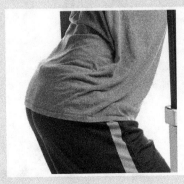 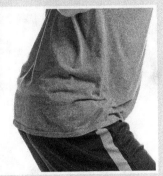

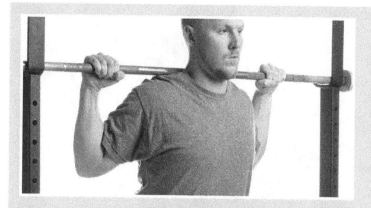

"Finally, try to 'wind' your elbows down under the bar, nestling it into your traps. Think 'weld the bar to your body' as you try to bend it over your back. If your wrists are hyperextended, return them to neutral; this will force your shoulders back, and lift your chest.

"Stand the bar up out of the rack. Take two steps back. Run your set-up checklist: back tight, glutes and abs locked, feet screwed into the floor. Squeeze the bar in your fists.

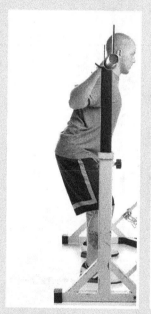
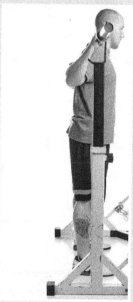
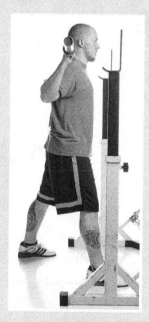
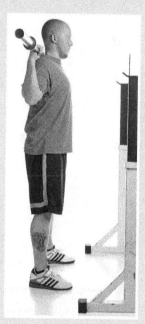

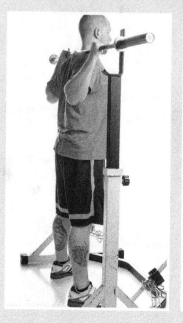
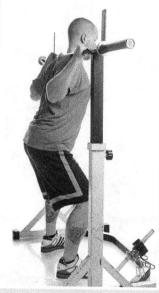

"For now, let's pretend you've just completed your set. When your set is finished, walk straight in until the bar hits the squat stand uprights, and then bend at the hips and knees to lower it into the cradles. DO NOT GO HUNTING FOR THE HOOKS.

"OK, step out from under the bar.

"Last week we discussed the Valsalva maneuver with regard to the deadlift. How do you apply this to the squat? Set up as we've discussed. After you walk the bar out of the rack, but before you initiate the squat, take a deep breath, apply Valsalva, and descend. Once you've stood back up, forcefully exhale, then inhale and hold again before starting your next rep.

"You must hold your breath through the entire movement. What does this sound like?" *(Squat, and then exhale as you stand, making a hissing sound.)* "Like a tire going flat, right? That's the sound of your spine losing support. If your spine feels unsupported (anthropomorphizing here) autogenic inhibition will cause you to miss the lift. So hold your breath and pressurize!

"Right! Back to the rack. With your arms straight, get your proper-width grip. Try to snap the bar in half. Pack your shoulders. Duck under the bar and nestle it into your traps. Get organized in a partial squat: weight just in front of the heels, knees out, hips back, chest up. Hollow out. Then stand up, and step out.

"Run your set-up checklist: feet shoulder-width and screwed into the floor, glutes and abs locked, back tight. Try gripping the floor with your toes; this will help keep your feet flat on the ground. Squeeze the bar tight in your fists as you pull your elbows down under the bar. This is **Back Squat Position 1 (BS 1).**

BS 1

"Take a deep breath and employ the Valsalva maneuver. Unlock your knees, then sit back. Push your knees out. This is **Back Squat Position 2 (BS 2).**

BS 2

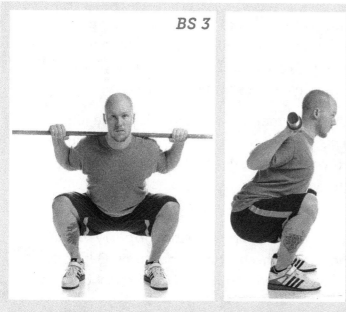

BS 3

"Sit straight down until the crease of your hip is below the top of your knee. Feet are flat, weight is in front of the heels, knees are out, chest is up, gaze is forward. This is **Back Squat Position 3 (BS 3).**

"In this position, your glutes are still firing! Don't go slack!

"Immediately rebound and stand up to **BS 2.** Concentrate on driving your shoulders into the bar, rather than pushing the ground away with your legs. This will help reinforce your Valsalva technique. BE EXPLOSIVE. Try to generate momentum out of the bottom of the squat that will carry you through the sticking point (where the bar often slows, about halfway up its return path).

"Squeeze your glutes to fully extend your hips and return to **BS 1**. Exchange breath. Reset, and repeat as required. "

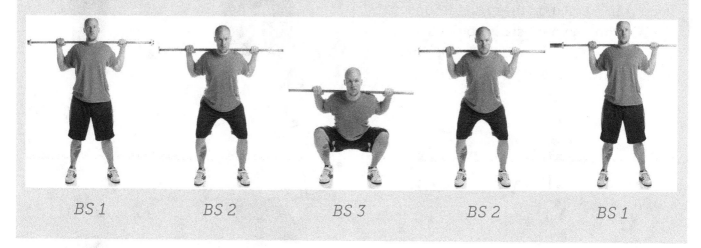

| BS 1 | BS 2 | BS 3 | BS 2 | BS 1 |

Positional Drills

"1! 2! 3! 2! 1!" Take athlete through each position in turn. Have them hold each position while you make necessary adjustments.

"1! 2! 3! Go!" Bring athletes into bottom position; when they look good, on your command "Go!", they return to **BS 1**.

"Five in the hole." This is "1-2-3-Go!" with a five second hold in the bottom position.

High Bar Back Squat Common Faults and Fixes

All of the common faults and fixes of the air squat (breaking at knees first, unable to maintain neutral spine position, spinal overextension, insufficient depth, weight on balls of feet, excessive foot turn out, knees cave in, etc.) also apply to the back squat, as well as the following:

1. Broken wrists.

Back Squat Position 1 violation. If the athlete holds the bar with wrists hyperextended, he's missing a chance to create some additional supporting tension in the upper torso. The bar should be held with wrists neutral or slightly goosenecked. This will force the shoulders back, which helps maintain thoracic extension.

 "Straight wrists!"

 Demonstrate proper BS 1.

 Adjust athlete into proper position by pressing the back of his hand away while pulling his wrists toward you. Some athletes, due to shoulder flexibility issues, will need to take a wider grip in order to maintain a neutral wrist.

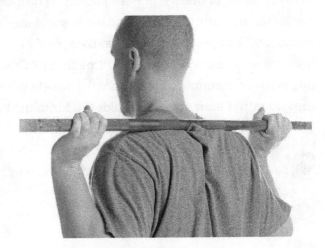

Fault

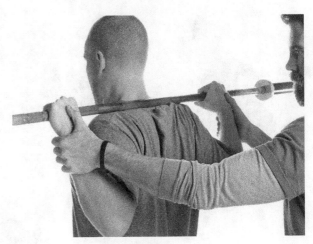

Tactile

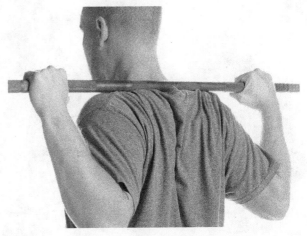

Correct BS 1

Back Squat Common Faults and Fixes, cont.

2. The guillotine.

Back Squat Position 2 violation. Bar moves far out in front of line of gravity, pressing down on trainee's neck. Occurs during eccentric phase of squat (descent) if athlete pushes hips too far back, or if he leans forward too much (not the same thing!). Occurs during the concentric phase (ascent) if athlete pushes hips up rather than driving shoulders up into the bar. Torso should be kept as vertical as possible.

 "Chest up!" or "Hips forward under the bar!"

 Demonstrate proper BS 2.

 With athlete holding in BS 2, adjust as necessary.

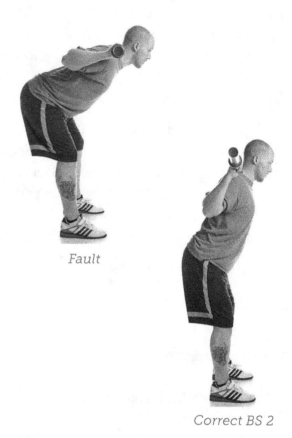

Fault

Correct BS 2

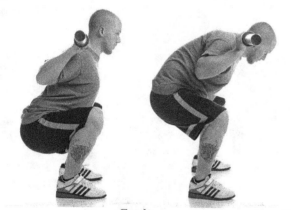

Fault

3. Back rounds on rising.

Back Squat Position 3 to Position 2 violation. If an athlete's back starts to round under load, it's because of fatigue, a lack of breath support, or a combination thereof. Remind the athlete that the muscles of the back alone are not enough to support the weight. He needs to recruit all of the musculature of the trunk and pressurize.

Also, remember there's no fixing this as it's happening; you can only head off trouble with the next rep.

 "Big breath! Lock it in!"

 Demonstrate correct transition from BS 3 to BS 2.

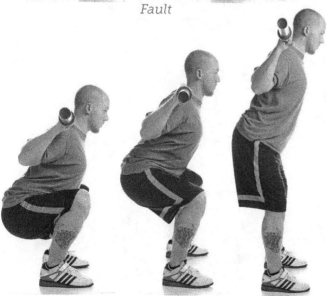

Correct transition from BS 3 to BS 2

Low Bar Back Squat Teaching Script

"Those athletes with tight ankles or long femurs and a short torso may find the low bar version of the back squat better suits them.

"Grab a piece of PVC pipe, lift it overhead, and place it on top of your traps. Here, below the nape of your neck, is where the bar would be situated for the high bar squat."

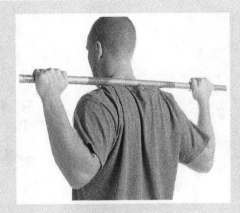

"For the low bar squat we're going to the hold the bar about two inches lower, so it's resting on top of your shoulder blades. It should fit securely into the 'divot' above the contracted deltoid muscle.

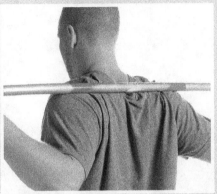

"Place your thumbs on the same side of the bar as your hands. Now slide your hands in toward your shoulders until your elbows are bent to about 60 degrees.

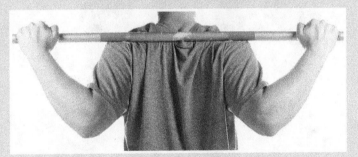

Straight wrists

"If your wrists are bent back, straighten them. Low bar squatting with bent wrists will force your arms to support the barbell, resulting in very unpleasant elbow pain.

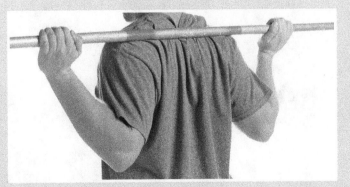

Bent wrists

"Now, the object of the low bar squat is the same as the high bar squat: lower and raise the bar in a straight line.

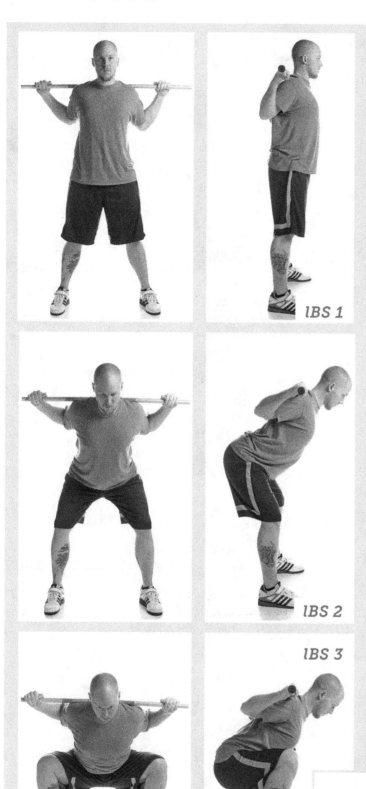

lBS 1

lBS 2

lBS 3

"With the bar held on top of the shoulder blades, you're going to have to really drive your butt back and push your knees out to keep the bar centered over your area of base. Keep your head in a neutral position; as your torso tilts, your gaze will move from the wall in front of you, to the floor about 4' in front, then back up the wall.

"Set up for the low bar squat as your would for high bar, the only exception being, you'll grasp the bar with your thumbs on the same side as your fingers. Walk the bar out and take your stance. The stance for the low bar squat is 2-3" wider than your high bar squat.

"Run your normal set up: abs on, butt tight, screw your feet into the floor. This is **Low Bar Back Squat Position 1 (lBS 1)**."

"Engage Valsalva.

"Now hinge your hips back. This is **Low Bar Back Squat Position 2 (lBS 2).**

"Instead of thinking 'down', just keep pushing your hips back and your knees out.

"Sit down until the crease of your hip just breaks parallel. This is **Low Bar Back Squat Position 3 (lBS 3).**

Notice the similarity between lBS 3 and DL 1. Low bar squatting is essentially deadlifting with a bar on your back. The hip drive is the same.

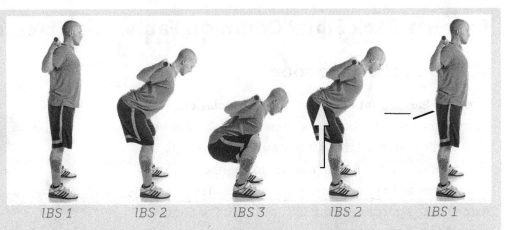

"To rise, push through the heels and drive your hips towards the ceiling. Your shoulders should rise at the same rate."

lBS 1   lBS 2   lBS 3   lBS 2   lBS 1

"Once the shins are vertical, change from driving the hips up to driving the hips forward until you've returned to **lBS 1**."

Positional Drills

"1-2-3-2-1." Take athlete through each position of the low bar squat. Have them hold each position while you make necessary adjustments.

"1-2-3-Go!" Bring athletes into bottom position; when they look good, on your command "Go!", they return to **lBS 1.**

"Five in the hole." This is "1-2-3-Go!" with a five second hold in the bottom position.

Low Bar Back Squat Common Faults and Fixes

1. Broken wrists.

Low Bar Back Squat Position 1 violation. In the low bar squat, good wrist position is critical; holding the bar with extended wrists will put a nasty strain on the elbow tendons. The bar should be held with wrists neutral. Rather than supported by the hands and arms, the bar is "pinned" to the back with the palms.

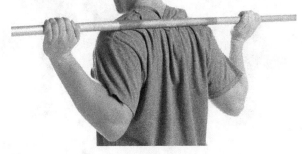

Fault

 "Straight wrists!"

 Demonstrate proper lBS 1.

 Adjust wrists into proper position.

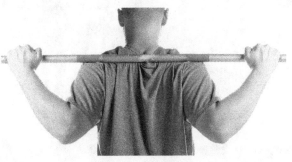

Correct lBS 1

Low Bar Back Squat Common Faults and Fixes, cont.

2. Lifting chest too soon.

Low Bar Back Squat Position 3 to lBS 2 violation. During the ascent, athlete lifts chest before shins have returned to vertical. Lifting the chest too soon limits the potential of the hips to produce force—the whole point of using low bar. Back angle must be maintained in the transition from lBS 3 to lBS 2. The shoulders should rise at the same rate as the hips.

 "Hip drive!" or "Six pack!"

 Demonstrate proper transiton from lBS 3 to lBS 2.

 Use the fist-on-tailbone demo from the "Hips start too high" deadlift fault and fix.

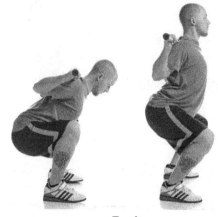

Fault

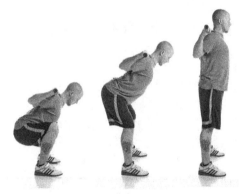

Correct lBS sequence

3. Hips rise too soon.

Low Bar Back Squat Position 3 to lBS 2 violation. Conversely, if the hips come up too fast, and the shoulders don't rise with them, the lifter will be put in a bad position—a good morning, for all intents. From here all they can do is lever up from their lower back. No bueno!

 "Chest up!"

 Demonstrate proper transiton from lBS 3 to lBS 2.

 Use the fist-on-tailbone demo from the "Hips start too high" deadlift fault and fix.

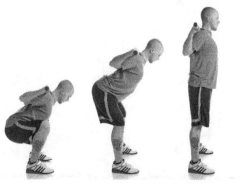

Fault

Correct lBS sequence

Spotting the Back Squat

"Sometimes a lift goes wrong. You descend too far, you lean too far forward, or it's just too damned heavy. Starting now, you'll practice what to do if you get into trouble with a back squat.

"Once you've realized that you're not going to be able to complete the lift, raise your chest, let go of the bar, and hop forward (in that order, but in extremely quick succession). As long as you have not already tipped too far forward, gravity will bring the bar down behind you and you'll be safely out of the way.

"Practice and experience are the only way to build confidence! Put some bumpers on the bar (not the 10lbs!) and bail out on purpose until you get a feel for it."

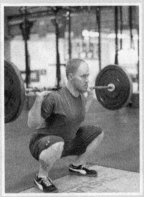 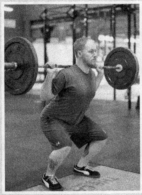 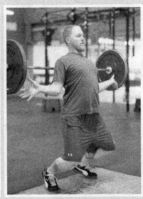 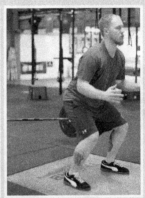

"For an extra margin of safety, use a spotter. If a lifter gets stuck, the spotter should grab the bar from above with a mixed grip, and help the lifter finish his rep. It should only take a few pounds of force. If worse comes to worst, once the lifter has let go of the bar, the spotter can pull it backward, allowing the spotter to escape forward. Before you start your set, let your spotter know if you prefer to bail out, or have him help you finish the rep!

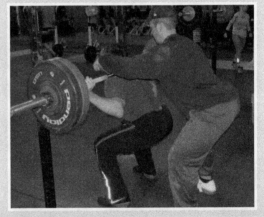

"For really heavy efforts, two spotters are better. Have them stand on either side of the lifter, with their hands cupped under the ends of the barbell sleeves. Designate one spotter the captain. Neither will put hands on the bar until the captain says so. The last thing you want is for one spotter to lift the bar, twisting it on the lifter's back. Once assistance has been rendered, all three walk the bar into the rack."

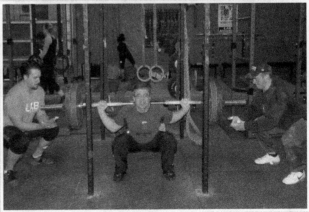

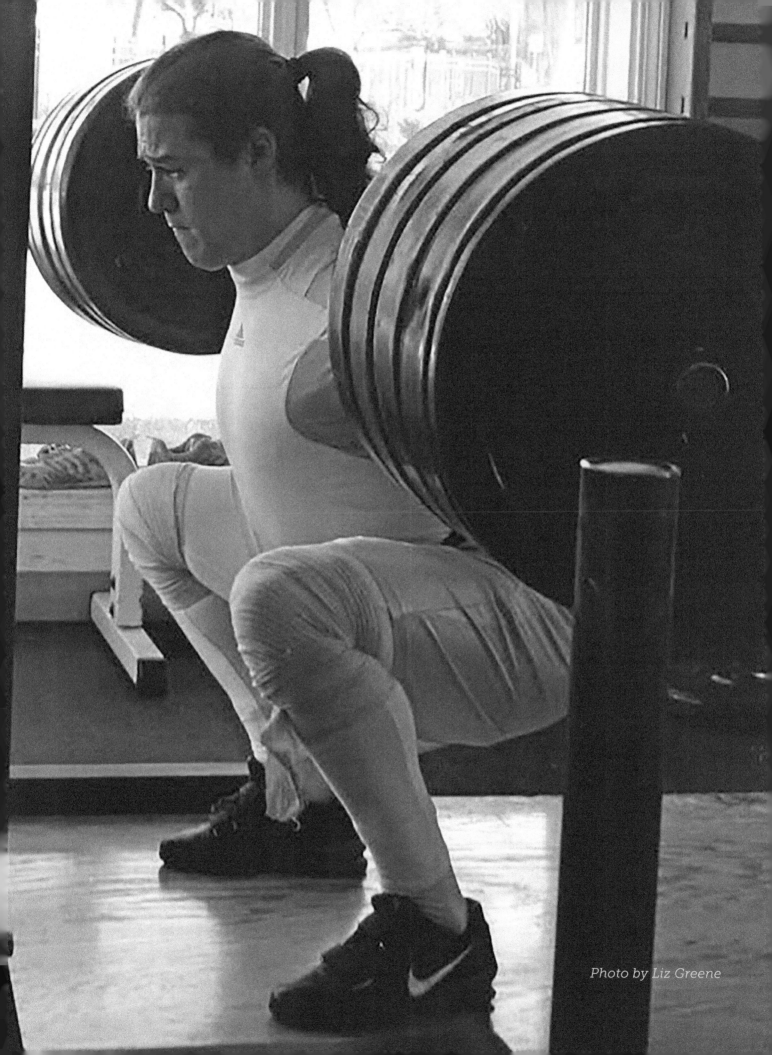

Photo by Liz Greene

FEET-ANCHORED SIT-UPS

Category: Hip and Trunk Flexion (seated)

Movement screen: N/a

Ability screen: Butterfly sit-up x 5

The feet-anchored sit-up, a variation on the classic 7th grade gym class exercise, is used when repetition cycle time is a concern. Rather than requiring the athlete to clasp his hands behind his head, he simply touches the ground behind his shoulders, then sits up to touch the dumbbells.

All three athletes of Team Space Monkey should be able to handle this one.

Feet Anchored Sit-up Teaching Script

"Place an Abmat on the floor with the logo upside down relative to you. Place two dumbbells side-by-side in front of it. (You'll need to use at least 25s). Have a seat on the floor with your tailbone at the edge of the mat. Wedge your feet under the dumbbells.

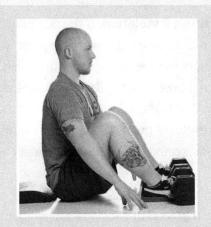

"Lie back until your shoulder blades are on the mat and the back of your head touches the floor. Extend your arms to-ward the ceiling. Bend your elbows to touch the floor just behind your shoulders. This is **Sit-up Position 1 (SU 1).**

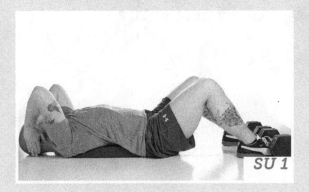

SU 1

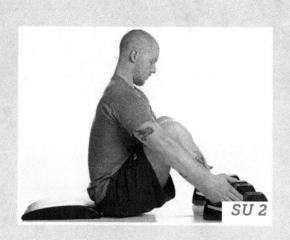

"Contract your abdominals to curl up your trunk. As your trunk moves to vertical, your hip flexors take over. Sit up tall to tap the dumbbells with both hands to complete the rep. This is **Sit-up Position 2 (SU 2)**."

Positional Drills

"1-2-1." Review positions of the feet-anchored sit-up one at a time, making corrections as necessary.

Feet Anchored Sit-up Common Faults and Fixes

1. Crunching.

Sit-up Position 2 violation. If the dumbbells are set too close to the Abmat, the athlete will not have to sit up completely in order to tap the dumbbells, leading to half-reps. Make sure the dumbbells are set at a distance such that the knees are bent at least 90 degrees, or have the athlete push his Abmat back until he is properly positioned. The torso must break vertical to the floor.

 "Push your butt back!" or "Chest to knees!"

 Demonstrate proper SU 2.

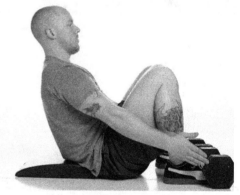

Fault

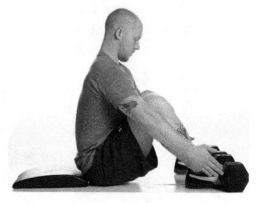

Correct SU 2

JUMPING MECHANICS

Category: Jump and Land

Movement screen: N/a

Ability screen: Air squat x 5

Don't take for granted that your trainees can perform even the most natural-seeming movements correctly. Although it seems like it should be as instinctual as walking, many trainees will lack the ability to take off and land in a two-footed jump, which makes exercises like broad jumps, box jumps, and, later, the clean and the snatch, problematic and possibly injurious.

The take-off for a jump involves hinging the hip and drawing back the arms. Jumping is explosively extending the knees and hips to propel the body into the air. Landing correctly demands the athlete re-establish contact with the ground in a well-organized, partial squat. Spend some time with your trainees working on this basic movement skill, and spare them an ACL injury later.

Harry and Amy will do fine with this. Tim almost has air squats—he's down to box squatting with one Abmat—but that's not enough. Without the strength and stability necessary for an air squat, I don't believe he can safely handle the ballistic forces created by jumping and landing. There's no rush. Jumping and landing can wait for a bit.

Jumping Mechanics Teaching Script

"Jumping and landing can be broken down into two familiar positions: the hip hinge and the squat.

"Your take-off is based on the hinge. Set your feet under your hips, screw your feet into the floor, brace your midline, and set your shoulders. This is **Jump Position 1 (JP 1).**

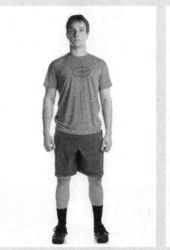
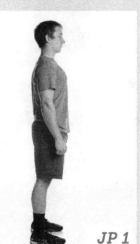

JP 1

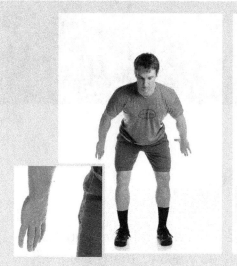

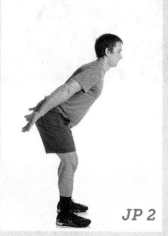

JP 2

"Unlock your knees and push your hips back, loading your hamstrings. Keep your shins as vertical as possible! Simultaneously draw back and internally rotate your arms (that is, turn your thumbs in). This is **Jump Position 2 (JP 2)**.

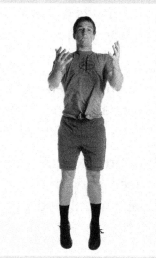

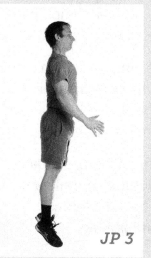

JP 3

"To jump, drive through the heels as you aggressively extend your knees and hips. Throw your hands forward as you externally rotate your arms. Make sure you are jumping from your heels, not your toes; although you may rise up onto the balls of your feet, that is not the primary locus of force application. This take-off is **Jump Position 3 (JP 3)**.

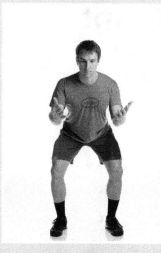

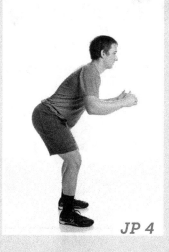

JP 4

"Land in a partial squat: feet screwed into the ground, knees out, hips back, shoulders back and down, hands out in front, palms angled toward ceiling. Hinging at the hip transfers the force of the landing into a posterior chain load, which protects the knees. This is **Jump Position 4 (JP 4),** the landing.

"Stand to return to **JP 1**.

"It's important to understand that the way you land depends on your position at take off. In other words, if your knees knock during the wind-up, you will almost certainly land with your knees caving in, predisposing you to injury."

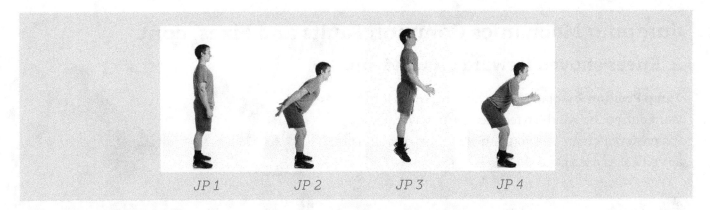

JP 1   JP 2   JP 3   JP 4

Positional Drills

"1-2-1." Have athlete practice winding up for the jump.

"1-2-Go! Freeze!" **Jump Position 3** is a passing position—there's no point in making the trainees pause while standing up on their toes. So a "Go!" from **JP 2** propels them straight through **JP 3**. However, there is good reason to make trainees freeze in **JP 4**, their landing. If they simply stand up back into **JP 1**, they'll have no idea if they landed correctly. Instead have them remain in **JP 4** while they self-assess. If they're not in an ideal position, fix it! With repetition, their positions will approximate this ideal with greater and greater precision. This in an idea we'll return to when working on the clean and the snatch.

Jumping Mechanics Common Faults and Fixes

1. Knees knock on wind-up.

Jump Position 2 violation. Valgus fault. Remember, the way an athlete takes off in a jump is the way he's going to land. As he pushes hips back to load hamstrings, he should simultaneously push out his knees to create torque at the hip. If he's unable to do so, he may have weak abductors and could benefit from X-band squats or other accessory exercises.

 "Screw your feet in!" or "Knees out!"

 Demonstrate a correct JP 2.

 Have athlete freeze in JP 2. Place your hands where you want athlete's knees to go. Tell him, "Push into my hands!"

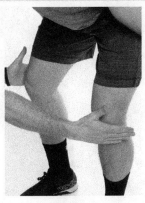

Tactile

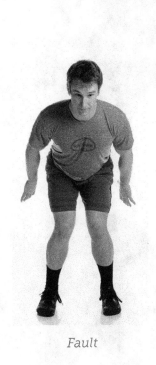

Fault

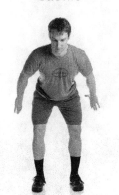

Correct JP 2

Jumping Mechanics Common Faults and Fixes, cont.

2. Knees shoved forward on wind-up.

Jump Position 2 violation. Shoving the knees forward during the wind-up reduces the involvement of the posterior chain. Tell your athlete to keep his shins as vertical as possible.

 "Hips back!" or "Shins vertical!"

 Demonstrate a correct JP 2.

 With your athlete in JP 1, place the back of your hand before his knee. Tell him, "Hinge back, but don't touch my hand!"

 Set up a utility bench and use it to block the trainee's knees as he practices hingeing from JP 1 to JP 2. *Only* hinging—make sure he understands he's not to try to jump!

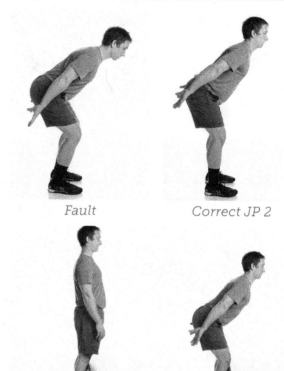

Fault   *Correct JP 2*

Orthosis

3. Thumbs out during wind-up.

Jump Position 2 violation. As the athlete hinges back in preparation for take-off, he must simultaneously draw his arms behind him and turn his thumbs in toward his centerline. This internal rotation at the shoulder creates tension that will be released in JP 3 as he swings his hands forward and externally rotates his arms.

 "Thumbs turn in!"

 Demonstrate a correct JP 2.

 Have your athlete freeze in his wind-up position (JP 2) and manually adjust his arms into the desired position.

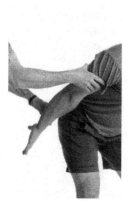

Fault

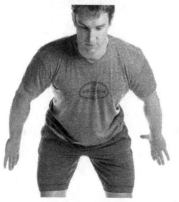

Tactile   *Correct JP 2*

Jumping Mechanics Common Faults and Fixes, cont.

4. Knees shoved forward on landing.

Jump Position 4 violation. Landing with the knees shoved forward puts excessive shearing force on the knee. Tell your athlete, "Make sure you land in a good partial squat, with shins as vertical as possible. Let the hips absorb the shock, rather than your knees."

 "Sit!"

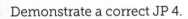 Demonstrate a correct JP 4.

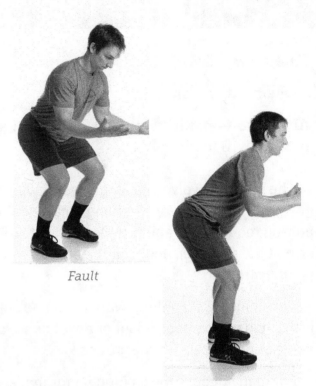

Fault

Correct JP 4

5. Knees knock on landing.

Jump Position 4 violation. Athlete lands jump with knees caving in. Emphasize to your athlete that the landing position is nothing other than the initial hinge of the squat: hips back and knees out. Remind him that "entering the movement tunnel" poorly means "exiting the tunnel" poorly.

 "Knees out!"

 Demonstrate a correct JP 4.

 Have your athlete freeze in his landing position (JP 4), place your hands where you want athlete's knees to go, and tell him, "Push into my hands!"

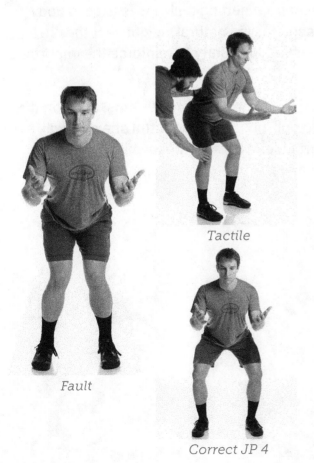

Tactile

Fault

Correct JP 4

PULL-UPS

Category: Pull to Object (strict, vertical)

Movement screen: N/a

Ability screen: Ring row x 10 (self- and band-assisted pull-ups), skinniest band-assisted pull-up x 10 (pull-up)

The pull-up involves hauling oneself, with an outside shoulder-width, pronated (palms away) grip, from a straight-armed hang, to a height at which one's chin is clearly above the bar. The pull-up requires the ability to flex and extend the elbows through a full ROM, externally rotate the arm at the shoulder, and maintain a neutral midline, not to mention a good deal of upper body pulling strength.

The chin-up is a pull-up with the palms supinated (facing in). Generally speaking, the hands will be closer together, about one foot apart, or whatever distance places the forearms at an angle perpendicular to the ground.

For many people, the limiting factor that keeps them from getting pull-ups is excess body weight; they might actually be able to do one, if it wasn't for the natural weight vest they're lugging around. I've always found the pull-up to be a useful opportunity to reinforce the importance of proper nutrition for success in MMGPP.

Harry is really excited for this. It's about time I let the Marine do some pull-ups! Amy, on the other hand, is intimidated. She'd very much like to do pull-ups, but is doubtful she ever will, even though she can do 5 piked ring rows without much trouble. We'll see! Meanwhile, Tim is perfectly content to keep working on his horizontal ring rows.

Pull-up Teaching Script

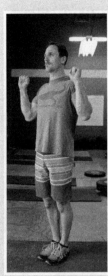
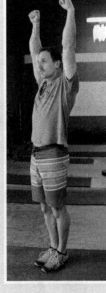
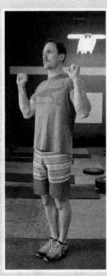

"Stand tall with feet together. Brace your midline by squeezing your butt and locking down your ribs. Pack your shoulders.

"Hold your fists just outside your shoulders. Push them straight up. That's how wide your grip should be on the bar. Curl your wrists slightly so that the knuckles of your little fingers are pointing at the ceiling.

"Take a deep breath and drive your elbows down until your hands are again outside the shoulders.

"Maintaining partial retraction and depression of your shoulder blades, straighten your arms again.

"This is the basic action of the pull-up."

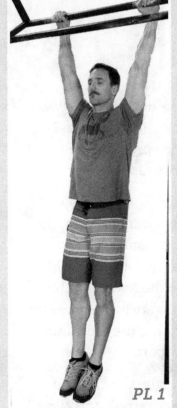
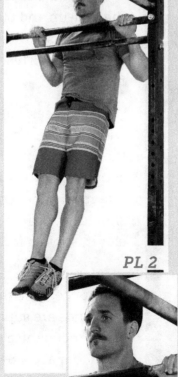

PL 1

PL 2

"Now we'll do it on the bar. Grasp the bar with a full, thumbs-around grip. ALWAYS thumbs around. This is for safety. Make sure your pinky knuckles point toward the ceiling. Squeeze your heels together and point your toes; keep your legs straight, midline braced, and shoulders active. This is **Pull-up Position 1 (PL 1).**

"Now drive the elbows down until your chin is clearly over the bar. This is **Pull-up Position 2 (PL 2).**

"Lower yourself back to PL 1.

Chin must clear the bar with neutral head position

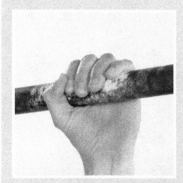

Eh, it's okay.

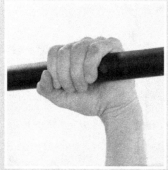

Legit!

"A little bit more about that grip: slightly 'goosenecking' the wrist so that the pinky knuckle is on top of the bar is what Dr. Kelly Starrett calls a 'pull-up hook grip.' It externally rotates the upper arm, which creates torque, and desirable stability, in the shoulder joint. This is a fine technical point, but it's the kind of thing that makes the difference between 'okay' and *'le git'*, which is French for, 'Actually cares about doing things correctly.'

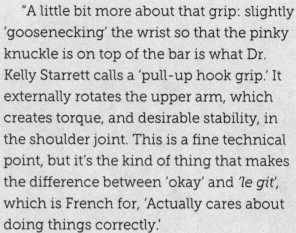
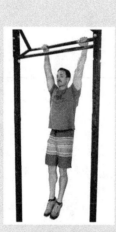

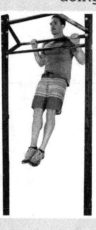
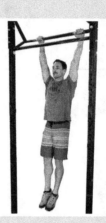

PL 1   PL 2   PL 1

"The most obvious difference between the pull-up and the chin-up is grip. The pull-up has the hands pronated, or palms facing away. The chin-up has your palms facing you.

"This necessitates a difference in grip width. For best mechanical advantage, at the top of the movement, the forearms should be vertical to the floor. For pull-ups, that means the hands are just outside the shoulders. Chin-ups require the hands be closer, about a foot apart.

"Many people find the the chin-up more accessible than the pull-up. When the hands are supinated, the biceps have a better mechanical moment arm, allowing them to make a better contribution to the movement, which makes chin-ups seem easier."

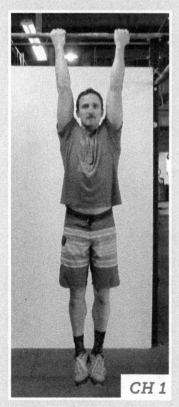

CH 1

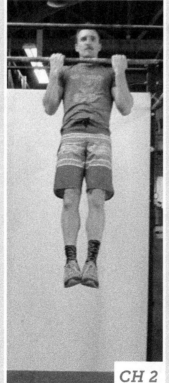

CH 2

Self-assisted pull-ups are an easy way for your trainees to begin working on the mechanics of the strict version of the movement. Unlike band-assisted pull-ups, the self-assisted pull-up offers no assistance out of the bottom position, where the primary challenge is generating enough force to overcome inertia and get moving.

However, they require very stable squat racks to be performed safely; not every gym will be equipped for them. If your gym is not, stick with the piked ring row.

"Set a barbell in a squat rack just below the height of your chin when you are standing. Take a pull-up or chin-up grip on the bar. Make sure you are positioned so you will be pulling the bar INTO the rack, and not AWAY. Squat down until your arms are straight. Feet may be together, or hip-width apart. This is **Self-Assisted Pull-up Position 1 (sPU 1)**.

"Using your arms only, pull yourself as high as you can. Then use your legs to help you get your chin cleanly over the bar. This is **Self-Assisted Pull-up Position 1 (sPU 2)**. Lower yourself to **sPU 1.**"

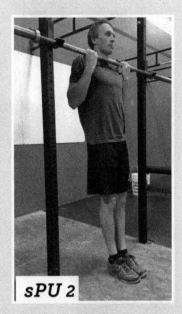

sPU 1   sPU 2

"If it's more comfortable, you can set your feet shoulder-width apart. And to to increase the challenge try lifting your toes so you are balanced on your heels, which can reduce the contribution of your legs."

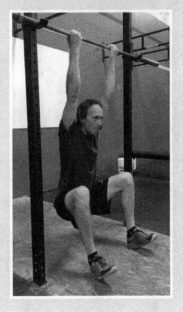
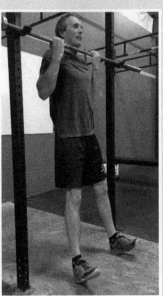

Using Assistance Bands for Pull-ups

! *NOTE: I like to teach the band-assisted pull-up after I've demonstrated and explained correct pull-up mechanics. You may prefer to teach assistance first, so no one feels left out—similar to how we used box squats before air squats. Either way, make sure your trainees understand all the points of performance for the pull-up before using assistance bands.*

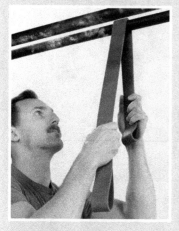
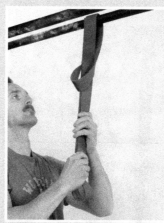

"Stand on a box tall enough to make getting in and out of the band relatively easy.

"Secure an assistance band by throwing it over the bar, and then pulling one end through the other.

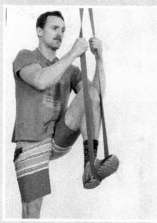
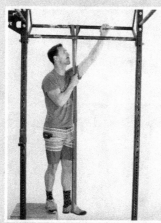

"Using the foot on the same side as the band, step into the band so that it comes across the center of the sole of the foot. Don't strain, and don't lean on the band as you stretch it—you may fall. Straighten the leg toward the ground. If the tension of the band makes straightening your leg difficult, use a thinner band. If that thinner band offers insufficient assistance, default back to piked ring rows.

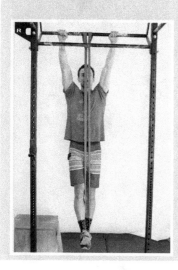
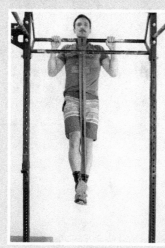

"Grip the bar securely and then step off the box, allowing your grip and the band to support your weight. Bring your feet together. The band should be centered on the chest. Pull your head back slightly but keep its position neutral. Execute pull-ups as instructed above."

"If your feet swing forward, so that you find yourself at an angle to the ground, squeeze your butt to get your feet back under you.

"When finished, step back on to the box with your free foot. Bend the knee of the banded leg, and withdraw the foot."

Assistance bands have their place, but it's important not to be overly reliant on them. Athletes should build strength for strict pull-ups through a combination of piked ring rows, jumping negatives, and band-assisted pull-ups. These various techniques can be employed during skills-based warm-ups, or on weighted pull-up strength days. Limit athletes to using assistance bands of 1" thickness or less. If they need more help than that, they don't need to be trying to do full pull-ups yet.

As far as metcon work goes: kipping on bands is absolutely *verboten*. However, I do allow those who have recently started doing kipping pull-ups (after earning the right by demonstrating 5 strict pull-ups), to finish workouts with band-assisted strict pull-ups when fatigue degrades the form of their kPL. (At that point, they're probably too tired to do many unassisted pull-ups.)

In your gym, you make the rules: just be aware that the assistance band can easily become a crutch that retards progress.

Pull-up Common Faults and Fixes

1. Midline breaks

Pull-up Position 1 violation. The athlete lifts his chest as his arms and back tire, basically attempting a ring row-style horizontal pull in mid-air. I'll expand the definition of this fault to include all attempts to gain some mechnical advantage, including bending at the knees, allowing the legs to sprawl out, and bicycling for elevation. Encourage your athlete to maintain a tight, efficient body position.

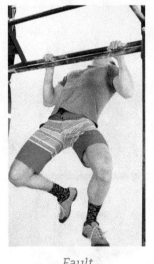

Fault

 "Hollow out!" or "Squeeze your glutes!" or "Feet together!" or "Long legs!" as appropriate.

 Demonstrate a correct transition from PL 1 to PL 2.

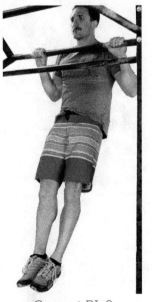

Correct PL 2

Pull-up Common Faults and Fixes, cont.

2. Chin fails to clear bar/athlete tilts head back to get chin over bar.

Pull-up Position 2 violation. At the top of the move-ment, the chin must be clearly over the bar for the rep to count—no reaching! The neck is part of the spine, and s/he shouldn't put needless strain on the cervical vertebrae in order to hit the standard.

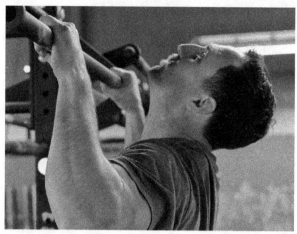

Fault

 If the fault results from insufficient effort, use "Pull harder!" or "Head neutral!" or "Chin over bar!" or "Drive elbows down!"

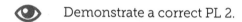 Demonstrate a correct PL 2.

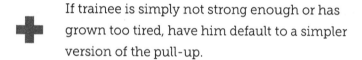 If trainee is simply not strong enough or has grown too tired, have him default to a simpler version of the pull-up.

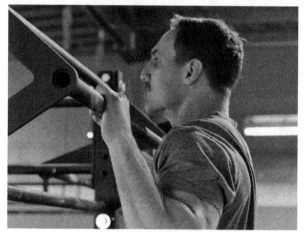

Correct PL 2

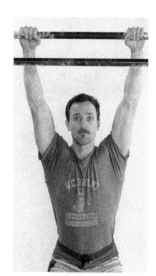

Fault

3. Arms fail to come to full extension.

Pull-up Position 1 violation. Elbows must be straight in PL 1.

 "Straight arms!"

 Demonstrate a correct PL 1.

 Grab on to athlete's legs and hang until his arms straighten.*

Correct PL 1

*Just kidding. Pants him instead. KIDDING!

Category: Push Object (vertical)

Movement screen: N/a

Ability screen: N/a

Being able to lift a heavy load from shoulder to overhead, or lower a load from arm's length overhead to the shoulders and chest, is a life skill. Think of shoving a carry-on bag into the overhead compartment of an aircraft, or pulling down a box of books from a closet shelf. The barbell press will teach your trainee how to organize his body into the positions that allow him to accomplish these actions safely and efficiently, and will greatly increase his overall pushing strength.

To press a barbell into proper position, the athlete must have full flexion of his shoulders, with the ability to maintain external rotation of the arms at the shoulder from initial position to finish. For those with limited range of motion, the barbell might not be the best implement with which to press; substitute dumbbells or kettlebells instead. You'll be able to suss out who needs a workaround during initial instruction with the PVC pipe.

With her flexibility and physical intelligence, I expect Amy will easily pick up the press. Harry and Tim both have shoulder flexibility issues, so time will tell if they get to work with the barbell

Press Teaching Script

"Stand with your feet under your hips, about 6-9" apart. Place a 5' length of PVC pipe on your traps, just below the nape of your neck. With a grip just outside shoulder-width, push the bar straight up to arms' length. 'Push up' through the shoulder blades, but don't actively shrug your shoulders up toward your ears. 'Snap' the bar in half by rotating your thumbs back. Brace your midline by locking in your glutes and abs. This is **Press Position 3 (PR 3),** overhead support, the finish position of the press.

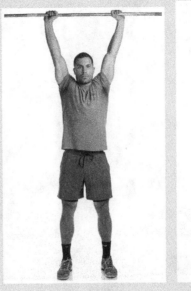
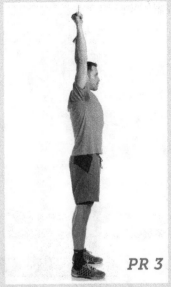

PR 3

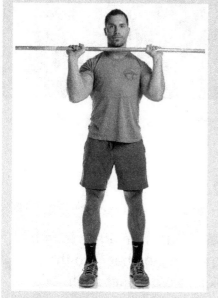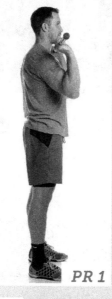

PR 1

"Now pull the bar down to your chest, just below your clavicles. Cant your elbows slightly in front of the bar. Make sure it's in your fists, across the center of your palms, and keep trying to 'snap' it in half, which in this position will draw your elbows in toward your ribs. Lock your midline, and screw your feet into the floor. This is **Press Position 1 (PR 1),** your start position.

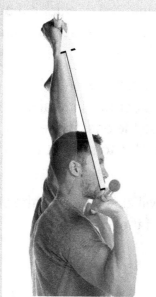

"As we've discussed before, we want to move this load as efficiently as possible. Right now, what's preventing this bar from traveling from **PR 1** to **PR 3** in a straight line? That's right—my face.

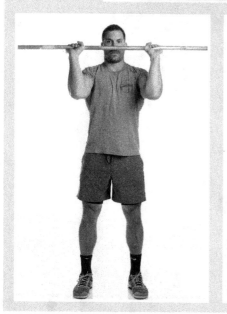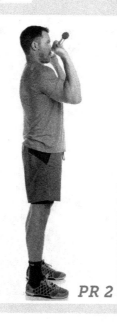

PR 2

"Pull your head back, giving yourself a sexy-looking double-chin. Push the pipe straight up so it's just in front of the tip of your nose. This is **Press Position 2 (PR 2).**

"Lower the bar to **PR 1**, allowing your head to return to neutral position. Practice this transition several times.

Positional Drills

"1! 2! 1!" Practice the transition from **PR 1** to **PR 2** and back. Make sure your athletes are pulling back their heads so that the bar rises in a straight line. Make sure that when the bar comes back to the starting position, the elbows are once again slightly in front of the bar.

"When you have a good feel for this, continue on from **PR 2** to lock out in **PR 3**. As the bar comes overhead, pull back until it lines up over the front of the heel (which, you'll remember, puts it in the line of gravity). Do NOT thrust your head forward. From its retracted position in **PR 2** your head should simply return to a neutral placement.

"Remember, in **PR 3** your shoulders should be externally rotated, the points of the elbows visible from the front. Then, as you return the bar to start position, keep trying to 'snap' it in half. This winds the lats back into tension as you return to **PR 1**."

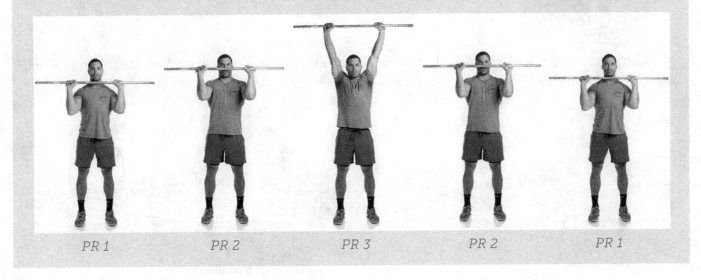

PR 1   PR 2   PR 3   PR 2   PR 1

Positional Drills

"1! 2! 3! 2! 1!" Drill the three poses of the press, making corrections as necessary at each position.

Setting Up for the Press

"As with the back squat, when setting up for the press it's imperative to create as much tension in the body as you can. In the process described below, as each body part is set in tension, it stays in tension, until the lift is completed. Don't slack!

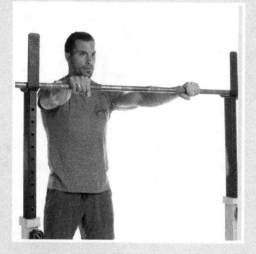

"With the barbell at upper chest-height in the squat rack, take a full-fist grip about half-a-thumb's distance out of the edge of the gnurling. Adjust as necessary so that your forearms are vertical in **PR 1.**

"With arms extended, 'snap' the bar in half by rotating your thumbs toward the ceiling. Walk in until your chest is almost touching the bar.

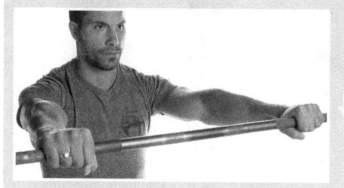
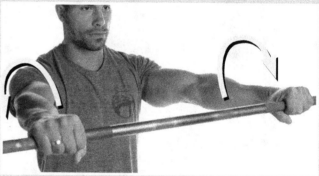

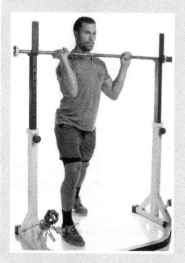
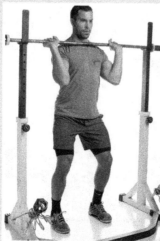

"Gripping the bar tightly, step forward and out with the right foot. Simultaneously, rotate the right elbow around and slightly in front of the bar. Imagine you are cranking your lat into tension, like winding up a clock.

"Repeat the process on the left side.

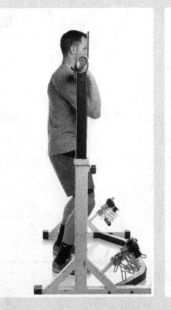
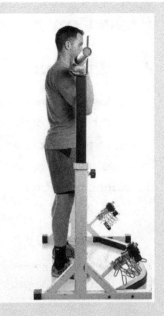

"Wedge your chest and shoulders up into the bar, 'hollow out' by bracing the midline, and then stand the bar up out of the rack.

"Take two steps back to clear the rack. IMPORTANT: don't relax your grip or drop your elbows as you take the bar out of the rack!

"You are in now in **PR 1**. Rapidly run your checklist (butt tight, abs locked down, feet screwed in), take a big breath, and go.

"Pro-tip: when doing multi-rep sets, when you are in **PR 3** of your first rep, exchange your breath, and on the next rep, touch-and-go at the bottom, pausing again at the top to rebreathe. This is more efficient than than letting the bar come to rest, rebreathing, and then having to overcome inertia to get it moving again."

Press Common Faults and Fixes

1. Bad set-up (low elbows).

Press Position 1 violation. Elbows must be slightly in front of bar, with forearms roughly pointing to bar's destination in PR 3.

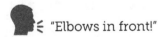 "Elbows in front!"

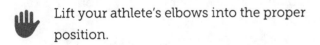 Demonstrate proper PR 1 elbow position.

Lift your athlete's elbows into the proper position.

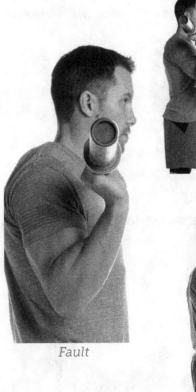

Tactile

Fault

Correct PR 1

Press Common Faults and Fixes, cont.

2. Bad rack position.

Press Position 1 violation. The bar must be held across the center of the palm, not back in the crooks of the fingers. If your athlete is unable to hold the bar in his palms and still get his elbows in front of the bar, consider using dumbbells instead.

 "Full fist grip!"

 Demonstrate proper PR 1 elbow position.

 Wrap athlete's fingers around the bar and adjust elbow position as necessary.

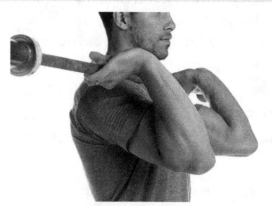

Fault

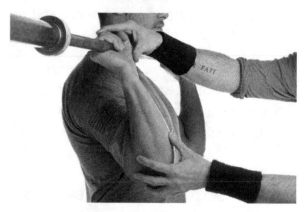

Tactile

3. Elbows flare out.

Press Position 2 violation. As the athlete presses up, his elbows twist out to the side. Elbow flare means the shoulders are internally rotating, which can lead to impingement, pain, and injury. The trainee must train to create torque to keep his shoulders in the best position.

 "Break bar in half!"

 Demonstrate proper transition from PR 2 to PR 3.

 A skinny band doubled-up and looped around trainee's arms below the elbows will teach him to keep his elbows in. Remind athlete to strongly retract his head as bar passes through PR 2 if he doesn't want his nose tweaked by the band.

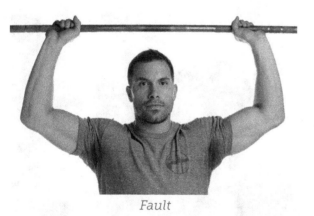

Fault

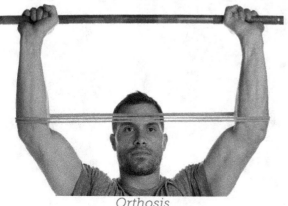

Orthosis

202

Press Common Faults and Fixes, cont.

4. Bar path not straight.

Press Position 2 violation. The bar must travel as straight as possible from start to finish positions. If your athlete doesn't pull his head back, he'll inevitably push the bar out around his face.

 "Sexy double chin!" or "Brush your nose!"

 Demonstrate proper transition from PR 1 to PR 2.

With your trainee in PR 1, stand with your palms directly in front of the bar. If the athlete ties to push the bar out, your hands will stop the bar's movement. The athlete will usually quickly make the necessary adjustments so that the bar can rise without hitting your hands.

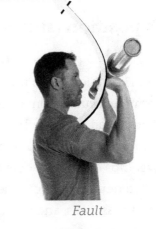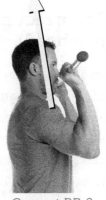

Fault *Correct PR 2*

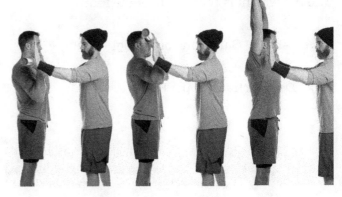

Tactile

5. Bar finishes out in front.

Press Position 3 violation. The bar must finish its travel in the frontal plane, or lined up over the front of the heel.

 "Pull back on the bar!" (Make sure trainee keeps abs engaged so he doesn't then execute an "arching back" fault [#8].)

 Demonstrate proper PR 3.

 With your trainee holding in PR 3, manually adjust bar into the correct overhead position.

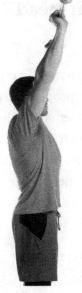

Fault

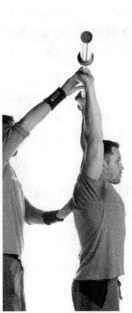

Tactile

Press Common Faults and Fixes, cont.

6. Incorrect finish position (ship's figurehead).

Press Position 3 violation. The athlete leans forward under the barbell, forming a curve from heels to hands, rather like the figurehead of a ship. Instead, the body should be locked straight, with hands stacked over shoulders over hips over knees over the front of the heels. To regain a neutral position, the athlete must engage the glutes and abs, and make sure the weight is centered over the foot.

 "Abs on! Glutes on!" or "Straight line!"

 Demonstrate proper PR 3.

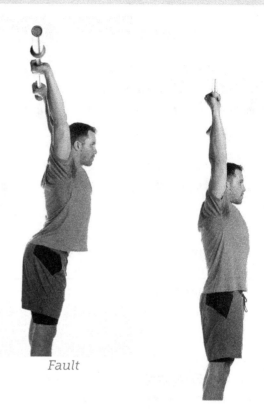

Fault

Correct PR 3

7. Incorrect finish position (head forward).

Press Position 3 violation. "Head through!" is a common cue meant to get the bar into the proper finish position, but often causes the athlete to snap his head forward and chin down. Instead, in the transition from PR 2 to PR 3, encourage the athlete to pull the bar back until it is over the front of the heel, as he returns his head and neck to a neutral position.

 "Pull back!" as bar comes overhead or "Head up!"

 Demonstrate proper transition from PR 2 to PR 3.

Fault

Correct PR 3

Press Common Faults and Fixes, cont.

8. Arching back.

Press Position 3 violation. Athlete leans back to get the bar into the line of gravity, breaking the midline, compressing his lower back. Cues and adjustment may fix this, but often the athlete is compensating for a lack of adequate shoulder flexion—which will probably take time and extracurricular mobility work to fix.

 "Abs on!" or "Six pack!"

 Demonstrate proper PR 3.

 A tap on the abs can get the trainee to pull his ribs down and return to a neutral midline.

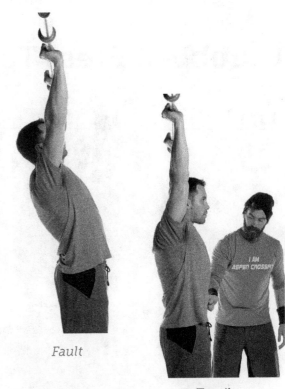

Fault

Tactile

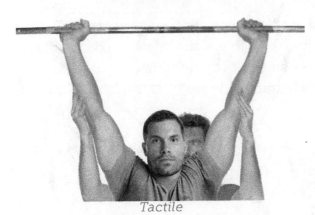

Fault

Tactile

9. Internally rotated overhead position.

Press Position 3 violation. When bar is held overhead, elbows are point out and back, rather than forward. For best stability, the athlete should continue to twist his hands into the bar, right hand clockwise, left hand counter-clockwise, as if he might snap it in half.

 "Snap the bar in half!" or "Armpits forward!"

 Demonstrate proper PR 3.

 As the athlete holds the bar in overhead support, grasp his arms above the elbows and gently rotate them into proper position.

Some trainees will lack the flexibility to get in a good set-up position for the barbell press, and/or to finish in a correct overhead support position. Rather than force these trainees into positions they may never be able to achieve (especially if they are middle-aged or older), teach them to use dumbbells to achieve the same training stimulus.

Dumbbell Press Teaching Script

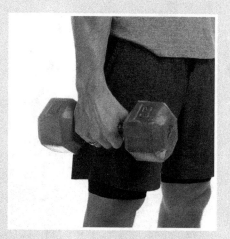

"Hold the dumbbell with the karate-chop knife edge of your hand against one head of the 'bell.

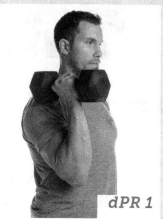

dPR 1

"Rack one end of the dumbbell on your shoulder with your forearm vertical and your elbow tucked in against your ribs. This is **Dumbbell Press Position 1 (dPR 1)**. *(Note: can also be performed with two dumbbells.)*

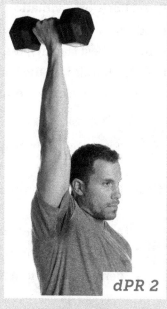

dPR 2

"Press the dumbbell straight up, maintaining external rotation on the arm. Do not pronate. Keep the dumbbells within the 'cylinder' of your body—that is, don't let it move laterally past your shoulder. Do your best to pull the dumbbell back until it is lined up over the front of your heel. This is **Dumbbell Press Position 2 (dPR 2).**

"Rack the dumbbell in **dPR 1** by pulling your elbow down and in tight to your ribs."

JUMPING PULL-UPS

Category: Hybrid (jump and land, pull to object [vertical, strict])

Movement screen: N/a

Ability screen: Static hang x 10 sec, jumping mechanics x 5

As a rapid full body up-and-down movement, the jumping pull-up can be a taxing conditioning tool. It should be noted that at high reps, the jumping pull-up has been cited as one possible cause of rhabdomyolysis, a relatively rare but still very dangerous condition in which muscles break down and spill their contents into the bloodstream. Use judiciously!

As a slow, controlled movement with a strong eccentric component, the jumping pull-up can help build strength for those working toward a strict pull-up. Those athletes will use jumping pull-ups with timed negatives on strength days, when more advanced athletes are doing weighted pull-ups. Be careful! Slow negatives are very potent, and can cause extreme soreness. Don't prescribe more than 25 reps (five sets of 5), and then only on days that include no other pulling movements, such as rowing or muscle cleans.

Tim's making great progress! He's ready to join Harry and Amy for this one.

Jumping Pull-up Teaching Script

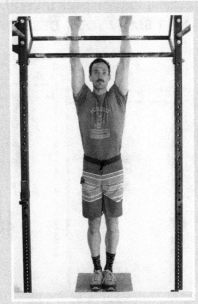

To use the jumping pull-ups for conditioning:

"Set up under the pull-up bar on a box, the height of which has the bar touching your forearm, about 2/3 of the way up from your elbow, when you hold your hands straight overhead.

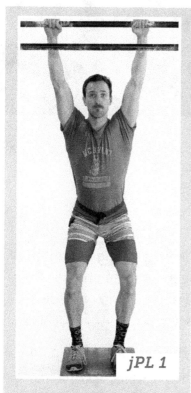

jPL 1

"Grasp the bar in a normal pull-up grip: thumbs around, hands outside your shoulders. With your shoulders actively locked down, squat until your elbows are straight. Heels should be hip-width, hips back and down. This is your starting position, **Jumping Pull-up Position 1 (jPL 1).**

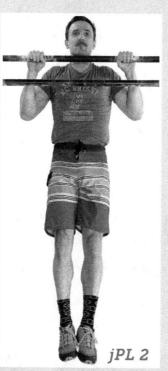

jPL 2

"Jump from the heels and then pull with your arms until your chin has cleared the bar. Your legs will be straight beneath you. This is your finish position, **Jumping Pull-up Position 2 (jPL 2).**

"Allow yourself to drop back into **jPL 1** without slowing your descent with your arms. I repeat: **DO NOT SLOW YOUR DESCENT**. Then immediately rebound into **jPL 2**. Cycle as required."

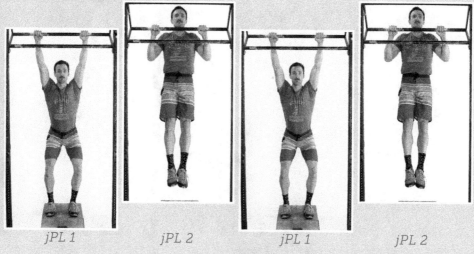

jPL 1   jPL 2   jPL 1   jPL 2

To use the jumping pull-up to build strength:

"Grasp the bar in a normal pull-up grip: thumbs around, hands outside your shoulders. With your shoulders actively locked down, squat until your elbows are straight. Heels should be hip-width, hips back and down. This is **Jumping Pull-up for Strength Position 1 (jPLs 1).**

"Bands offer the most assistance at the bottom position, so it's often the last part of the movement to get strong. We'll start this version of the jumping pull-up with an isometric pull to improve your starting strength.

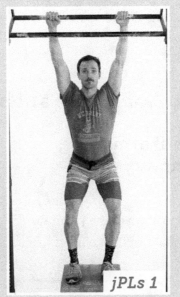

jPLs 1

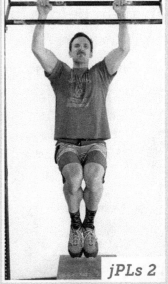

jPLs 2

"Pick your feet up off the box and pull as hard as you can for 1 second (count *'One-one-thousand!'*). Assuming you lack the strength to do a strict pull-up, your elbows will flex, and your shoulders may adduct a little, but not much more will happen. This is **Jumping Pull-up for Strength Position 2 (jPLs).**

"Reset yourself in **jPLs 1**, then immediately jump from your heels . Pull until your chin has cleared the bar. Legs will be straight beneath you. This is **Jumping Pull-up for Strength Position 3—jPLs 3.**

"Hold this position for one second (if possible), then take 3 full seconds to lower until you are in a straight-arm hang (**jPLs 3.4**). Count them out—and be honest! Then reset in **jPLs 1.** You can also try working a 90 degree bent arm static hang. Mix it up and experiment."

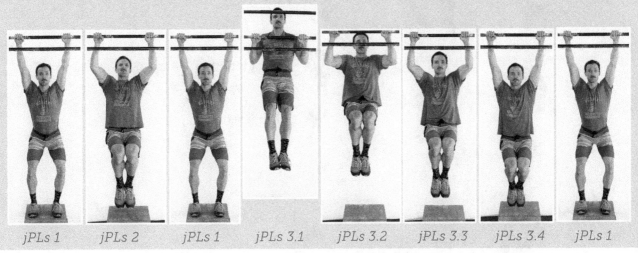

| jPLs 1 | jPLs 2 | jPLs 1 | jPLs 3.1 | jPLs 3.2 | jPLs 3.3 | jPLs 3.4 | jPLs 1 |

DO NOT allow athletes to do slow negatives for high reps! Excess volume will make them debilitatingly sore. Three to five sets of five reps is plenty for a day's training.

Jumping Pull-up Common Faults and Fixes

1. Not squatting until arms are straight before jumping.

jPL 1 violation. In the first position of the jumping pull-up, the athlete must squat until the elbows are straight.

 "Straight arms!" or "Squat lower!"

 Demonstrate a correct jPL 1.

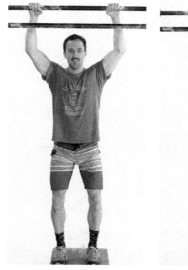
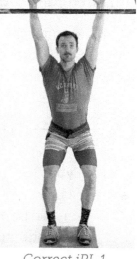

Fault   *Correct jPL 1*

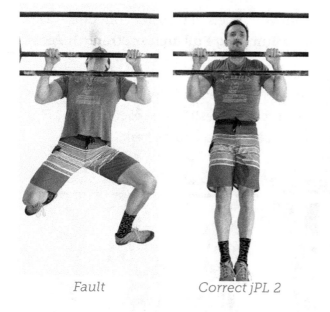

Fault   *Correct jPL 2*

2. Vertical sprawl.

Jumping Pull-up Position 2 violation. Athlete fails to reach the top position of the jumping pull-up in an organized fashion—midline breaks, feet flail about, etc. This will make it more difficult to land in a well-organized jPL 1.

 "Feet together!" "Abs on!" "Neutral chin!" etc.

 Demonstrate a proper jPL 2.

DOUBLE-UNDERS

Category: Monostructural (jump rope)

Movement screen: N/a

Ability screen: Jumping mechanics x 5

Double-unders, a jump rope sprint in which the rope passes under the feet twice on every hop, develop stamina, endurance, coordination, balance, and timing. However, achieving consistent double-unders often takes a LOT of practice and can be frustrating for new trainees, so from the start, assure them that being able to do double-unders is really fun, and the weeks and maybe months of practice will be worth it.

If an athlete is physically capable of jumping rope, there is no scale or substitute for double-unders. No number of single bounces will get an athlete double-unders...only trying and failing, trying and failing, until success is achieved.

Tim has started to get the hang of jumping-and-landing, so I'm going to let him try to learn to skip rope. Athletic prowess is not a guarantee of double-under success, we'll see how Harry and Amy do...

Double-unders Teaching Script

"When learning double-unders, it's better to work with a plastic or vinyl rope than a wire rope. Wire ropes are lighter, which make them faster, but a little more difficult to learn with.

"It's important to you select a rope that's the correct height. Pick up a rope, step one foot in the center, and hold the handles up by your armpit. The top of the handles should reach the top of your shoulder.

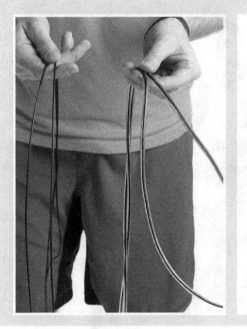
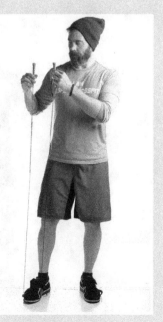

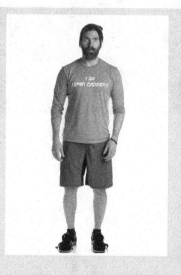

"We'll start with the basic bounce. Set your feet hip-width, then stand tall. Brace your midline, pack your sholders. Get up on the balls of your feet.

"Execute a little jump, 1-2" off the floor. Land on the balls of your feet, pushing your knees out. Rebound by pushing off the ground with your knees and ankles. Keep your midline stable. Do ten without stopping.

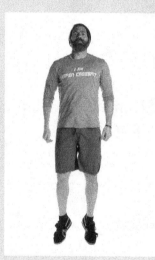
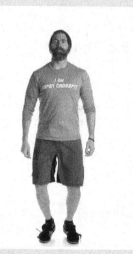
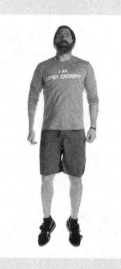
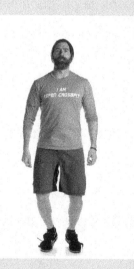

DU 1

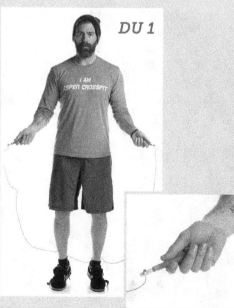

"Okay, pick up your rope. Brace your midline. Keep your elbows against your sides, and hold the rope with your thumbs pointing down and aligned along the handles of the rope. Once again bring your feet under your hips. Stand up on the balls of your feet, but keep your knees soft. This is **Double-under Position 1 (DU 1).**

"Lift the rope so that it hangs somewhere between the back of your knees and your ankles.

"When I say 'GO!', swing the rope around vigorously and execute a two-footed hop over it. Listen for the *thwack* of the rope on the ground—that's your signal to jump. Ready...go!

"If you successfully skipped the rope, now try to get five in a row. When you get twenty in a row, you're ready to try for a double-under.

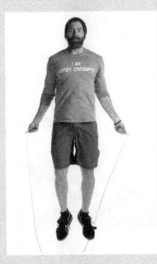 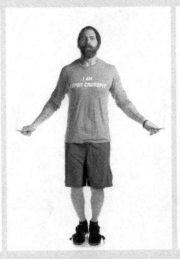 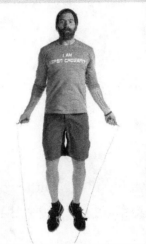 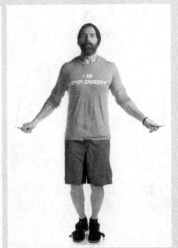

"If your basic bounce looks like this (*demonstrate basic bounce*)...

"Your double-under looks like this—that is, the same as your basic bounce, but with twice as much altitude (3-4"). This is necessary to create sufficient hang time so the rope can get around twice on one jump. In the air, you're in **Double-under Position 2 (DU 2).**

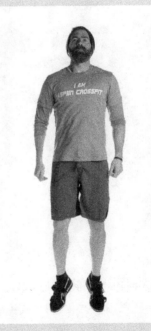 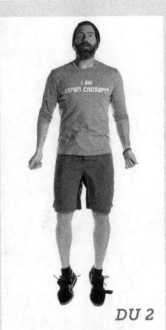

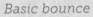

DU 2

Basic bounce   Super bounce

"Call it a super bounce. Notice that nothing about my body position changed. I didn't start pulling my knees high, I didn't start kicking my feet back. And I avoided the dreaded pike at the hips, also known as 'the flipper.' I simply pushed off a little harder with my ankles.

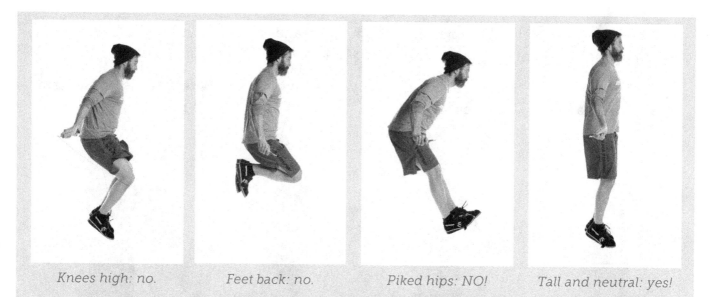

Knees high: no. *Feet back: no.* *Piked hips: NO!* *Tall and neutral: yes!*

"As I jump, I find it helpful to make a little sound effect to myself to help illustrate how long I need to be in the air to successfully double-under, like this: *BOING! BOING! BOING!* Try it!

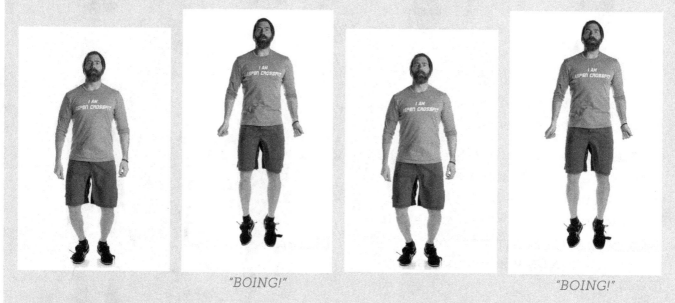

"BOING!" *"BOING!"*

"The action of the double-under comes from the wrist. Pretend to hold a fork in your right hand and mime whisking an egg, rotating your hand counter-clockwise—that'll give you the general idea.

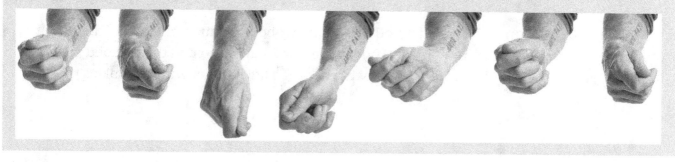

"Hold a second imaginary fork in your left hand and whisk clockwise at the same time to get a feel for the double-under rope spin—two small sharp circles from the wrist to get the rope whistling around: *tsch tsch, tsch tsch*. If you marry this with the super bounce, it's like this: *BOING tsch tsch BOING tsch tsch*. The sound effects begin a split second after you leave the ground. First let's try it without the rope. Get in **DU 1.** One my go, do five basic bounces, and then five super bounces. As you super bounce, flick your wrists, visualizing yourself spinning the rope around you twice for every super bounce. *BOING tsch tsch BOING tsch tsch* etc.

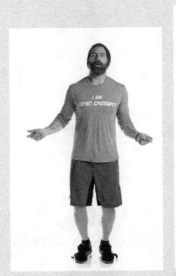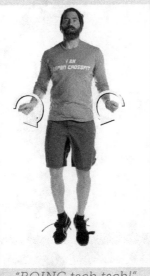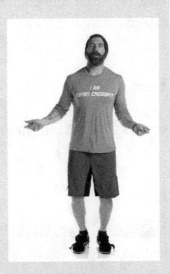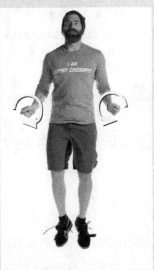

"BOING tsch tsch!"   *"BOING tsch tsch!"*

"Now let's try it with the rope. Execute three single-unders and then one super bounce with a double-under. If you miss, try again. If you manage it, then go for two double-unders in a row. If you get two, go for ten. Stay relaxed. STAY RELAXED, DAMMIT!"

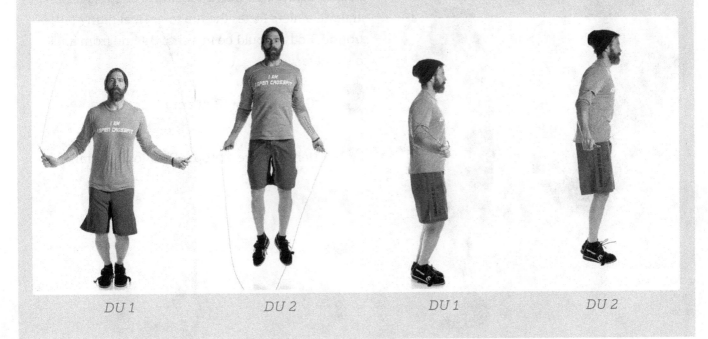

DU 1   DU 2   DU 1   DU 2

Double-unders Common Faults and Fixes

1. Kicking back or knees high.

Double-under Position 2 violation. Kicking back and pulling the knees high have the same effect: even if the athlete gets the rope around twice, the athlete will land too hard and never get off the ground in time for the next rep. Remind him to stand tall and bounce from the balls of the feet, to land lightly and immediately rebound.

 "Stay tall!" or "Long body!"

 Demonstrate a correct DU 1 to DU 2 transition.

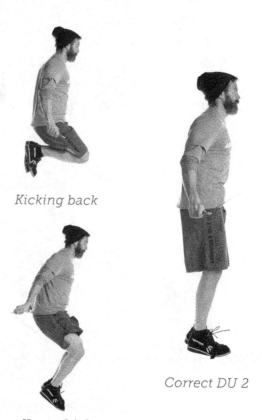

Kicking back

Knees high

Correct DU 2

2. Piking.

Double-under Position 2 violation. Keeping legs straight, athlete flexes the hip to get feet high off the ground. Body should be in a straight line from ankle to shoulder.

 "Glutes on!" or "Butt tight!"

 Demonstrate a proper DU 1 to DU 2 transition.

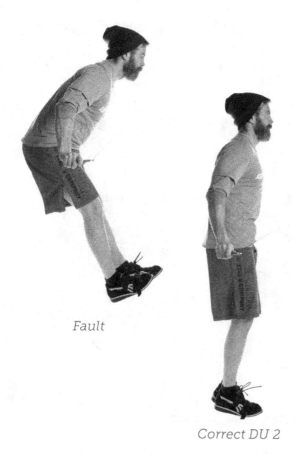

Fault

Correct DU 2

Double-unders Common Faults and Fixes, cont.

3. Shot in the back (midline breaks).

Double-under Position 2 violation. Trainee arches his back, surrendering midline stability.

 "Abs on!" or "Six pack!" or "Tall and neutral!"

 Demonstrate a correct DU 1 to DU 2 transition.

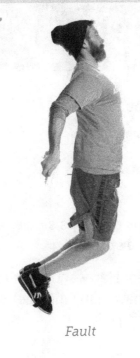

Fault

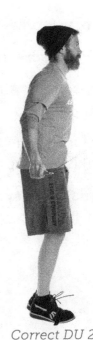

Correct DU 2

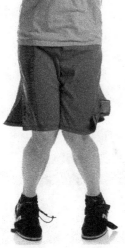

Fault

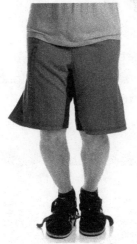

Correct DU 2

4. Knees cave in on landing.

Double-under Position 1 violation. Knees knock on landing. Explain to your athlete that he must keep his glutes actively engaged to externally rotate the femurs, and defeat the tendency to commit a valgus fault.

 "Glutes on!" or "Butt tight!"

 Demonstrate a proper DU 1 to DU 2 transition.

FORWARD LUNGES

Category: Single-leg Squat

Movement screen: Samson stretch

Ability screen: Air squat x 5

The forward lunge helps develops single-leg strength and teaches a position fundamental to the Turkish get-up and the split jerk.

This is still easy stuff for Harry and Amy. I'm going to let Tim try it, but I'll keep a careful eye on him. If need be, I can have him lunge between two boxes, in case he needs some help with balance.

Forward Lunge Teaching Script

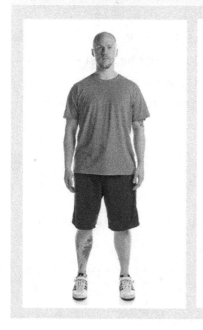 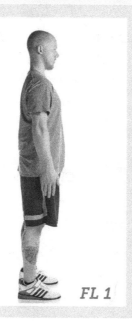

FL 1

"Begin by standing with feet hip-width, feet screwed in to the deck, midline braced, shoulders packed. This is **Forward Lunge Position 1 (FL 1).**

"Keeping your torso vertical, step one foot forward and slightly out. At this point, your feet are shoulder-width apart. Lower yourself until the knee of the rear leg 'kisses' the ground. The forward step should be long enough that when the trailing knee makes contact, the knee of the leading leg lines up over its ankle. This is **Forward Lunge Position 2 (FL 2).**

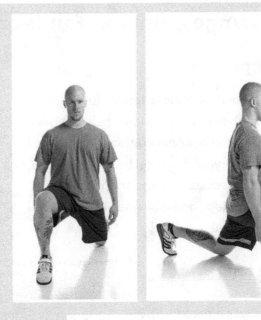

"The rear leg should be up on the ball of the foot, with the heel kicked out. (This is similar to the rotation of the rear leg at the finish of a baseball bat swing.) This slightly internally rotated position will keep the hips 'squared' in the direction of travel, making the whole position more stable.

"Next, simultaneously pushing off the rear toe and down through the front heel, and without pressing on the legs with the hands, step up and forward so that the rear foot lines up with the forward foot, again with a hip-width stance. You've returned to **FL 1.**"

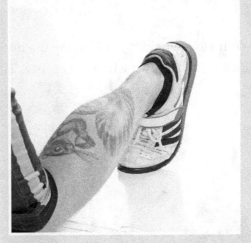

If you've swung a baseball bat, you know how to kick out your heel.

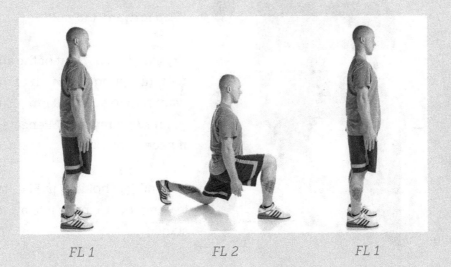

FL 1   *FL 2*   *FL 1*

Forward Lunge Common Faults and Fixes

1. Short steps.

Forward Lunge Position 1 violation. Failing to step forward far enough results in the knee being shoved ahead of the toe in the bottom position. This is undesirable for the same reason we don't want to see it in a squat—it puts unnecessary stress on the knee. The knee of the forward leg should be lined up over the ankle, the shin vertical.

 "Longer step!"

 Demonstrate a correct FL 2.

 With athlete holding in FL 2, tap the heel of the leading foot to move it to the proper distance.

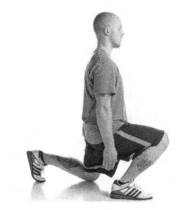

Fault

Tactile

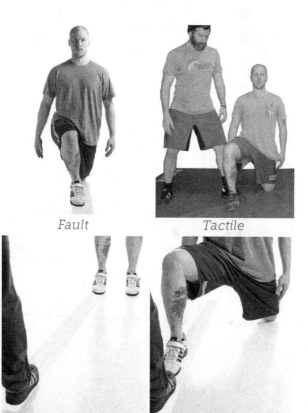

Fault *Tactile*

Correct FL 2 w/ visual referrent

2. Tightrope walking

Forward Lunge Position 2 violation. If the athlete steps in rather than out, he draws his feet into a single line, robbing himself of lateral stability.

 "Step forward and out!"

 Try standing in front of the athlete with one foot indicating the width of the stride you want him to take. Tell him, "Step forward and in line with my foot." Repeat for the other side if necessary.

 With athlete holding in FL 2, tap the heel of the leading foot to move it to a shoulder-width stance.

Walking Lunge Common Faults and Fixes, cont.

3. Torso lean.

Forward Lunge Position 2 violation. Athlete tilts forward, breaking the neutral midline rule. Upper body should be kept vertical.

 "Torso vertical!" or "Chest up!"

 Demonstrate a correct FL 2.

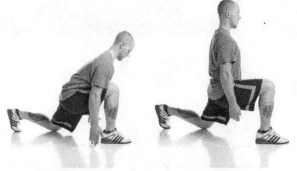

Fault   *Correct FL 2*

4. Pushing on legs with hands.

Forward Lunge Position 2 to Position 1 transition violation. Tired athletes will attempt to assist their lunge return by pushing on their thighs. NO REP!

 "No hands!"

 Demonstrate a proper FL 2.

Fault   *Correct FL 2*

5. Incomplete knee and hip extension.

Forward Lunge Position 1 violation. Athlete "sloshes" forward without coming to a full stand. For best training effect and for the rep to count, knees and hips must completely extend between steps.

 "Stand up!"

 Demonstrate a correct FL 1.

 Hold your hand at the athlete's approximate height and encourage him to hit it with the top of his head as he passes though FL 1.

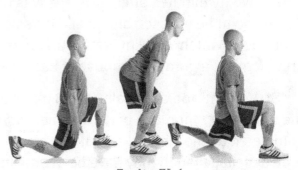

Faulty FL 1

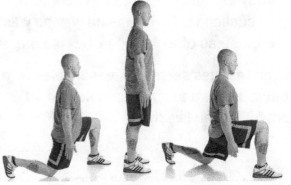

Correct FL 1

"ST. VINCENT"

For our second benchmark workout, I've chosen "St. Vincent". "St. Vincent" is composed of two movements, double-unders and sit-ups, in a descending ladder of reps: 49, 39, 29, 19, 9.

If you have double-unders, "St. Vincent" is hard, fast fun requiring seven minutes or less to complete. If you don't have double-unders, well...

This is one of those "learn from my mistakes" stories. Back in 2008, when my first gym had been open for just a few months, "St. Desiree Nosbusch Vincent" came up in my programming for the first time. One of my clients, Mike, had recently gotten the knack of double-unders, and was particularly excited when he saw the WOD on the whiteboard; this would be the first workout he'd be able to perform as prescribed.

But twenty minutes after "GO!", he was only halfway through his set of thirty double-unders. By this point he was screaming and cursing on every missed rep. It was both excruciating and hilarious to watch, and I'm pretty sure there's still a black cloud of obscenities hanging over our first location, a grimy warehouse in Easthampton, MA.

"St. Vincent" took Mike almost 28 minutes. (Again, this was 2008, "Death before DNF!" was the rallying cry for many of us, and *mea culpa*.) I knew something wasn't right about that. He'd completed all the work, sure, but this workout was supposed to be *intense*. Half an hour of jump rope self-flagellation may have been grueling, but it was hardly intense.

A guy like Mike took the 145 double-unders and sit-ups written on the whiteboard as a personal challenge. There was no way he was going to quit until he was done. But what if, I wondered, instead of a challenge, he was presented with a test? One with a time limit?

Ten minutes seemed a reasonable cut-off. Based on that, I figured a logical way to schedule double-under and sit-up couplets of 49, 39, 29, 19, and 9 reps. Next time I programmed "St. Vincent," it looked like this:

"By the Numbers Testing 'St. Vincent'"

AMRAP :90 double-under attempts. If you get 49 successful double-unders before time is up, move on to...
AMRAP :90 sit-ups. If you get 49 before time is up, move on to...
AMRAP :75 of double-under attempts. If you get 39 before time is up, move on to...
AMRAP :75 sit-ups. If you get 39 before time is up, move on to...
AMRAP :60 double-under attempts. If you get 29 before time is up, move on to...
AMRAP :60 sit-ups. If you get 29 before time is up, move on to...
AMRAP :45 double-under attempts. If you get 19 before time is up, move on to...
AMRAP :45 sit-ups. If you get 19 before time is up, move on to...
AMRAP :30 double-under attempts. If you get 9 before time is up, move on to...
AMRAP :30 sit-ups. If you get 9 before time is up, you're done.

If an athlete completes the work assigned within an interval, he immediately moves on to the next exercise. If not, when the instructor calls "SWITCH!", the athlete writes down how many reps he did get, and then advances. If he finishes before time is up, he records his time to completion. If not, he writes down total double-unders/total sit-ups, with an eye to beating those numbers the next time "St. Vincent" pays a visit.

No matter what happens, the whole ordeal is over in ten minutes. I'll never again have to behold the horror of a half-hour "St. Vincent"!

CUSTOMIZING "ST. VINCENT" FOR ATHLETES OF VARYING ABILITY LEVELS

Some people get double-unders almost immediately. Most, though, struggle with them for a long time. Weeks, months, or even a year or two. Amy is one of those people who gets a double-under on her first attempt, and before that first session was over she was getting 10 in a row. Harry, much to his disgust, is still only able to string together 2 or 3 at a time.

Both athletes will be well-served by our time-delimited approach to "St. Vincent". My prediction is that Amy will actually complete the WOD before time is up and be able to record an "as Rx'd" score. If "St. Vincent" started with sit-ups, then Harry might have a shot at finishing, too, because he'll knock them out so quickly he'd have an extra 30 seconds or more to use for double-unders. But alas, the WOD starts with double-unders.

Tim has never skipped rope before, not even as a kid. Just jumping and landing safely and efficiently is a challenge for him. So although it's not part of the "official" movement hierarchy, I have him practice jumping up and down while spinning the rope with one hand held out to the side. He's going to practice timing his jump to the crack of the rope on the ground. When he gets that down, he can graduate to attempting single skips.

As far as his sit-ups go, speed is not of the essence for Tim, so today I assign him butterfly sit-ups. I decide to cap the volume, too, just to err on the side of caution. His version of "St. Vincent" will have him practicing his rope skips when the others are doing double-unders, and he'll do 20 sit-ups during his first effort, 16 in the second, 12 for the third, 8 for the fourth, and 4 for the fifth. If he finishes his sit-ups before time is up, he's to rest until it's time to jump rope again.

"3...2...1...GO!"

Harry

Harry, as fit as he his, struggled with this one. Doing a combination of singles, double-unders, and missed attempts at double-unders, at 1:28 into the workout he had managed to complete 31 DUs. At 1:29 the call came to "Switch!" He wrote down his score, and proceeded to crank out 49 to-standard sit-ups in 40 seconds. When he stood and picked up his rope, he had the remaining time allotted to sit-ups (about 50 seconds) plus the next double-under section (75 seconds) to get 39 double-unders. This time, in spite of an aggravating series of missed attempts, he got 33 double-unders. At 2:45 he began his second set of sit-ups. After that, he got all of his double-unders. As sit-ups were never the problem, it's unsurprising that his final score was 104/145.

Amy

Amy, despite having just learned double-unders at our last class, managed to get all 49 DUs in the first 90 seconds of the workout. She got all her sit-ups, too, although it took most of the allotted time. From there, even though her sit-ups continued to be slow, she was able to use the extra time from every double-under set to get her reps in. In the end, she got the only Rx'd "St. Vincent" time of the group: 8:15. Impressive!

Tim

After his first couple of sets of jumping practice, I told Tim to switch to trying to get some jump rope singles. And he did! In his last 30 seconds on the rope he even got 5 singles in a row. On the sit-up front, he had a little more trouble. Even with the constrained volume, by the time he got to his third round of sit-ups—the set of 12—he was slowly down and having trouble completing reps. I did want him to get in at least 50 sit-ups today, so I tied a 1/2" band to the pull-up bar and handed him the loose end. As he sat back, tension was put on the band that aided him in the concentric part of the movement. That way he was able to keep moving continuously for the entire10 minutes. By the end he was pouring sweat and breathing hard, but definitely happy! Especially when I promised him that next time he'd be allowed to do as many sit-ups as he could.

FRONT SQUATS

Category: Squat

Movement screen: Elbows-up wall squat test

Ability screen: Back squat x 5

The front squat is an air squat with a barbell resting on the front of the shoulders. It develops anterior chain leg strength, and is a foundational movement for the clean and the thruster.

Not everyone can or should front squat, at least initially. Like the back squat, the front squat has a simple movement screen: the *Elbows-up Wall Squat Test.* To perform the Elbows-Up Wall Squat Test, have your athlete stand half a foot's length from the wall. Tell him to interlace his fingers behind his head, so that his elbows are pointing forward, just shy of touching the wall.

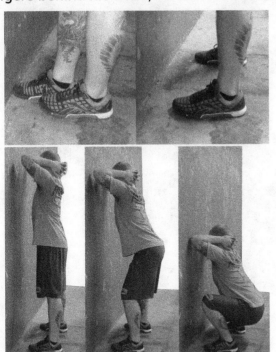

Then have him squat. If he fails—that is, if his elbows hit the wall and then force him to stop or fall back— let him move back two inches and then try again. If he still can't make it down and up without falling over, he's probably not ready to front squat, and should be prescribed mobility homework, while continuing to train with barbell back squats and dumbbell squats. Note that these screens aren't meant to embarrass anyone, only to help you (and your athlete) understand if he's actually ready for the movement.

It's also possible you'll have a trainee who has a mature enough squat, but lacks the flexibility to hold a barbell in front rack position. For someone like that, alternative versions of the front rack are explained at the end of the chapter.

This athlete is cleared to front squat.

When I teach the front squat to a group, the athletes use light barbells:15kg for men, 8kg for women. PVC pipe doesn't cut it. Virtually no one has the flexibility to adopt a good rack position with PVC, and holding the bar down with your chin is not only uncomfortable, it's senseless, as it's not how the movement is practiced.

Harry and Amy are both ready for the front squat. Tim, who by the end of last week got his first full air squats, can work on dumbbell squats today.

Front Rack Teaching Script

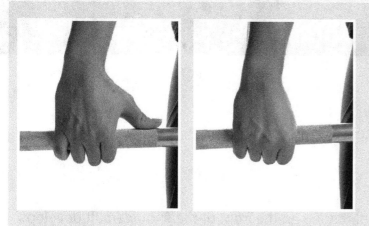

"Go ahead and pick up your barbells. Place the tips of your extended thumbs right at the edge where the gnurling meets the smooth center section of the bar. Then wrap your thumbs around your fingers to make a fist. This is our default grip width—we'll adjust it as necessary.

"Now curl the bar up to rest on your shoulders. Elevate and protract your scapulae. Lift your elbows until they are pointing straight ahead, allowing the bar to roll back onto your fingertips.* (If you have the flexibility, you can use a full fist grip—this will prove very useful later when we learn thrusters.) The bar should be sitting between the peak of the deltoids and the throat.

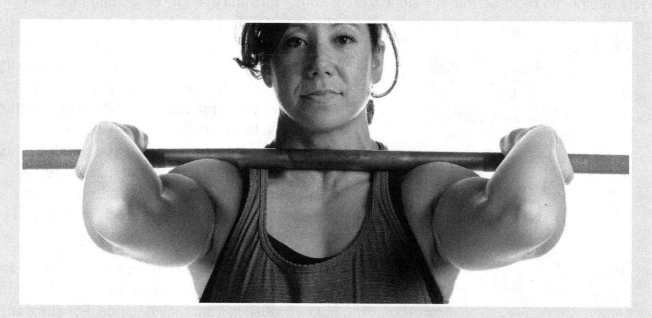

"Understand that you are NOT holding the bar with your hands; the bar should be sitting on the torso, with your hands 'babysitting' the bar. Remember, DO NOT pack your shoulders. Elevate and protract. Then tighten the upper back to create stability."

If an athlete can't front rack with all four fingers under the bar, set that as a goal and prescribe mobilizations as appropriate.

Front Squat Teaching Script

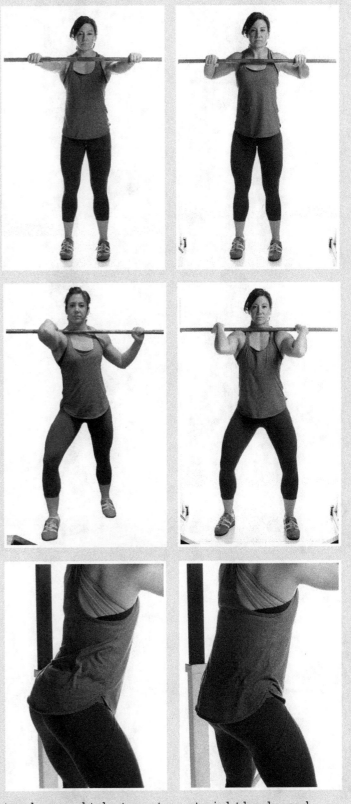

"To set up for the front squat with the bar in the rack, begin by taking your proper width, thumbs-around grip on the bar. Attempt to snap the bar in half by rotating your thumbs toward the ceiling.

"Step straight up to the bar.

"Step forward and out with the right foot, simultaneously rotating your right elbow around the barbell until it is pointing straight ahead and the barbell is firmly seated on the shoulder.

"Match it on your left side.

"For a strong front rack set-up, you must create torque in the shoulder by applying rotational force against the fixed point where your fingers are trapped beneath the bar. Rather than think about 'pushing' your elbows up, 'pull' them up by strongly contracting the muscles of your upper back.

"At this point, you should be in a partial front squat. Your lower back may be hyperextended—squeeze your glutes and lock down your abs and stack your spine under the bar.

"Wedging your shoulders up into the bar, stand up and take two steps straight backward. You're almost ready to start the lift!

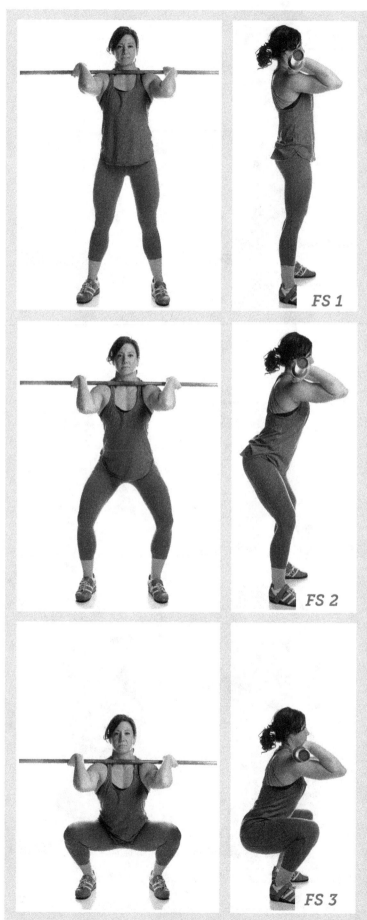

FS 1

FS 2

FS 3

"Stand with feet shoulder-width apart. Weight should be on center of foot with a slight emphasis on the heel. Screw your feet into the floor. Brace your midline. Tighten your upper back to pull your elbows up until your upper arms are parallel to the floor. This is **Front Squat Position 1 (FS 1).**

"Engage the Valsalva maneuver by taking a big breath and pressurizing.

"Then, keeping your chest up and elbows pointing forward, unlock your knees and sit your hips back. Push your knees out. This is **Front Squat Position 2 (FS 2).**

"Sit down over your heels until the crease of your hip is below the top of your knee. Knees track over toes or slightly outside, back is straight, elbows are high. This is **Front Squat Position 3 (FS 3).**

"In deep front squats, it's fine if the knees push out in front of the toes, as long as the shared center of mass of the athlete and the barbell remain balanced in the line of gravity.

"Once you've hit legal depth, drive your elbows up until you have returned to **FS 2.**

"Bring your hips forward to complete the repetition in **FS 1.**"

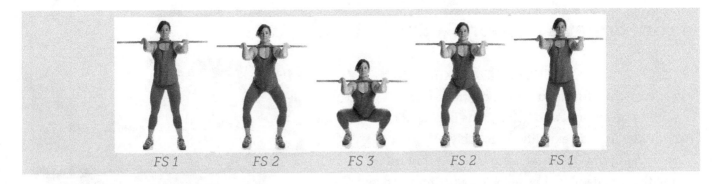

FS 1   FS 2   FS 3   FS 2   FS 1

Positional Drills

"1! 2 ! 3! 2! 1!." Take your athletes through each position of the front squat. Have them hold each position while you make necessary adjustments.

"1! 2! 3! Go!" Bring athletes into bottom position; correct their position as necessary. When they look good, on your command "Go!", they return to **FS 1**.

"Five in the hole." This is "1! 2! 3! Go!" with a five second hold in the bottom position.

Front Squat Common Faults and Fixes

All of the common faults and fixes of the air squat—breaking at knees first, unable to maintain neutral spine position, spinal overextension, insufficient depth, weight on balls of feet, excessive foot turn out, knees cave in—also apply to the front squat, as well as the following:

1. Low elbows.

For optimal stability and to avoid injury, the humerus should be more or less parallel to the floor at every stage of the front squat. An athlete's inability to keep the elbows high could have one (or more) of many causes.

A. INCORRECT GRIP. If the athlete is unable to lift her elbows high in FS 1, check her hands. If she's holding the bar in a full-fist grip and is relatively inflexible, that might be the problem. Have her relax her fists and let the bar roll back on her fingertips. (Note that ideally she could hold the bar in her fists and still keep her elbows high, a requirement for the thruster.)

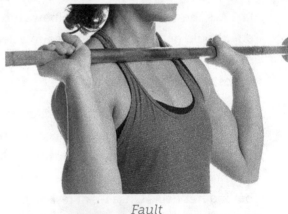

Fault

 "Bar back on fingertips!"

 Demonstrate proper FS 1.

 Adjust hands and elbows into proper position.

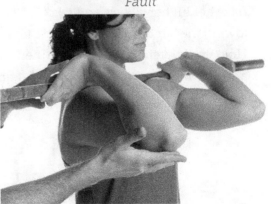

Tactile

Front Squat Common Faults and Fixes, cont.

B. LACK OF LAT AND SHOULDER FLEXIBILITY. If your athlete is unable to front rack the bar while standing up straight and holding the bar on her fingertips, lack of flexibility is probably the culprit. Sometimes light PNF stretching can help, but more often this issue will not be resolved with simple fixes. Some people, especially the middle-aged, will never be able to hold the bar in a good front rack position, and indeed will injure themselves if they insist on performing front squats. Substitute back squats or dumbbell squats instead.

 "Elbows up!" or "Pull elbows high!"

 Demonstrate a correct FS 1.

With your trainee holding in FS 1 (or set up in the rack in preparation to take the bar out), instruct her to resist as you lightly press down on her elbows. Hold for a count of 10, then relax. Ask the athlete to pull her elbows higher—she should get at least another couple degrees of ROM. Repeat this PNF stretch 3-4 more times at each new elevation.

While mobilization techniques are outside of the scope of this book, here's an easy way to stretch an athlete's front rack position. Have her press a barbell overhead, then lower it behind her neck. Once it's at rest on the traps, have her lift her elbows and relax her grip, allowing the bar to roll back on their fingertips. Hold this stretch for 30 seconds, then regrip and rest with bar on traps. Repeat 3-4 times.

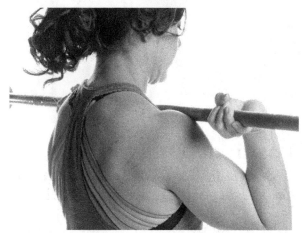

Fault

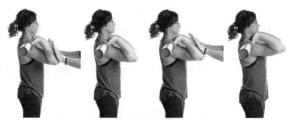

Tactile PNF stretch

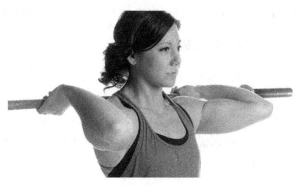

Orthosis

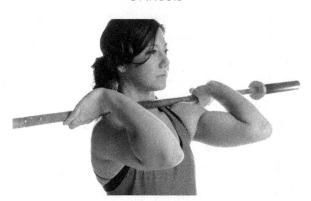

Correct FS 1 rack position

Front Squat Common Faults and Fixes, cont.

C. MOTOR CONTROL. If your athlete has a decent rack position in FS 1, but her elbows drop as soon as she hinges back into FS 2, it's likely a motor control issue. To keep her elbows high, she needs to maintain tension in her upper back as her hips hinge. Cueing during execution of the squat will be ineffective; either remind her when she's standing tall, or have her perform the "1-2-3-2-1" positional drill, fixing her while she holds in FS 2.

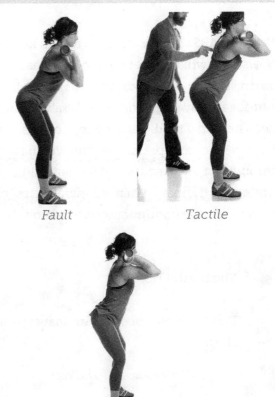

Fault   *Tactile*

 "Tight back!" or "Pull your elbows to the ceiling!"

 Demonstrate a correct FS 2.

 Tap your athlete between the shoulder blades to remind her to tighten her upper back and pull her elbows up.

Correct FS 2

D. LACK OF THORACIC MOBILITY. A second cause of elbows dropping during the descent is an inability to extend the thoracic spine. It will be glaringly obvious in FS 3—an otherwise sound squat will be marred by a rounded upper back. Cue as you can, but if the t-spine is a problem, only extra mobility work will improve matters.

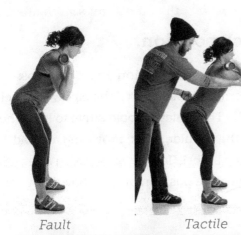

Fault   *Tactile*

 "Chest up!"

 Demonstrate a proper FS 2.

 With the athlete holding in FS 2, try pressing with one hand at the base of the shoulder blades, lifting at the elbow with the other, and if necessary, creating a fulcrum at the tailbone by blocking it with your fist.

Have athlete practice front squatting with her elbows touching a wall.

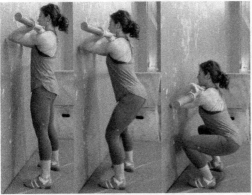

Orthosis

Front Squat Common Faults and Fixes, cont.

E. WEAK ABS. If your athlete is able to keep her elbows high while descending in the squat, but slumps when she hits bottom or starts to rise, it's likely she's not adequately employing the Valsalva maneuver to keep her torso rigid. Between reps or sets, remind her how to brace and pressurize. The breath must be held throughout the execution of the rep. (Although, for optimal performance in metcons, athletes must learn how to breathe continuously while strongly braced.)

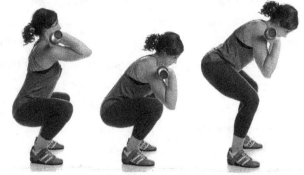

Faulty sequence

 "Big breath! Hold it!"

 Demo taking a deep breath that expands the chest.

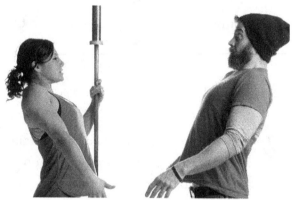

Demo how big a breath you want your athlete to take

2. Bad rack position.

Front Squat Position 1 violation. Front rack position can be compromised even if the elbows are held relatively high. The athlete should strive to keep the chest up and the shoulders out, providing a broad platform for the barbell. Ideally, arms are in line with the wrists. If not, the position of the elbows can point to the cause.

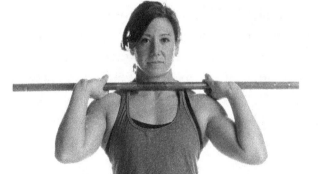

Fault

A. ELBOWS FLARING OUT. If the athlete's grip is too close, the shoulders will internally rotate, the chest will cave in, and the elbows will flare out. Remind your athlete that her grip should be at least thumb's width out from the gnurling of the bar.

 "Wider grip!"

 Demonstrate a proper FS 1.

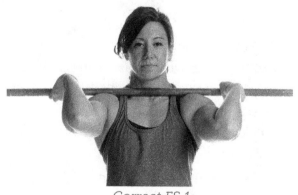

Correct FS 1

Front Squat Common Faults and Fixes, cont.

B. ELBOWS POINTING FORWARD, BUT HANDS TWISTING OFF BAR. If the grip width is correct but the hands are twisting off the bar, it's likely the upper arms are internally rotated—that is, turned in toward the centerline. Part of a good rack position is being able to strongly externally rotate the humerus even with the elbows flexed and the hands pinned.

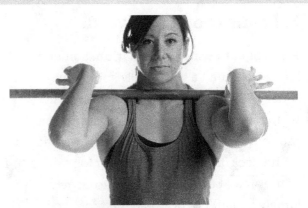

Fault

 "Inside of your arms up!"

 Demonstrate correct external rotation of arms in front rack position.

 Gently turn athlete's upper arms (left arm clockwise [relative to you], right arm counter-clockwise) to indicate desired position.

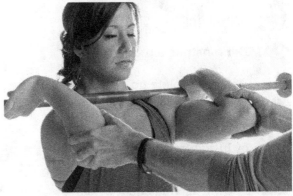

Tactile

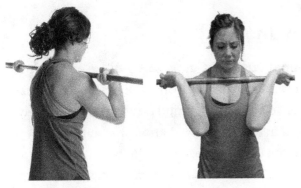

Internal rotation of shoulders tends to dump elbows toward centerline.

C. ELBOWS POINTING IN. If the bar is centered on the hand with all four fingers under the shaft, but the elbows are point in, that means that the shoulders are internally rotated, which inhibits creating the torque necessary for stability and that supports thoracic extension.

 "Tight upper back!" or "Pull elbows high!"

 Demonstrate a proper FS 3.

 A skinny band looped around the shoulders can act as a "bar bra", encouraging athlete to keep shoulders back.

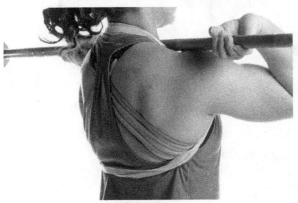

Orthosis

Front Squat Common Faults and Fixes, cont.

3. Leans too far forward.

Front Squat Position 3 violation. Sometimes an athlete may exhibit a technically sound but "immature" squat—that is, she may be able to squat below parallel with knees pushed out and a straight spine, but has a pronounced forward lean. With the bar racked in front of the neck, this lean puts the bar too far out in front of the area of base. Your ability to correct this *in situ* is largely a matter of how bad the problem is.

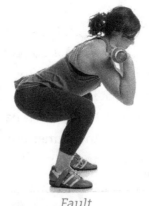
Fault

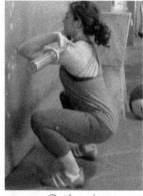
Orthosis

 "Chest up!"

 Demonstrate a proper FS 3.

 With the athlete holding in FS 3, try creating a fulcrum at the tailbone by blocking it with your knee, and bringing her torso to vertical by lifting from her elbow.

 Elbows-up Wall Squat w/ bar.

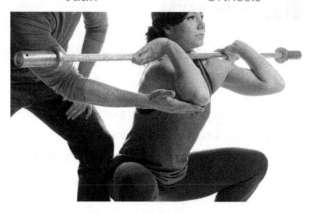
Tactile

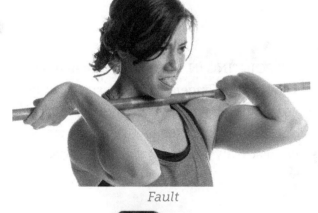
Fault

4. Choking out.

Front Squat Position 1 violation. Athlete complains barbell is choking her. In front rack position, the barbell will sit close to the carotid artery, and it's entirely possible that a trainee could knock herself out by allowing the barbell to press on the neck and occlude the carotid for even a few seconds. To avoid this, the athlete must push her shoulders up into the bar and use breath support.

 "Push your shoulders into the bar!"

 Demonstrate a proper FS 1.

 With athlete holding in FS 1, manually adjust her position.

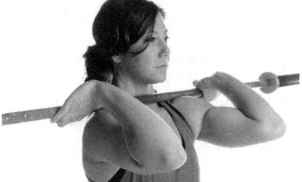
Correct FS 1

Bailing Out of the Front Squat

"Bailing out of the front squat is easy. If something goes wrong, simply drop your elbows and step back. Gravity will take care of the rest. Never use a spotter for front squats.

"Practice and experience are the only way to build confidence! Put some bumpers on the bar (not the 10lbs!) and bail out on purpose until you get a feel for it."

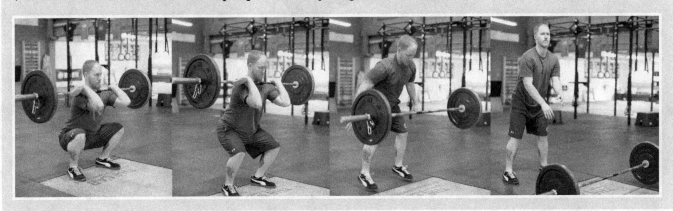

Front Rack Position Alternatives

Long experience has taught me that some athletes simply do not and will not ever have the flexibility to front squat without significant discomfort. Here are a couple alternate methods for loading the anterior side of the body in the squat.

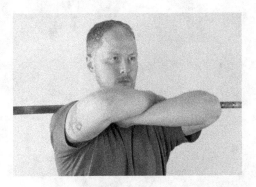

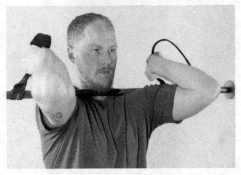

GENIE SQUAT. With the bar racked at chest height, have the athlete set up in a partial squat under the bar, with the bar on his shoulders and his arms out straight. He then folds his arms to bring his right hand to his left shoulder, and his left hand to his right. He may, if he wishes, hook his fingertips around the bar.

STRAP IT ON. If you have canvas lifting straps, you can tie them around the bar. Have the athlete set up as in the Genie squat, then grasp the ends of the straps near the knot and pull. The tension will help keep his elbows high, while taking the strain off his wrists.

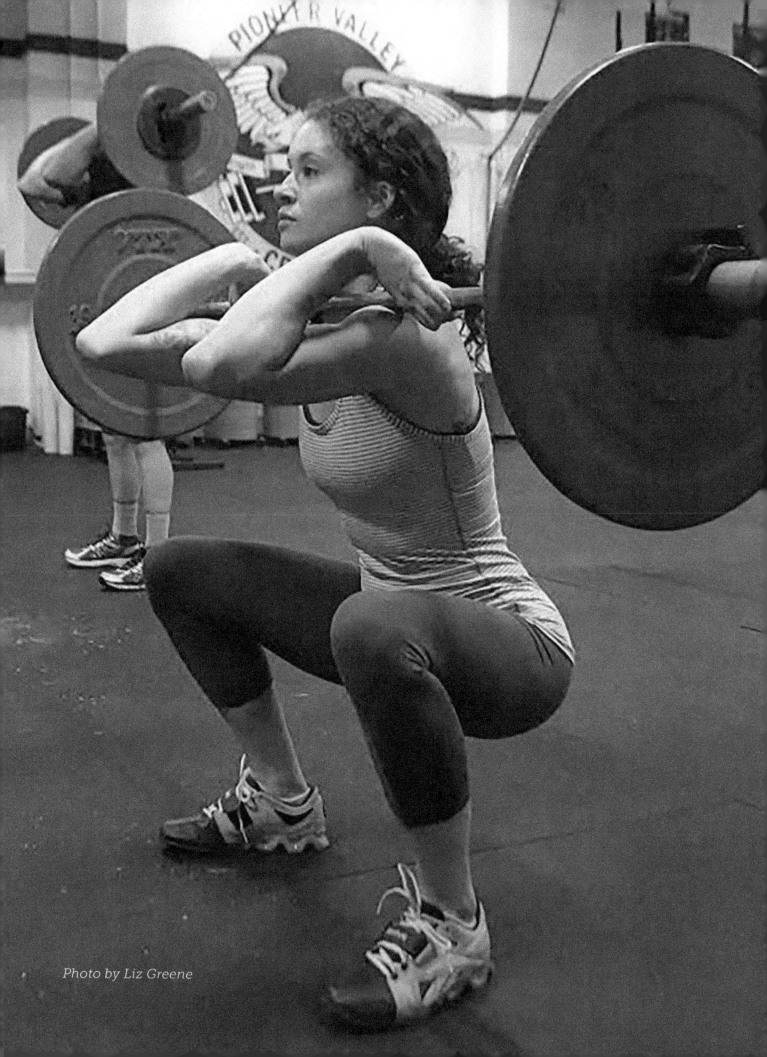

Photo by Liz Greene

KNEES-TO-ELBOWS

Category: Hip and Trunk Flexion (hanging, bent knee)

Movement screen: N/a

Ability screen: Feet-anchored sit-up x 5 (supine knee draw), supine knee draw x 5 (incline knee raise), high incline knee raise x 5 (knees-to-elbows)

"Knees-to-elbows" couldn't be more self-explanatory: hanging from the bar with arms and legs straight, the athlete raises his bent legs until his knees touch his elbows, then lowers them until they are straight again. This requires considerable grip and abdominal strength. However, the knees-to-elbow cannot be accomplished purely through trunk flexion. No matter how strong your abs are, if you don't have the strength to extend the shoulder while hanging suspended, thus lifting the chest, you'll never get near a good knee-to-elbows finish position.

Although largely supplanted by the toes-to-bar in modern MMGPP programming, the strict knees-to-elbows is a necessary step in the progression toward skin-the-cats and ultimately front and back levers.

Out of the three members of Team Space Monkey, only Harry currently has sufficient upper body strength for a strict knees-to-elbows. Amy and Tim will end up sticking with one of the exercises that progress toward the full movement.

Knees-to-Elbows Teaching Script

The exercise progression toward the strict knees-to-elbows begins with the supine knee draw.

"Have a seat on the floor about 2' in front of a stable post. Assume a supine position. Reach overhead, grasp the post with both hands, and then scoot forward until your arms are straight. Legs should be extended in front of you, with feet together and toes pointed. Contract your abdominals to hollow out. This is **Supine Knee Draw Position 1 (sKD 1).**

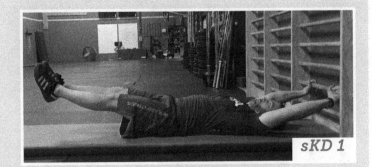

sKD 1

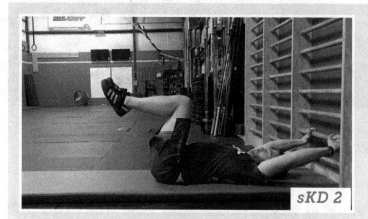

sKD 2

"Grasping the post to help keep your trunk anchored, draw your knees toward your chest. When your hips have fully closed, continue to pull your knees in, flexing the trunk so that your hips leave the ground. This is **Supine Knee Draw Position 2 (sKD 2).**

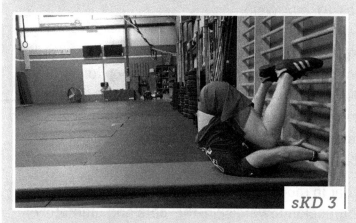

sKD 3

"If possible, continue curling thr trunk until your knees touch your elbows. This is **Supine Knee Draw Position 3 (sKD 3).** If this position is uncomfortable due to neck compression, don't worry about bringing knees all the way to elbows.

"Extend the hips and knees to return to **sKD 1**. Take care to maintain abdominal tension throughout the movement. "

The jump in difficulty between the supine knee draw and the knees-to-elbows is quite drastic. The incline knees is a great way to bridge the gap. It increases the challenge of the supine knee draw by gradually moving the torso towards vertical. Use stall bars and an incline board, or you can build an incline by propping one end of a utility bench on bumpers in front of a post.

Have a seat on an incline board or bench. Assume a supine position. Reach overhead, grasp the post with both hands, and then scoot forward until your arms are straight. Legs should be extended in front of you, with feet together and toes pointed. Contract your abdominals to hollow out. This is **Incline Knee Raise Position 1 (iKR 1).**

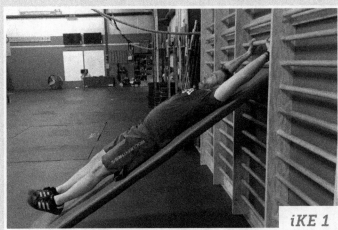

iKE 1

Grasping the post to help keep your trunk anchored, draw your knees toward your chest. When your hips have fully closed, continue to pull your knees in, flexing the trunk so that your hips leave the board. This is **Incline Knee Raise Position 2 (iKR 2).**

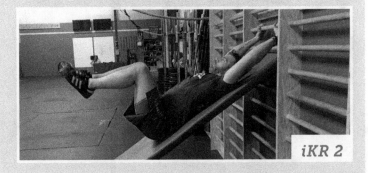

iKR 2

Continue curling the trunk until your knees touch your elbows. This is **Incline Knee Raise Position 3 (iKR 3).**

Return to **iKR 1.**

Once you can do 10 Incline Knee Raises at a given angle on the board, raise the board up, increasing your torso angle relative to the floor, to make the exercise more challenging.

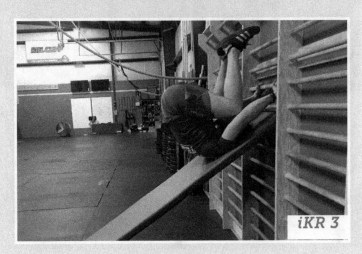

iKR 3

If your gym doesn't have stall bars and improvising an incline board with materials at hand seems impractical, you can use the hanging knee raise as a progression between supine knee draw and knees-to-elbows. While the incline knee raise has the benefits mentioned earlier, the hanging knee raise teaches the first two positions of the knees-to-elbows, and builds grip strength, besides.

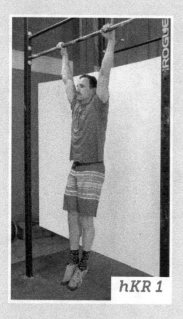

hKR 1

"To do a hanging knee raise, begin in an active hang from the pull-up bar: hands shoulder-width in a pull-up hook grip, shoulders active, abs and glutes locked in, legs straight, feet together. This is **Hanging Knee Raise Position 1 (hKR 1).**

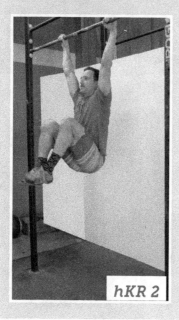

hKR 2

"Keeping your legs together and your midline braced, pull the knees as high as possible. This is **Hanging Knee Raise Position 2 (hKR 2).**

"Extend the hips and knees to return to **hKR 1**. Take care to maintain abdominal tension throughout the movement.

"Finally, by recruiting the lats, we'll turn this movement into the knees-to-elbows.

"To execute a full knees-to-elbows, begin with **hKR 1** and **hKR 2** (now **Knees-to-Elbows Position 1 [KE 1]** and **Knees-to-elbows Position 2 [KE 2]**). Then,

"As the knees pass the waist, push down on the bar to lift the chest toward the ceiling.

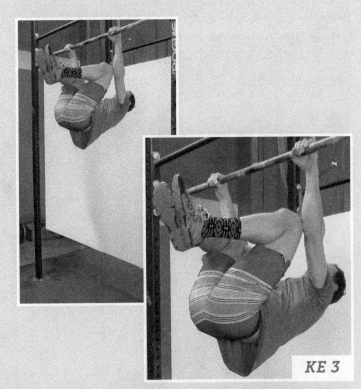

"This additional elevation allows you to bring the knees to touch the points of your elbows. This is **Knees to Elbows Position 3 (KE 3)**.

"Make sure your gaze travels from looking forward to looking at the ceiling as your head, remaining in a neutral position, moves in line with your body."

"Flex the shoulders and extend the hips and knees to return to **KE 1**.

KE 3

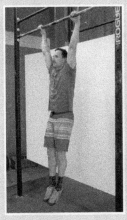
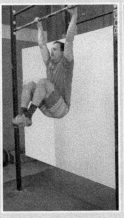
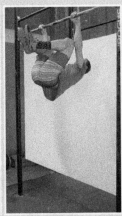
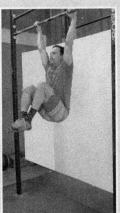
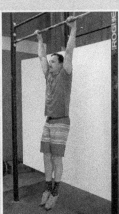

KE 1 *KE 2* *KE 3* *KE 2* *KE 1*

Positional Drills

"1! 2 ! 3! 2! 1!" Take athletes through each position of the knees-to-elbows. Have them hold each position while you make necessary adjustments.

Knees-to-Elbows Common Faults and Fixes

1. Pendulum swing.

Knees to Elbows Position 1 violation. If your athlete begins to swing back and forth under the bar, stop him with a hand on his hip. Then teach him to stop himself by putting a toe down on a short box placed beside him. To prevent a swing from starting, tell him to concentrate as he lowers himsef on squeezing the bar tight, and maintaining tension in the lats.

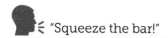 "Squeeze the bar!"

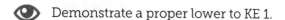 Demonstrate a proper lower to KE 1.

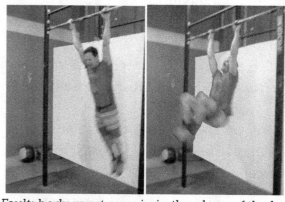

Fault: body must remain in the plane of the bar

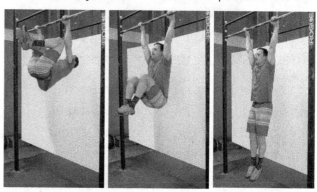

Grip the bar tightly and lower under control.

2. Knees to armpits.

Knees to Elbows Position 3 violation If knees fail to make contact with elbows, usually the athlete needs to more strongly engage the lats to close the angle between arms and torso and lift the chest. In experienced athletes, this happens due to fatigue; in newer athletes, it's caused by a lack of trunk strength.

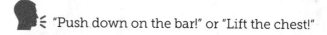 "Push down on the bar!" or "Lift the chest!"

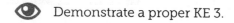 Demonstrate a proper KE 3.

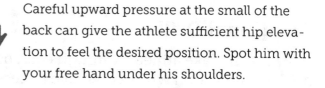 Careful upward pressure at the small of the back can give the athlete sufficient hip elevation to feel the desired position. Spot him with your free hand under his shoulders.

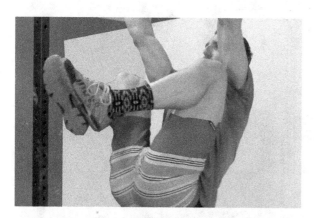

Fault: Lats insufficiently engaged

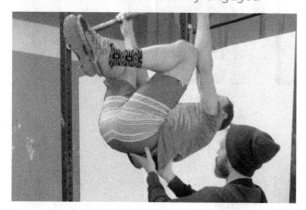

Tactile

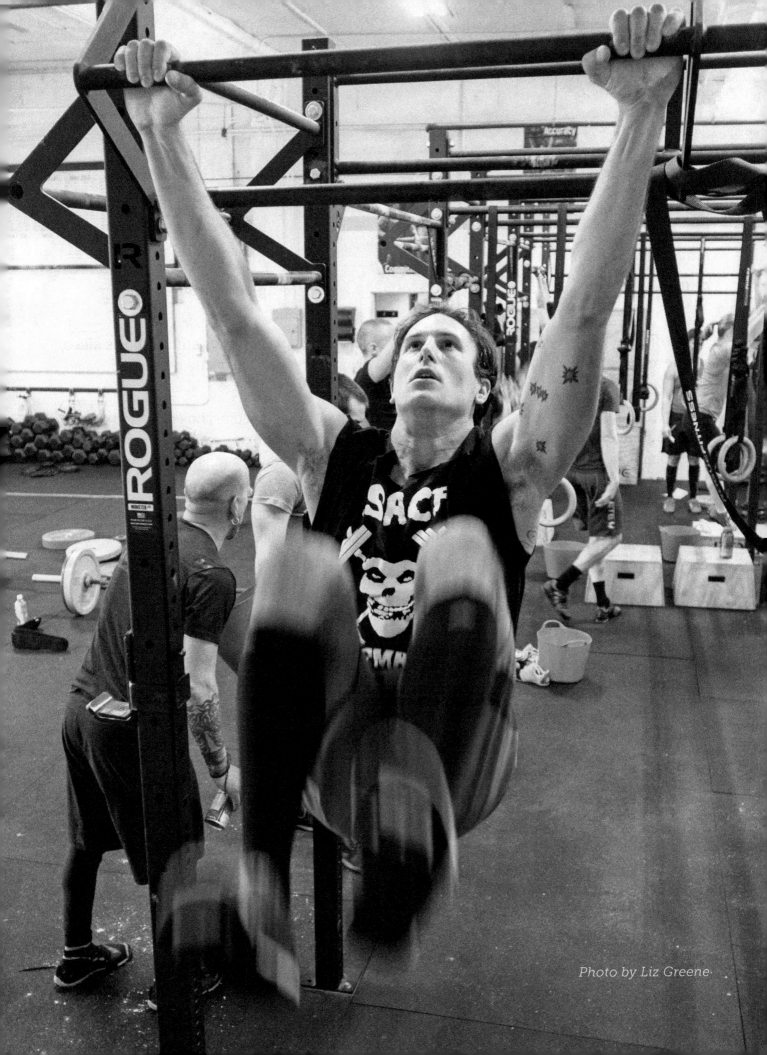

Photo by Liz Greene

DIPS

Category: Push Away from Object (vertical)

Movement screen: N/a

Ability screen: N/a (parallette dip), parallette dip x 10 (box dip), box dip x 10 (bar dip)

The dip teaches how to keep your shoulders stable under load with the arms at one's sides, and develops the ability to produce force in a downward direction to elevate oneself above an object.

We teach three exercises in a progression toward dips: parallette dips, box dips, and stationary bar dips. Virtually every trainee, no matter how weak or deconditioned, can find in one of these movements an appropriate level of stimulus. Make sure your athletes master the basic concepts of the dip at each level of complexity before allowing them to attempt the next.

Predictions for today? Harry will go all the way through the progression. Amy will probably find box dips pose enough challenge, and for the forseeable future, Tim will be doing his dips on parallettes.

Parallette and Box Dip Teaching Script

The exercise progression toward the dip begins with the parallette dip.

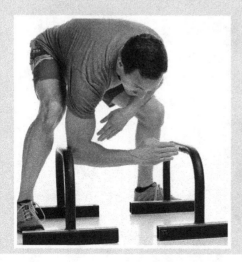

"Set the parallettes approximately shoulder-width apart. You can also measure the distance using the point of your elbow to the tip of your finger.

"Crouch between the parallettes, then grasp them with a full-fist grip about midway on the horizontal bar. Pull your shoulders back and down. Keeping your arms straight, twist your hands into the bars, right hand clockwise, left counterclockwise. Then walk your feet forward until your knees are bent at 90 degrees. Your hips should be under your shoulders. This is **Parallette Dip Position 1 (pDP 1).**

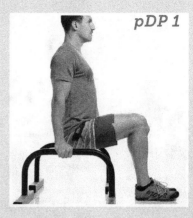

pDP 1

"Hinging back at the hips, lower yourself until your buttocks touch the ground. Keep your shoulders locked back and down. This is **Paralllette Dip Position 2 (pDP 2).**

"Using as much leg assistance as necessary, push yourself back up to **pDP 1**.

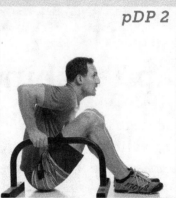

pDP 2

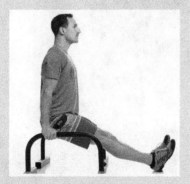
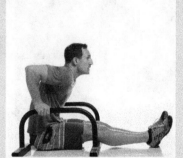

"If this is relatively easy, straighten your legs and try again.

"If that was still too easy, set a pair of boxes approximately shoulder-width apart. Start with the 24" side up; later you can progress to 20".

"Crouch between the boxes, then place your hands palm down atop them. Screw your hands into the box top, right hand clockwise, left hand counterclockwise. Pull your shoulders back and down. Your hips should be under your shoulders. Walk your feet forward until your knees are straight. Point your toes. This is **Box Dip Position 1 (bDP 1).**

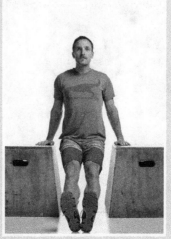
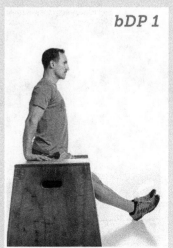

bDP 1

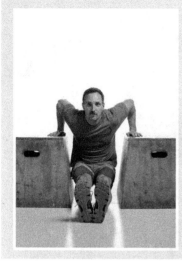
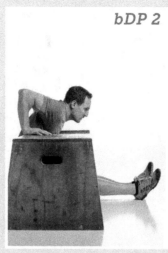

bDP 2

"Hinging back at the hips, lower yourself until your elbows are higher than your shoulders. Keep your shoulders packed back and down. Forearms should be vertical, hands in line with hips. This is **Box Dip Position 2 (bDP 2)**.

"Push yourself up to **bDP 1**."

Bar Dip Teaching Script

Competence with strict dips on the stationary bar are necessary before an athlete can safely begin working on ring dips. If your gym doesn't have stationary bars...get some. Beyond being safer than band-assisted ring dips, they're great for exercises like weighted dips.

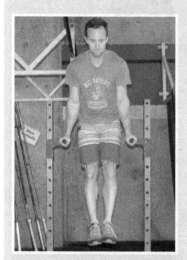
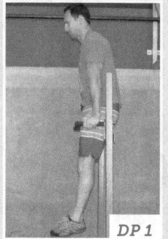

DP 1

"Grip the bars with thumbs around. Step up into **Dip Position 1 (DP 1)**: arms locked straight, shoulders over hands, hands twisting into the bars (right hand clockwise, left hand counterclockwise), shoulders packed, hollow body position, legs straight and feet together, slightly in front of the body. Keep the toes pointed—it takes slack out of the body, and promotes better control.

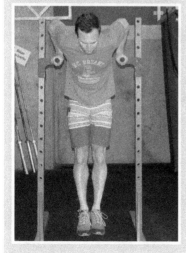
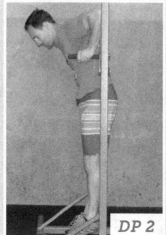

DP 2

"Lower your center of gravity until you reach end ROM—generally speaking, elbows higher than the shoulders. The torso will lean forward slightly. Forearms should be vertical, hands in line with hips. If hollow body position is maintained, at this point the feet will point at the floor. This is **Dip Position 2 (DP 2)**.

"Push to return to **DP 1**. Do not allow midline to break, and keep the elbows from flaring out."

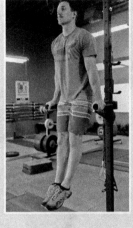 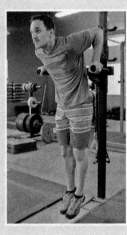 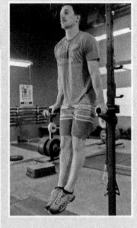

DP 1   *DP 2*   *DP 1*

Dips Common Faults and Fixes

1. Partial ROM

All dips Position 2 violation. If athlete's elbows are not slightly higher than the shoulders at the bottom of the movement, cue him to dip deeper. If this is too difficult, default to an easier variation.

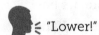 "Lower!"

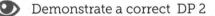 Demonstrate a correct DP 2

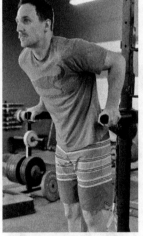 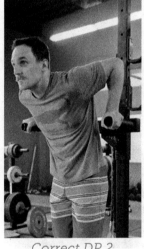

Fault   *Correct DP 2*

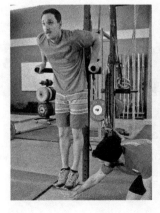 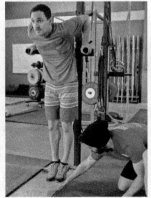 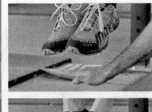 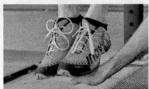

Give the athlete a target by putting the back of your hand at the height to which he should lower his feet.

Tactile

Dips Common Faults and Fixes, cont.

2. Head fault

All dips Position 2 violation. As torso tilts forward into Position 2, athlete keeps his gaze forward, bending his neck and violating the neutral midline rule. In Position 2, gaze should be on floor with neck in line with the spine.

 "Lower!"

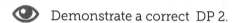 Demonstrate a correct DP 2.

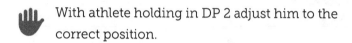 With athlete holding in DP 2 adjust him to the correct position.

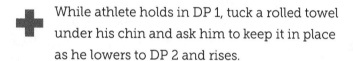 While athlete holds in DP 1, tuck a rolled towel under his chin and ask him to keep it in place as he lowers to DP 2 and rises.

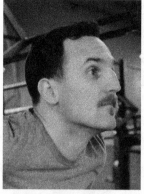

Fault

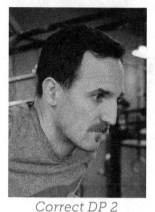

Orthosis

Correct DP 2

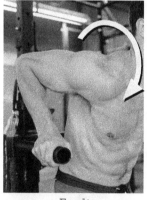

Fault

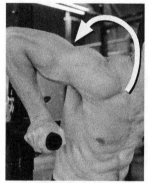

Correct DP 2

3. Shoulder dump

In Position 2 (pDP 2, bDP 2, DP 2), the bottom of the movement, if the shoulders round forward, it's because the athlete is missing internal rotation. If the missing ROM isn't too great, it can be countered with conscious recruitment of upper back; if not, extra mobilization work will be required.

 "Shoulders back and down!"

 Demonstrate a proper 2nd position of the dip.

 A skinny band looped around the shoulders can act as a "scapular bra", encouraging athlete to keep shoulders back.

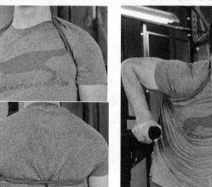

Orthosis

Dips Common Faults and Fixes, cont.

4. Spinal overextension (ship's figurehead)

Dip Position 2 violation. As the athlete tires, he hyperextends his spine in an attempt to turn the vertical push of the dip into a horizontal effort, a sort of mid-air push-up. Usually there's a fair amount of kicking and squirming involved as well, anything to gain a little mechanical advantage. For optimal training benefit, athlete must be disciplined about maintaining a hollow body position and pushing down in line with the torso.

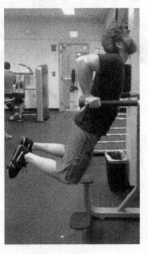

Fault

 "Abs on!" or "Legs straight beneath you!"

 Demonstrate a correct transition from DP 2 2 to DP 1.

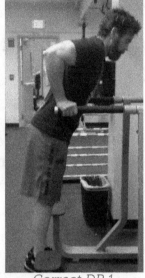

Correct DP 1

5. Hands behind hips.

Parallette or Bar Dip Position 2 violation. Generally you'll only see this with parallette or box dips, or when an athlete is scaling bar dips with a band: at the bottom of the movement, his hands are behind his hips, not in line. This is a positional mistake that must be corrected before the athlete can progress.

 "Hands line up with hips!"

 Demonstrate a proper Position 2 of the dip.

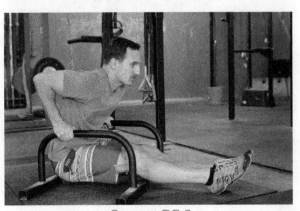

Fault

Correct DP 2

Category: Push Object (horizontal)

Movement screen: N/a

Ability screen: N/a

The bench press is the great developer of horizontal pushing strength. Lying supine on a bench, the athlete takes a bar from the rack, lowers and raises it a set number of times, then returns it. The bench press requires the ability to maintain the entire body in tension under load, especially the scapulae, which must be strongly retracted and depressed throughout the lift.

For reasons of safety and efficiency, we teach how to spot for the bench alongside how to actually perform the movement.

All of Team Space Monkey should be able to handle the bench press. They all have good unassisted push-ups. If you have light enough barbells (every gym should have some 15lbs bars), the bench press is accessible even to those who don't yet have push-ups.

Bench Press Teaching Script

Running your athletes through the basics of the set-up position while they are still standing tall can help them understand what they need to do on the bench.

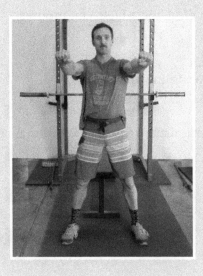

"Take a wide stance.

"Raise your arms straight hands up in front of you, make fists, and slightly extend your wrists.

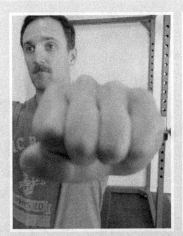 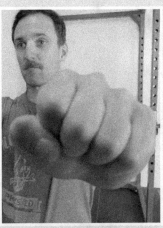

"Rotate your thumbs a quarter turn toward the ceiling.

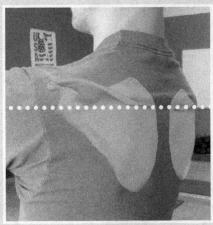 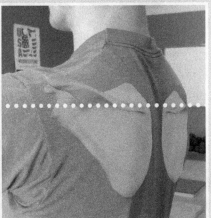

"Pull your shoulder blades back and down.

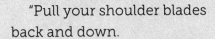

"Squeeze your butt and lock your abs in.

"Screw your feet into the floor.

"If you were lying on your back with your knees bent at 90°, you'd be set up for the bench press.

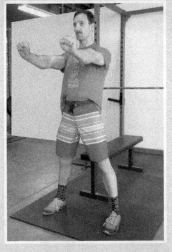

"Now, lie down on the bench with your eyes 'south' of the bar. This will help you avoid accidentally hitting the hooks of the rack during the concentric phase of the lift.

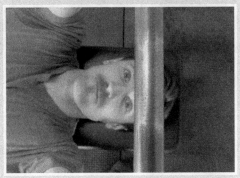

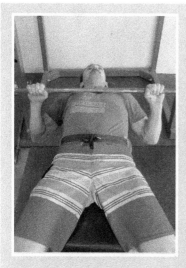
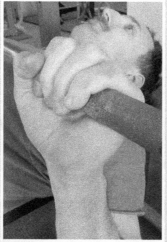

"Take your grip. It should be just wide enough so that at the bottom of the lift, your forearms are perpendicular to the floor. You may have to experiment a bit to find the proper width for you.

"Use a full-fist grip, with the bar centered across the palm. Let your wrists extend to about 45°.

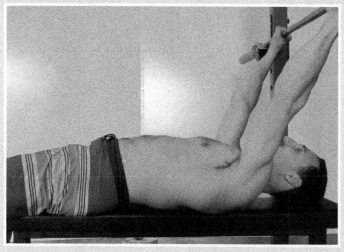

Shoulder blades neutral

"Strongly retract and depress your shoulder blades. This will lift your chest up toward the bar (happily enough, shortening the ROM).

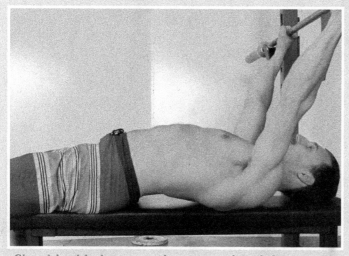

Shoulder blades strongly retracted and depressed. Lumbar curve is accentuated, but not exaggerrated. Don't compress the spine.

"Try to snap the bar in half by rotating your thumbs in toward your face.

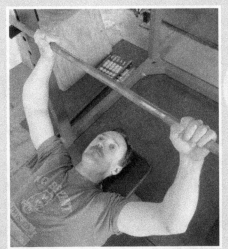 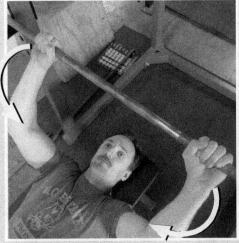

"Screw your feet into the floor, and drive your heels into the ground. You have now created two arcs of tension: one from the heels to the buttocks, and another from the buttocks to the back of the shoulders.

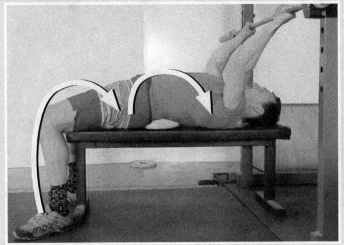

Arcs of tension: heels to butt, butt to shoulders

"To take the bar out of the rack, the spotter comes into play. The spotter takes a two-handed, alternating grip on the bar. The lifter counts to three: 'One, two, three!' and on 'Three!' together the spotter and the lifter take the bar out of the rack.

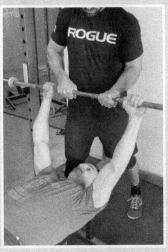 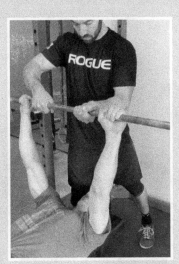

"One...two..." *"...three!"*

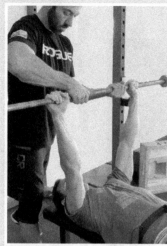

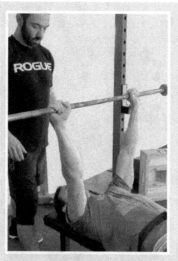

"Got it?"   *"Got it!"*

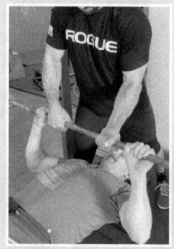

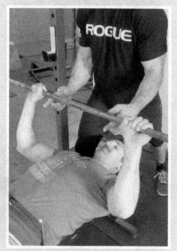

If lifter is in trouble, grab the bar. Otherwise...   *"It's all you, bro!" = NO REP*

"The lifter keeps his elbows locked, while the spotter helps guide the bar out to where the lifter's arms are perpendicular to the floor. The spotter asks, 'Got it?' and when the lifter answers in the affirmative, the spotter takes his hands off the bar.

"The spotter will not touch the bar again until the set is complete, UNLESS: 1) the lifter asks for help, 2) the bar stalls in the concentric phase of the lift and then begins to descend, 3) one arm pushes higher than the other, putting a lot of torque on one shoulder and possibly leading to injury, or 4) the instructor on the floor bellows 'TAKE IT!'. In the absence of any of those three scenarios, allow the lifter to battle for his last rep, even if it seems to take forever. Touching the bar invalidates the rep. When his elbows finally lock out, grab the bar and pull it straight back into the uprights.

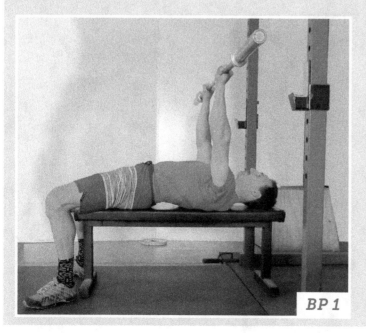

BP 1

"With the bar held in a full-fist grip, arms perpendicular to the floor, arms externally rotated and shoulder blades retracted and depressed as strongly as possible, abs and glutes locked, and heels driving into the ground, you are now in **Bench Press Position 1 (BP 1).**

"Stare through the bar at the ceiling. You will maintain this sight picture throughout the movement. Do not follow the bar with your eyes.

"Take a deep breath and employ the Valsalva maneuver.

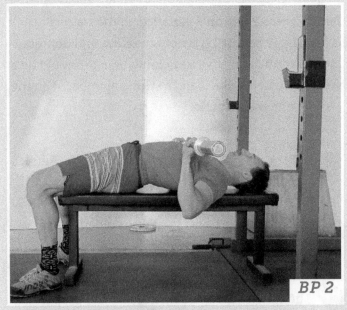

BP 2

"Continuing to try to snap the bar in half, pull the bar down to the chest just below the nipple line. Your forearms are vertical. This is **Bench Press Position 2 (BP 2).**

"As soon as the bar makes contact with the chest, immediately drive up as hard and fast as possible to return to **BP 1**.

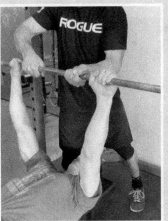
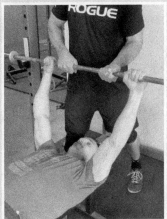

"When the lifter finishes his set, the spotter grabs the bar, and together they bring it straight back to the rack. The lifter only bends his elbows to lower the bar after it makes contact with the uprights. DO NO GO HUNTING FOR THE HOOKS."

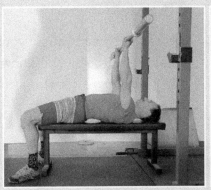
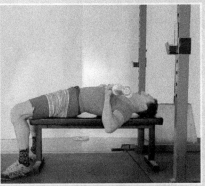
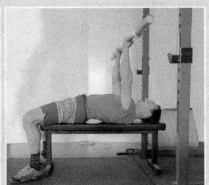

BP 1   BP 2   BP 1

Bench Press Common Faults and Fixes

1. Weak set-up.

Bench Press Position 1 violation. If the trainee's back is flat on the bench, he is not retracting and depressing his shoulder blades sufficiently. There should be a visible rise in the chest and a strong arch between the t-spine and the tailbone.

 "Back tight!" or "Pack the shoulders!" or "Retract and depress!"

 Demonstrate how to retract and depress shoulder blades.

 With athlete in BP 1, reach under him to lift him by the thoracic ribs into the proper position.

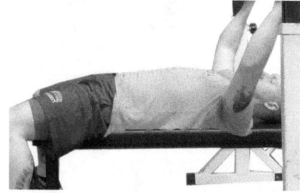

Fault

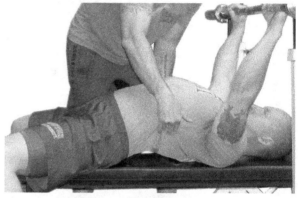

Tactile

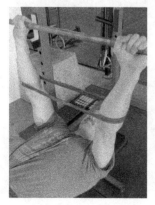

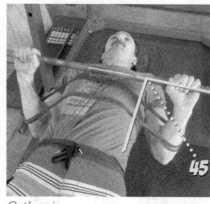

Fault

Orthosis

2. Elbows flare out.

Bench Press Position 2 violation. Upper arms should remain at approximately 45 degrees out from the body. Athlete needs to create external rotation.

 "Snap the bar in half!"

 Demonstrate a proper upper arm angle in BP 2.

 Loop a skinny band about your athlete's arms below the elbow to help him learn to keep his arms from flaring out.

Bench Press Common Faults and Fixes, cont.

3. Incorrect bar path.

Bench Press Position 2 violation. The bar should touch the torso between the xiphoid process and the nipple line. Explain to the athlete whether you want the bar to make contact lower on the chest (toward the feet), or higher on the chest (toward the head).

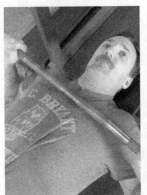 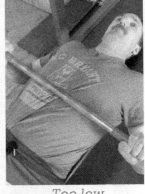

Too high   *Too low*

"Lower!" or "Higher!"

Demonstrate a correct BP 2.

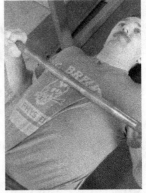

Just right

4. Feet come off floor.

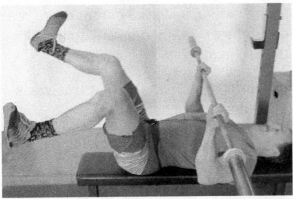

Fault

Bench Press Position 2 violation. This is the classic flailing "dying cockroach", when during maximum efforts feet lose contact with ground, decreasing stability and efficient force production. Emphasize that although the athlete is supine, the feet are still the base of the body. Even if the body is supported by the bench, the heels must be actively driven into the floor to create maximal tension.

"Drive your heels down!"

Demonstrate a correct BP 2.

If athlete's legs are not long enough to reach the floor, place a bumper plate under each foot for him to brace against.

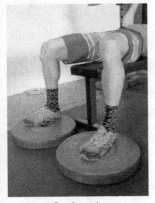

Correct BP 2   *Orthosis*

KIPPING PULL-UPS

Category: Pull to Object (kipping)

Movement screen: N/a

Ability screen: Static hang x 10 sec (kip swing), kip swing x 10 and pull-up x 5 (kipping pull-up), kipping pull-up x 10 (chest-to-bar pull-up)

There are two schools of thought regarding the kipping pull-up. One recommends and teaches a kipping pull-up based on the shoulder extension and flexion of the kip swing, with the body held in a tight hollow position. More traditionally, the kipping pull-up is powered by the extension of the hips, similar to the action of the kettlebell swing. We'll discuss both.

Either way, instruction begins with the kip swing. The kip swing teaches the athlete to maintain a tight, hollow body position while flexing and extending the shoulders. It can also help develop shoulder flexibility and conscious activation of the muscles that stabilize the shoulder. Even those who can't yet do strict, unassisted pull-ups can benefit from learning the kip swing. Beyond being the necessary first step in developing a kipping pull-up, later it will prove foundational to the kipping toes-to-bar and kipping muscle-up. It's worth getting in weeks or months of practice on the kip swing before introducing kipping versions of strict movements—maintaining the rhythm of the swing without "pendulum-ing" back and forth can be quite challenging!

We program kip swing practice as a regular part of our warm-ups. Those athletes too weak and/or overweight to kip swing should continue working on their static hang.

A final note: because the kipping pull-up uses the power of an explosively extending hip to propel the body upward, it's accessible to athletes who lack the strength to perform strict pull-ups. The kipping pull-up is a useful conditioning tool, but it's not a substitute for strict pull-ups! The kipping pull-up puts a huge load on the shoulders, especially during the descent, and if an athlete lacks the strength to do a strict pull-up, he's also missing the stability necessary to buffer those forces. Require your athletes to demonstrate at least five strict pull-ups before allowing them to do kipping pull-ups. A baseline of ten is even better.

Oh, Team Space Monkey? Harry is chomping at the bit to do some kipping. Amy can learn to kip swing, but with only one strict pull-up under her belt, that's as far as it'll go today. Tim can work on his scapular pull-ups and ring rows.

Kip Swing Teaching Script

Here are two methods to teach the kip swing. The first is based on flexion and extension of the shoulder.

"Stand tall with your feet together. Raise your arms straight overhead.

"Press your arms down about four inches. Can you feel your lats activating to extend your shoulders? Reach back up, then press down again until you can. This is the back end of the kip swing, **Kip Swing Position 1 (KS 1)**.

"Now pull your arms back as far as you can. At this point, you should feel a strong stretch through the pectorals, the anterior shoulder, and the biceps. This is the forward part of the swing, **Kip Swing Position 2 (KS 2)**.

"Okay, now hang from the pull-up bar with active shoulders, midline braced, legs straight, feet together.

"Squeeze the bar tightly. Contract your lats to partially close your shoulder joint. Hinged at the shoulder, your torso and legs come forward. This is **KS 1**.

"Keeping your shoulders active, allow yourself to swing forward into an arch. Now your torso and legs point back. This is **KS 2**.

"As you transition from **KS 1** to **KS 2**, allow your hands to relax as they rotate around the bar. Tighten your grip as you return to **KS 1**.

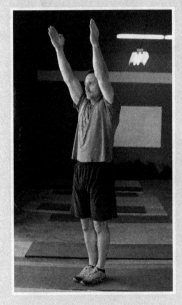 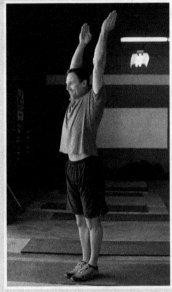

Back swing   Forward swing

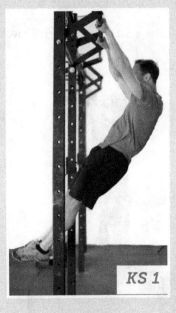 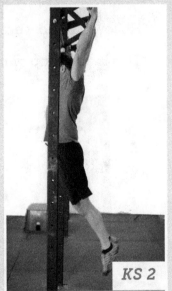

KS 1   KS 2

"Repeat this cycle, each time pushing down a little bit harder on the bar during the back swing. You should start gaining some altitude, with your arms getting closer and closer to parallel to the floor."

The second method is based on two gymnastics exercises: the hollow rock, and the superman.

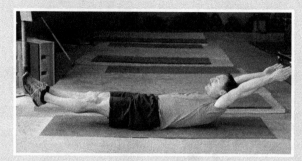

Hollow body hold

"Have a seat on the floor, then lie back. With your feet together, legs straight, arms stretched overhead next to your ears, contract your abdominal muscles hard enough to press your lumbar vertebrae to the floor and lift your feet and hands a few inches off the ground. This position is called the 'hollow body hold'.

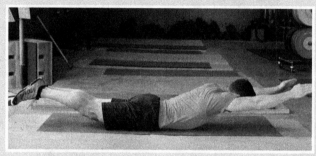

Superman hold

"Keeping your arms and legs out-stretched, roll over on your stomach. On my command 'Go!', I want you to contract all the muscles from your butt to your neck, pulling your arms and legs from the floor. This is called a 'superman'. Ready? Go!

"Now hang from a pull-up bar: pronated grip on the bar with pinky knuckles slightly rolled over, shoulders active, abs on, glutes on, legs straight, feet together, toes pointed.

"Hollow out. Now execute a superman. Hollow! Superman! Hollow! Superman!

"This is also a kip swing."

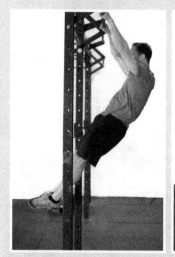 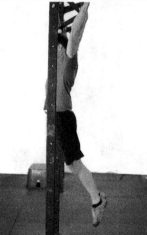 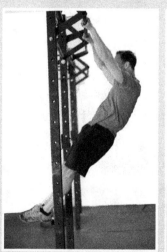 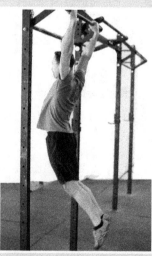

Hollow!	*Superman!*	*Hollow!*	*Superman!*

"Next we'll build on this swing to create the CrossFit-traditional, hip drive-based kipping pull-up."

Kipping Pull-up Teaching Script

"Hang from the bar with active shoulders, midline braced, legs straight, feet together. Imagine you have only one joint: your shoulders.

"Contract your lats to partially close your shoulder joint and swing your torso back and legs forward. This is **Kipping Pull-up Position 1 (kPL 1).**

"Keeping your shoulders active, allow yourself to swing forward into an arch, your legs trailing back. This is **Kipping Pull-up Position 2 (kPL 2)."**

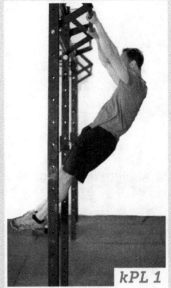 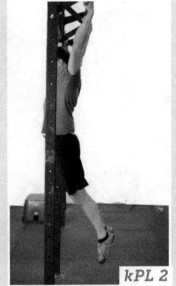

Positional Drills

"1! 2! 1! 2!" Cycle between these two positions, getting a feel for generating momentum while keeping the swing centered on the plane of the bar. Do not hold positions.

"The next step is to introduce, during the back swing of Position 1, a knee raise. This closes the hip slightly. Make sure the knees are bent, with your feet under you. Raising the knees with your legs straight will tilt you backward toward the floor. This is **Kipping Pull-up Position 3 (kPL 3)."**

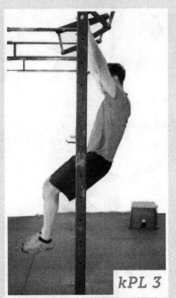 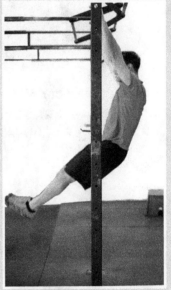

Knees bent: good!   *Knees straight: bad!*

Positional Drills

"2! 3! 2! 3!" Cycle between these two positions, getting a feel for generating momentum while keeping the swing centered on the plane of the bar. Do not hold positions.

"For the next part, we're going to come down off the bar to lie on the floor. We'll practice explosively extending the hip out of **Kipping Pull-up Position 3**.

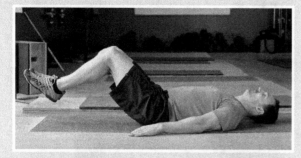

"Get supine. Arms by your sides, legs out straight, feet together.

"Draw your knees toward your hip; stop with your femurs at about 45 degrees. Your feet should be about 6 inches off the floor. This is a good approximation of **Kipping Pull-up Position 3**.

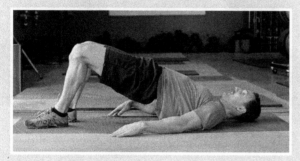

"Aggressively pop your hips toward the ceiling, driving your feet powerfully into the floor. When you're hanging from the bar, this will be **Kipping Pull-up Position 4 (kPL 4).**

"This is how you use your hips to propel yourself toward the bar in a kipping pull-up. Be sure you are not first stomping down your feet and *then* driving your hips up! The action must be initiated by the hip.

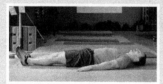 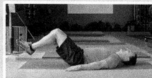 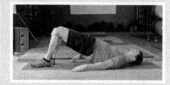

"Back to the bar. We're going to cycle twice between **kPL 1** and **kPL 2** (hollow, arch), then twice between **kPL 3** and **kPL 2** (hollow w/ knees up, arch), then hit **kPL 3** and **kPL 4** in rapid succession. Properly implemented, the 'hip pop' should propel you up toward the bar."

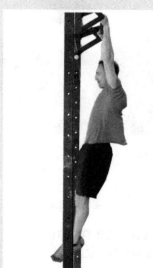 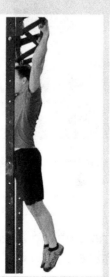 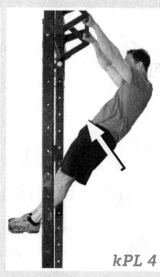

kPL 4

Hollow, arch   *Knees up*   *Pop hips*

Positional Drills

"1! 2! 1! 2! 3! 2! 3! 2! 3! 4!" Kip swing x 2, kip swing w/ knee up x 2, hip pop. Do not hold positions.

"Once you've a feel for the hip pop, add a pull with your arms to get your chin clearly over the bar. Maintain a neutral head position. This is **Kipping Pull-up Position 5 (kPL 5).** Voila! You have a kipping pull-up.

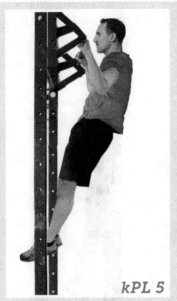

kPL 5

"The last step is, after your pull over the bar, do a push-up off the bar to get yourself back into the swing. This returns you to **Kipping Pull-up Position 1,** alebit with more shoulder extension—let's call it kPL 1(e).

"From here, swing forward into **kPL 2** to cycle the movement."

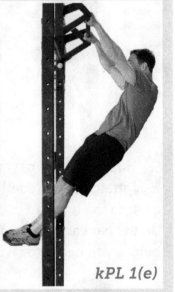

kPL 1(e)

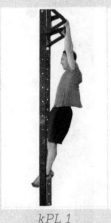 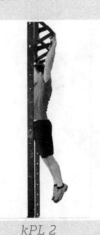 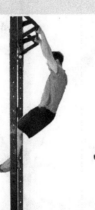 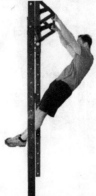 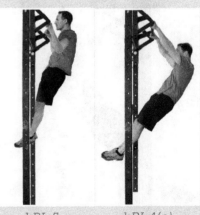

| *kPL 1* | *kPL 2* | *kPL 3* | *kPL 4* | *kPL 5* | *kPL 1(e)* |

Positional Drills

"1! 2! 1! 2! 3! 4! 5!" Initiate with a kip swing, pop your hip and get your chin over the bar.

"1! 2! 1! 2! 3! 4! 5! 1! 2! 3! 4! 5! 1! 2! 3! 4! 5! 1!" Initiate with a kip swing and then do 3 kipping pull-ups. Do not hold positions.

The Gymnastics Kipping Pull-up

The gymnastics version of the kipping pull-up is both simpler and more demanding than the traditional kipping pull-up. It's powered entirely by the kip swing—no hip drive at all.

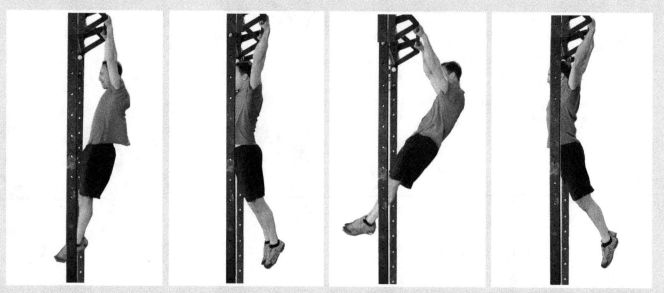

"Hop up on the bar and get organized: pull-up hook grip, active shoulders, midline braced, legs straight, feet together, toes pointed. Initiate a kip swing, your arms and torso/legs pivoting around the fulcrum of your shoulders. Build the amplitude of your swing by pushing down on the bar each time you hollow out. Notice that that there's a split second of weightlessness before you begin to swing forward into the arch. Use that time to regrip.

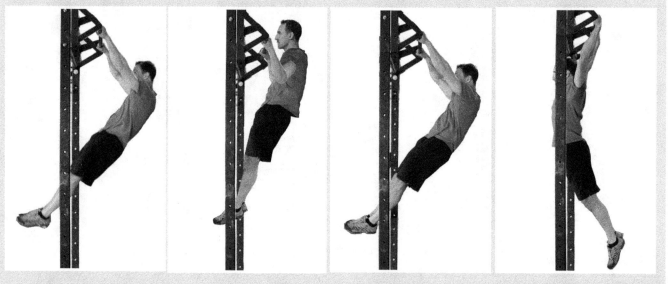

"Try it again. This time, when you feel that brief weightlessness, pull your chin over the bar. Hold that position! You should still be in a tight, hollow body position with toes pointed and head neutral, with your chin clearly over the bar. When your position is correct, forcefully push yourself back to swing forward and down into the arch. Move back into the hollow to cycle. (When cycling, don't hold at the top!)"

The Chest-to-Bar Pull-up

"The chest-to-bar pull-up was introduced in order to make it easier to judge pull-ups in competition. Nothing changes in terms of positions from the kipping pull-up; one simply drives more powerfully with the hip and pulls a little harder with the arms. For the rep to count, the bar must make contact with the athlete's body somewhere south of the clavicles."

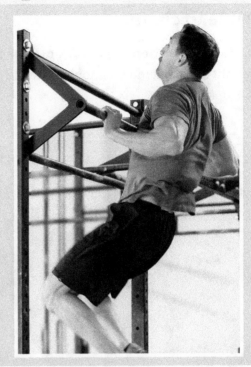

Kipping Pull-up Common Faults and Fixes

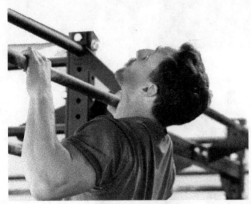

Fault

1. Reaching with chin.

Kipping Pull-up Position 5 violation. An athlete who fails to pull hard enough will throw his head back in an attempt to satisfy the "chin over bar" standard. The athlete should maintain a stable midline with a neutral head position. Cue him to drive his elbows down a little harder; this should provide the necessary extra pulling power to help him hit a proper kPL 5. If he can't do it, have him default to strict or band-assisted pull-ups.

 "Neutral chin!" or "Don't reach!"

 Demonstrate a correct kPL 5.

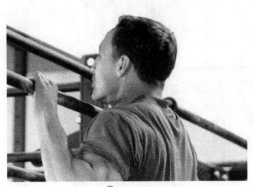

Correct

Kipping Pull-up Common Faults and Fixes, cont.

2. Unable to chain.

Kipping Pull-up Position 1(e) violation. If the trainee doesn't actively push off the bar into kPL 1(e) he'll drop straight down, killing the momentum of his swing and making it impossible to chain together kipping pull-ups.

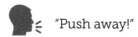 "Push away!"

 Demonstrate a correct transition from kPL 5 to kPL 1(e) to kPL 2.

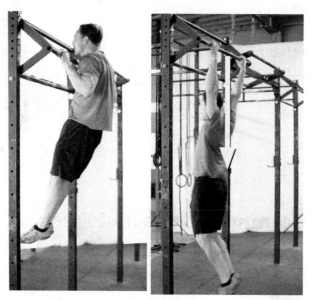

Fault: after completing rep, athlete drops straight down

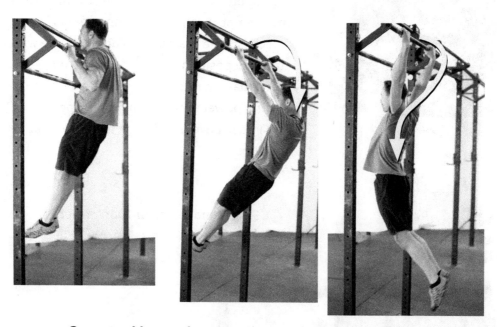

Correct: athlete pushes away to move back into the swing

Kipping Pull-up Common Faults and Fixes, cont.

3. Arms don't straighten.

Kipping Pull-up Position 2 violation. Elbows must straighten completely at the bottom of the pull-up. Shoulders should remain active.

 "Straight arms!" or "Relaxed biceps!"

 Demonstrate a correct kPL 1.

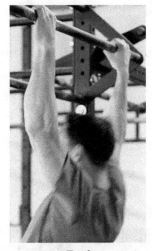

Fault

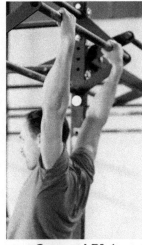

Correct kPL 1

4. Astronaut kip / Pendulum swing.

Kipping Pull-up Position 3 violation. The athlete fails to keep his feet underneath him while raising his knees into kPL 3. Allowing the feet to come up in front throws off the athlete's balance, tilting the him toward parallel to the floor and making what should be a vertical pull, horizontal. From there, he'll then begin to swing like a pendulum from the bar, which will prevent him from stringing pull-ups together.

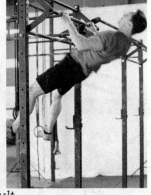

Fault

 "Knees up, feet down!" or "Squeeze your knees together!"

 Demonstrate a correct transition from kPL 2 to kPL 3.

 Block your athlete's legs with your extended arm. He'll kick you a couple times but he'll quickly learn how to keep his feet under himself and his torso vertical as he shifts into kPL 3.

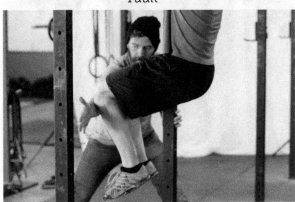

Tactile

Kipping Pull-up Common Faults and Fixes, cont.

5. No hip drive.

Kipping Pull-up Position 4 violation. Sometimes a trainee will have a difficult time figuring out how to fire his hips to help lift himself up to the bar. Instead, he'll swing back and forth, and then do what is essentially a deadhang pull-up to get his chin over the bar.

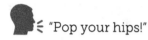 "Pop your hips!" Demonstrate a correct transition from kPL 3 to kPL 4.

Take the athlete back to the floor to repeat the hip drive drill.

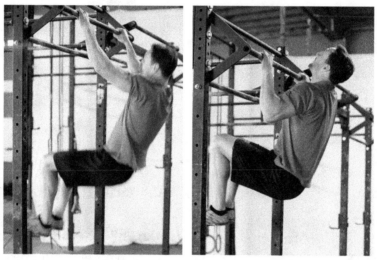

Fault: athlete fails to extend hips, uses arms only

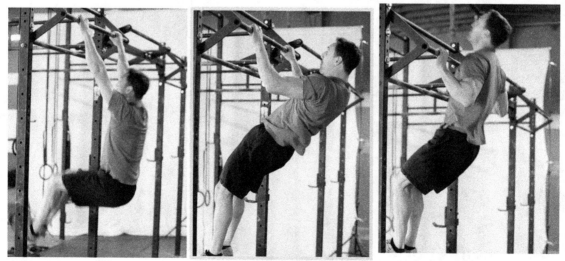

Correct: "snapping" the hip open drive the body upward

Category: Monostructural (run)

Movement screen: N/a

Ability screen: Jumping mechanics x 5

Some people love to run. Some people hate running with the heat of a thousand suns. But either way, if you're going to do MMGPP, you're going to run: blazing 100m sprints, 800m slogs in the middle of long WODs, seemingly endless 5k efforts. So if there's no avoiding it, your athletes may as well do it correctly. And that's going to take some instruction and some practice, because for such a natural movement, running gives the average athlete a lot of trouble. I believe we can blame this on the modern running shoe, which, based on a misunderstanding of the biomechanics of the running gait, encourages bad technique.

When human beings walk, one foot is always on the ground. The leading foot makes contact at the heel, the foot goes flat to support the body's weight as the opposite foot travels forward, and then what was the leading foot—now trailing—rises onto the ball of the foot as the other heel makes contact.

If you conceptualize running as a sped-up form of walking, with higher impact forces due to increased velocity, it would make sense to design a running shoe with a built-up, padded heel. But running is not fast walking. Running is, in fact, a sort of controlled falling forward while hopping from foot to foot. When an athlete is running, only one foot is in contact with the ground at a time, and the athlete spends nearly as much time in the air as he does in contact with the earth. And like the bounce we used for skipping rope, in the running stride the lead leg should impact the ground on the back half of the ball of the foot. This is called a mid-foot strike.

I don't dogmatically insist that all of my athletes adopt a midfoot strike—if someone is an experienced runner and has a heel-striking stride that works well, more power to her. But for non-runners and those complaining of chronic injuries from running, learning the midfoot strike will be a vast improvement over their default motor patterns.

What follows are a few simple drills you can use to get your athletes working on a midfoot strike. This is a quick, fast, and dirty approach; there are seminars you can take, certifications you can earn, that will delve substantially deeper into gait analysis, technique drills, etc. But if your goal is simply to get new athletes running efficiently enough to get the most out of their MMGPP workouts, this progression works well.

No escape, Team Space Monkey! Some will go faster, some slower—but everybody runs today.

Running Teaching Script

"Set up as you would to skip rope: feet under hips, up on the balls of your feet, midline stabilized. Now bounce, leaving the ground an inch or two. Feels pretty good, right? Your ankles and knees do a good job of absorbing the force of your impact on the ground.

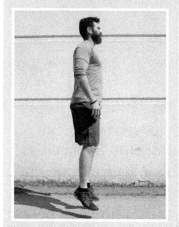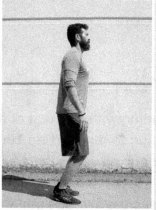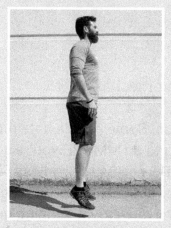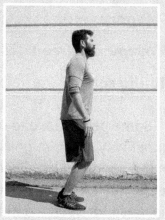

Bouncing on the balls of the feet feels natural.

"Now rest. Get your weight back on your heels...and bounce. What do you think? Kind of sucks, right? You can feel the shock travel up through your legs into your hips and lower back.

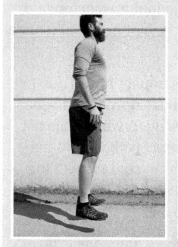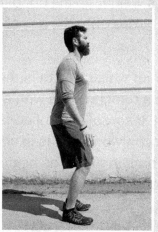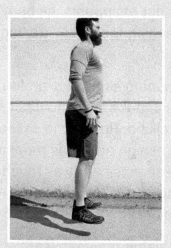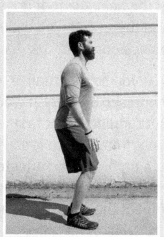

Bouncing on the heels does not. Ouch!

"That's what's happening when you heel-strike during a run. If you need to be further convinced, take off your sneakers and try running around the gym with your usual heel-striking stride. I'd be willing to bet that you won't take more than three or four steps before you shift to what we'll call a mid-foot strike: keeping your heels elevated, your feet will make contact with the ground just behind the ball of your foot, with your toes slightly raised out of the way and your ankles and knees absorbing the impact. This is how the human body has evolved to run.

1. Heel strike zone

2. Mid-foot strike zone

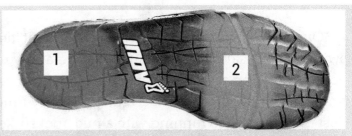

"Let's go back to that bounce. If I start bouncing, and then incline forward just a little bit, I begin to travel. I'm not bunny hopping—that is, I'm not propelling myself forward with my jumps. But as I lean, my torso acquires moment and gravity starts pulling me toward the ground. As soon as I stand vertical again, I stop falling forward. You try it! Bounce three times straight up and down, lean forward and allow yourself to travel for three bounces, then arrest your progress by resuming an upright stance. Travel across the room like that, and then come back. Ready? Go!

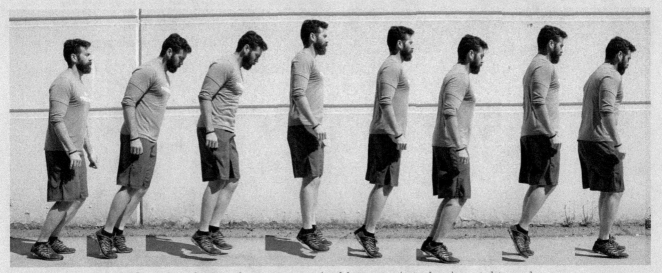

Leaning forward turns a vertical bounce into horizontal travel

"Now we have to learn the 'figure four' position. Engage your hamstring and hip flexor in equal measure to lift your heel until your shin is parallel to the floor, around the height of the knee of your standing leg. The weight of your body is balanced just behind the ball of the supporting foot.

"This is **Run Position 1 (RN 1).** Note that if you just contract the hamstring without sufficient engagement of the hip flexor, you'll draw your heel to your butt, and if you fire your hip flexor without any hamstring, you'll pull your knee to the height of your hip.

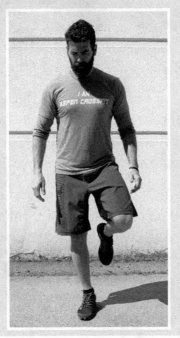
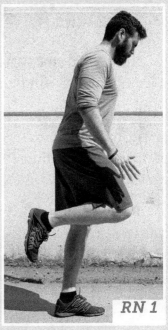

RN 1

271

"Once you've found the right balance and hit 'figure four', try it on the other side. Then keep switching back and forth, gradually accelerating until you are hopping from foot to foot. When you're bouncing at the same speed we practiced earlier, allow yourself to tilt forward and travel, still drawing up the heel and knee every time your weight shifts to your supporting leg. Just like that, you're running with a mid-foot strike!

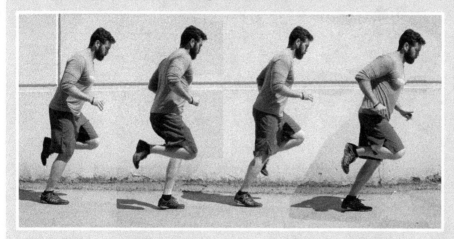

"Remember that every time your foot hits the ground you are landing a jump, so stay up on the balls of your feet. To increase your running speed, simply use the draw of the supporting leg moving toward **RN 2** as a chance to 'pull' at the ground, propelling you forward.

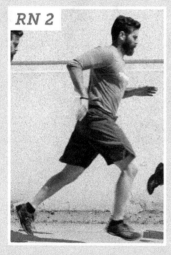

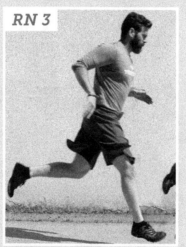

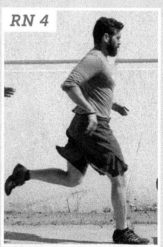

"**Run Position 2 (RN 2)** happens just before the rear foot leaves the ground after the pull. The leading foot is swinging forward.

"**Run Position 3 (RN 3)** sees the runner briefly airborne. The knee of the leading leg has lifted, bringing the shin vertical to the ground. The leading foot is dorsiflexed (toes up) in anticipation of landing. (The example photo shows the runner perhaps a tenth of a second after this ideal pose.)

"**Run Position 4 (RN 4)** has the leading foot making contact with the ground with the ball of the foot, and the trailing leg drawing toward the figure four of **RN 1**.

"So, put very simply, those are the below-the-beltline mechanics of an efficient running stride. But what should be happening above the waist?

"Do your best to keep your midline stable, just as we've practiced with most other movements: glutes on, abs on, shoulders back and down. Concentrate on staying neutral, and it will be easy to avoid leaning back and dampening the efficiency of your stride (and probably giving yourself some serious back pain).

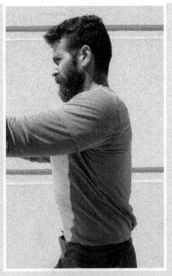 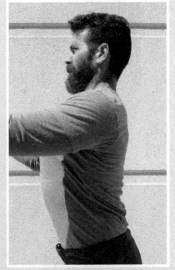

Braced: good!   *Unorganized: bad!*

"Allow your arms to travel forward and back. Keep your elbows to about 90 degrees flexion, fingertips lightly touching your thumb. As your arm travels behind your body, slightly internally rotate it (that is, turn your thumb in toward your centerline), and conversely, as it travels in front, slightly externally rotate it (thumb away). Resist the impulse to rotate your torso back and forth.

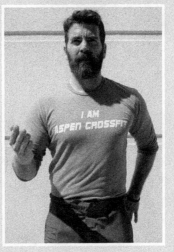 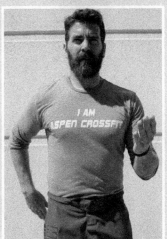

"The last thing I'd like you to keep in mind is that the positions of the run do not change, whether you're pacing yourself through a 5k or sprinting 100m. Foot strike, torso lean, and arm swing all stay the same. Simply increase the cycle time to go faster."

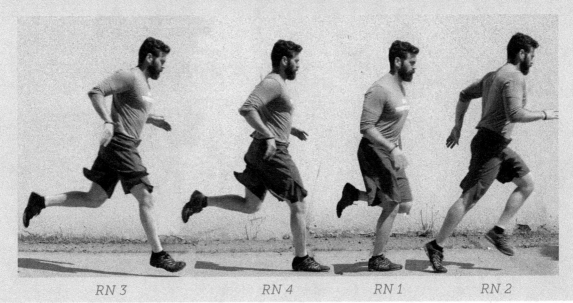

RN 3   RN 4   RN 1   RN 2

Running Common Faults and Fixes

1. Slapping the ground.

Running Position 3 violation. Athlete lands on his heel, the rest of his foot smacking the ground afterward.

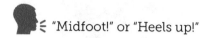 "Midfoot!" or "Heels up!"

 Demonstrate a correct transition from RN 3 to RN 1.

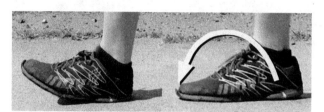

Fault: heel strokes first, then foot slaps down

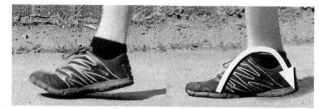

Correct RN 3: foot makes contact just behind ball of foot and heel eases down

2. The Tom Cruise (leaning backward).

Global position violation. Athlete must lean forward in order to take advantage of the "controlled fall" of an efficient running stride. Often leaning back is caused by inadequate engagement of the abs.

 "Abs on!" or "Six pack!"

 Demonstrate a correct RN 1

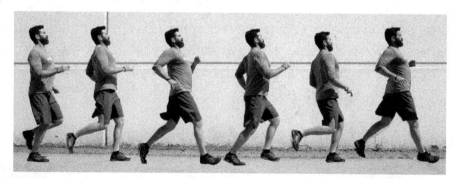

Leaning back is inefficient. Running is a controlled falling forward.

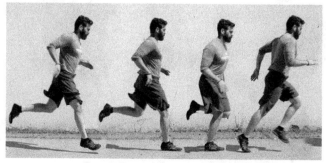

Correct running sequence

Running Common Faults and Fixes, cont.

3. Center of gravity does not rise (speed walking).

Running Position 2 violation. Heel strikers are prone to a kind of sloshing shuffle that is little more than speed walking. Remind your athlete that the run is a sort of continuous forward jump. If his center of gravity does not rise and then descend on every stride, if his feet are not briefly out of contact with the ground, he is not really running.

 "Drive up off your toe!" or "Get some air!"

 Demonstrate a correct transition from RN 1 to RN 2 to RN 3.

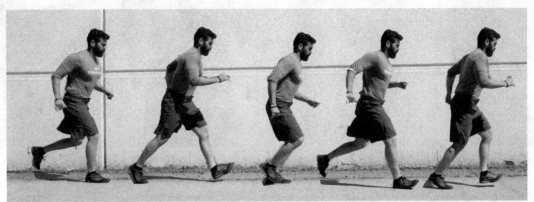

If you don't get airborne on every stride, you're speed walking, not running.

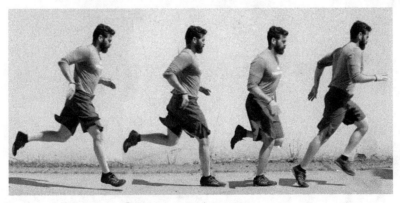

Correct running sequence

Running Common Faults and Fixes, cont.

4. Rotating from the hips.

Global position violation. When running, the athlete should maintain a stable and neutral midline. The arms must travel back and forth to counterbalance the legs, but the torso should remain facing forward, not rotating left and right on the mediolateral axis.

 "Abs on!" or "Arms only!"   Demonstrate a correct arm swing for the run.

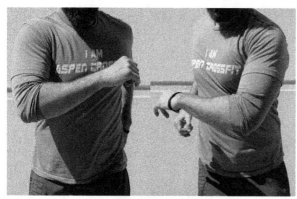

Fault: torso rotates on axis, arms swing across body

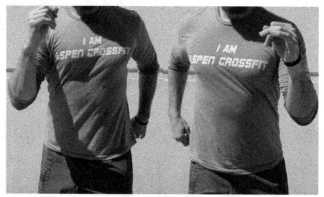

Spine should remain rotationally neutral, with arms swinging forward and back

THE KETTLEBELL SWING

Category: Kettlebells

Movement screen: Deadlift Position 2 test (Russian swing), supine shoulder flexion test (American swing)

Ability screen: N/a (Russian swing), Russian swing x 5 (American swing

The two-handed kettlebell swing comes in two varieties: Russian and American. Both are built on the hinge, a rapid flexion and extension of the hip that causes the 'bell, held with relaxed arms, to rise. The Russian-style swing brings the 'bell to about the height of the chest/chin. It's the basis of the one-handed swing, the kettlebell clean, and the kettlebell snatch.

The American swing brings the kettlebell straight overhead, which nearly doubles the distance it travels when compared to the Russian swing, and requires (theoretically) more power to be produced by the hip on every swing. Because the American swing puts a high demand on the athlete's shoulder flexion, it is not appropriate for some athletes.

Athletes should master the Russian swing before attempting to go overhead.

Harry's missing shoulder flexion, so he'll be confined to the Russian swing. Amy's swung kettlebells in her bootcamp classes, so hopefully she'll get to try the American version. And Tim...oh, Tim. Tim's rDLs are improving, but he doesn't have a full deadlift yet. I'm going to teach him the Russian swing, but I'll probably have to rig an orthosis so he can safely take the kettlebell from the floor.

Russian Swing Teaching Script

"Stand tall. Put two fingers in the crease of each hip.

"Unlock your knees, then push your hips back until your torso is about 135° to the ground. Your shins should remain perpendicular to the ground. Now stand.

"Hinge and stand again. This is the basic action of the swing. It's not a pelvic thrust—you are not sending force forward. You are driving your head toward the ceiling.

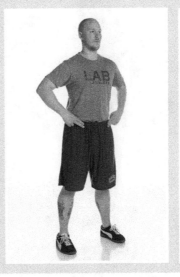
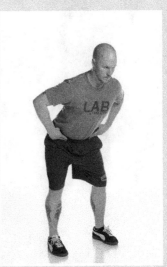

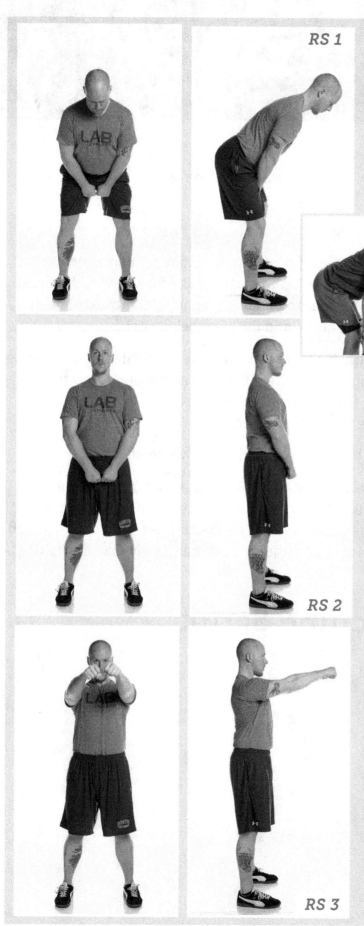

RS 1

"We're going to learn the positions of the swing with an imaginary kettlebell. Stand tall, with a shoulder-width stance. Grip the floor with your toes. Brace your midline. With arms straight, bring your fists together. Hinge back, drawing your fists back between your thighs. This is **Russian Swing Position 1 (RS 1).**

"Notice the similarity to **Deadlift Position 2**—the shins are vertical, the knees bent, the back angle virtually the same.

"Stand straight up, squeezing your butt and your abs so that you don't overextend the spine. Your hands should be in front of your groin, with your elbows tucked into your sides. At this point, the power generated by the rapid acceleration into extension of knee and hip has yet to fully transfer to the 'bell. This is **Russian Swing Position 2 (RS 2).**

RS 2

"Raise your arms until your hands are about in line with your chin. Keep your arms relaxed. Keep your shoulder blades partially retracted. This is **Russian Swing Position 3 (RS 3).**

RS 3

278

"Drop your hands to return to **RS 2.** When you feel your upper arms on your ribcage...

"Hinge back to **RS 1.**"

| RS 1 | RS 2 | RS 3 | RS 2 | RS 1 |

Positional Drills

"1! 2! 1! 2!" Have your athlete practice the hinge and stand. Make sure the knees bend but do not come forward in the hinge. This drill can also be performed with the kettlebell to get a feel for how the hip "pop" can make the kettlebell "float."

"1! 2! 3! 2! 1!" Practice the positions of the Russian swing one at a time, making corrections as necessary.

Hiking the Kettlebell into Play

"Now set a light kettlebell on the floor 6" in front of you.

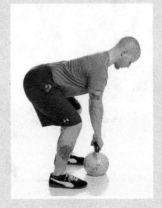
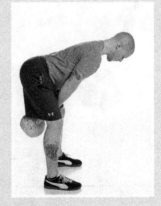

"Screw your feet into the floor, brace your midline, and set your shoulders back and down.

"Keeping your arms straight, hinge back and then bend your knees until you can grasp the kettlebell handle. Try to snap the handle in half by rotating your thumbs away from your face.

"To initiate the swing, hike the kettlebell back between your legs by driving up your hips and pulling back with your arms. Then stand up aggressively. The force of your hip extension will swing the 'bell forward and up. If you are using a heavy kettlebell, you may need to do a half-swing to get the bell moving before you can safely execute a full swing.

"Allow the bell to fall back all the way into **RS 2** before hinging back into **RS 1**. As you exhale sharply, aggressively drive up through **RS 2** to **RS 3**. The bell will feel weightless for a split second; use this time to reset your midline bracing. Make sure your abs support your back during the kettlebell's descent. When you've completed your set, return to **RS 1**, and then, keeping your back straight, bend your knees to return the kettlebell to its initial position, the 'hike'.

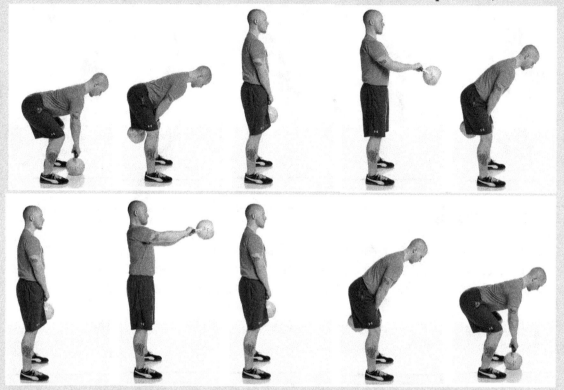

American Swing Teaching Script

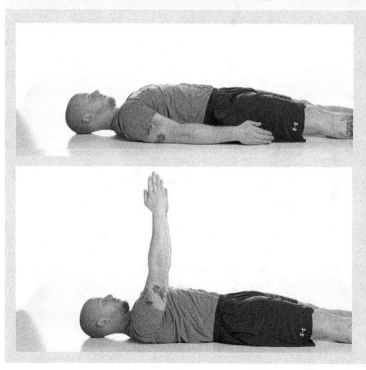

Many trainees will lack the shoulder ROM to execute the American swing safely. Here's how to figure who should (and shouldn't) practice the American swing.

"Have a seat on the floor. Now lay back, arms by your side, legs straight, feet together. Lift your arms until they are perpendicular to the floor. Seat your shoulders back and down.

"Strongly contract your abs to pull your ribcage toward your pelvis.

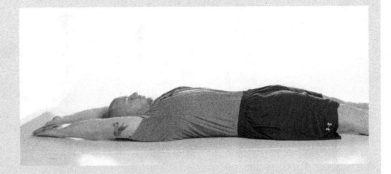

"Now bring your arms overhead until your hands touch the floor. If they can touch the floor, try to put the back of your hands on the floor and then bring your hands together.

"If you can accomplish this without surrendering a neutral midline (that is, without your ribs lifting), you have the flexibility necessary to perform the American swing safely.

"However, if you can't get your arms to the floor, or must lift your chest to do so, you should stay with the Russian swing until you've developed better mobility.

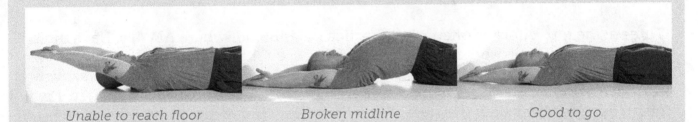

Unable to reach floor   *Broken midline*   *Good to go*

"The American swing adds a fourth position to the three positions of the Russian swing, which are now **American Swing Position 1 (AM 1), American Swing Position 2 (AM 2), American Swing Position 3 (AM 3).**

"With your midline braced, two-hand press a kettlebell straight overhead. Fists should be over shoulders over hips over heels. Squeeze the handle of the kettlebell tight, and try to snap it in half by rotating your thumbs back. This is **American Swing Position 4 (AM 4).**

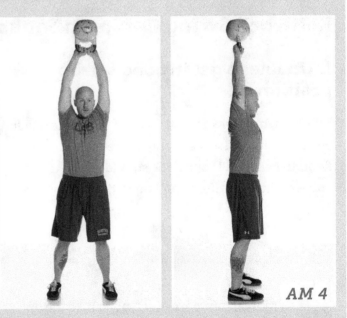

AM 4

"Allow your arms to fall back through **AM 3** and **AM 2**.

"Hinge back into **AM 1**, and snap the hips forward to send the 'bell back overhead.

"For the American swing, we begin with the same hike-and-half-swing that we used to initiate the Russian swing. The half-swing is even more important now, as it's not advisable to try to swing a heavy kettlebell overhead from a dead stop on the floor. Overcome inertia in stages."

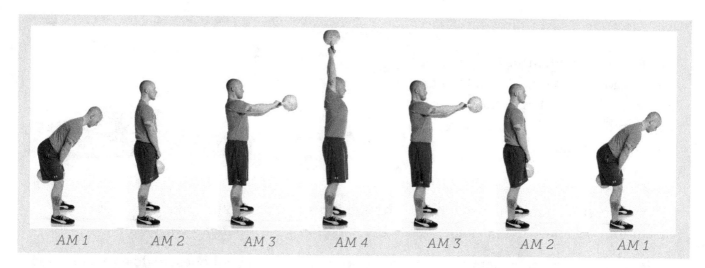

AM 1   AM 2   AM 3   AM 4   AM 3   AM 2   AM 1

Positional Drills

"1! 2! 3! 4! 3! 2! 1!" Drill all four positions without a kettlebell.

"Three at the top." Athletes often need practice to figure out where **AM 4** is. Have them press a light kettlebell overhead with two hands, hold for a count of three before allowing it to drop, then swing it back overhead for another three count. This is a great way to groove a good pattern and memorize a correct finish position. Make sure they don't initial the hinge back until they feel their upper arms contact their ribs.

Kettlebell Swing Common Faults and Fixes

1. Unable to get in good set-up position.

Athletes who have difficulty setting up for the deadlift will have similar issues taking the kettlebell from the floor: the back will round, the shoulders will droop, and weight will shift forward on to the balls of the feet.

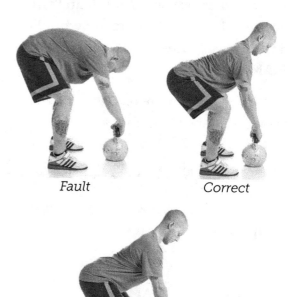

Fault   Correct

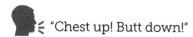 "Chest up! Butt down!"

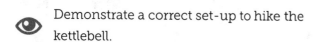 Demonstrate a correct set-up to hike the kettlebell.

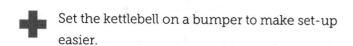 Set the kettlebell on a bumper to make set-up easier.

Orthosis 1

282

Kettlebell Swing Common Faults and Fixes, cont.

2. Bad pick up/put down.

Set-up violation. An ahlete who may have no flex-ibility issues affecting his set-up may still pick up or put down the kettlebell with a rounded back out of sheer carelessness. Remind him he can get hurt put-ting down a weight improperly just as easily as he can picking it up.

 "Chest up!" or "Hike it!" or "Angry gorilla!" and demonstrate that the correct pick up position looks alot like the stance of a silverback gorilla.

 Demonstrate a correct pick up and put down.

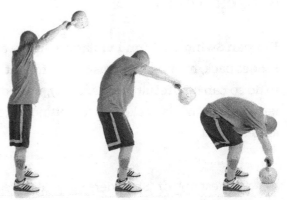

Bad put down (reversed: worse pick up!)

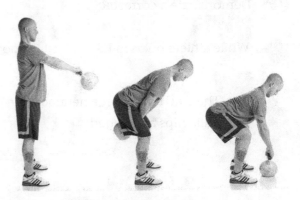

Good put down

3. Two-handed Snatch

American Swing Position 3 violation. In an effort to go faster, some athletes abbreviate the swing by pulling the kettlebell straight up. As Jeff Martone says (roughly), "Whatever it is, it's not a swing." Call it a two-handed kettlebell snatch and save it for competitions, when cutting corners is okay. To get the best training ROI, arms must remain straight throughout the swing, with the path of the bell an arc.

"Straight arms!" or "Long arc!"

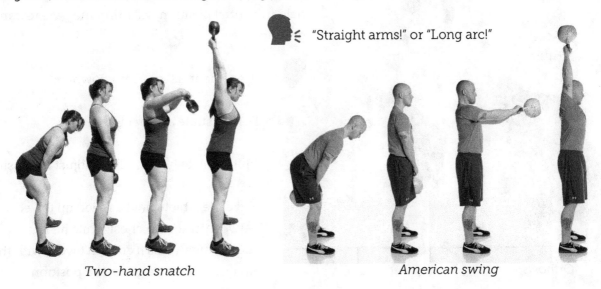

Two-hand snatch   *American swing*

Kettlebell Swing Common Faults and Fixes, cont.

4. Back rounds.

Russian Swing Position 1 violation. As the athlete hinges back, he must keep his spine straight. Failure to do so can be a result of inflexibility, neglecting to keep the shoulders packed, or forgetting to keep the abs engaged.

 "Chest up!" or "Shoulders packed!" or "Abs on!"

 Demonstrate a correct RS 1.

 While athlete holds in RS 1, adjust his position.

 Use "The Tail" to reinforce neutral spine position while hips are hinged.

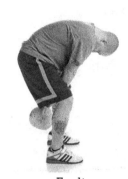
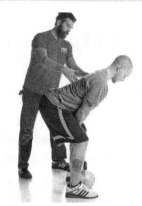

Fault   *Tactile*

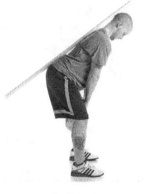
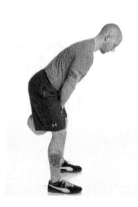

Orthosis   *Correct RS 1*

5. Heads up!

Russian Swing Postion 1 violation. At the bottom of the swing, the athlete cranes his neck to keep his gaze directed forward. The neck is part of the spine, and should stay in line with the spine. With the hips hinged back and the torso leaning foward, a head held in neutral position will bring the gaze toward the ground.

 "Head neutral!" or "Chin down!"

 Demonstrate a correct RS 1.

 While athlete holds in RS 1, adjust his position.

 Have the athlete hold a rolled up towel between chin and chest while he Russian swings. (This fix doesn't work with the American swing's overhead position.)

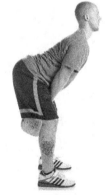
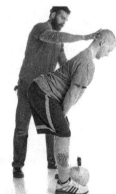

Fault   *Tactile*

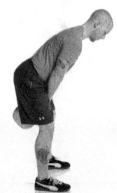

Orthosis   *Correct RS 1*

Kettlebell Swing Common Faults and Fixes, cont.

6. Squatting the swing.

Russian Swing Position 1 violation. The most common error I've seen is powering the swing with a knee bend rather than a hip hinge. On the downswing, the athlete will bend his knees and allow them to come forward over his toes, putting slack on the hamstrings and robbing himself of the potential force generated by a posterior chain drawn into tension.

 "Hips back more!" or "Shins vertical!" or "Knees don't come forward!"

 Demonstrate a correct RS 1.

Stand to athlete's side and place the back of your hand in front of his knee while he is standing. Tell him, "Don't touch my hand!" and have him swing until he moves correctly.

Place two utility benches about 12-18" apart (depending on size of trainee). Have him set up with his knees touching the benches, then practice his swing. If he tries to send his knees forward, the benches block them.

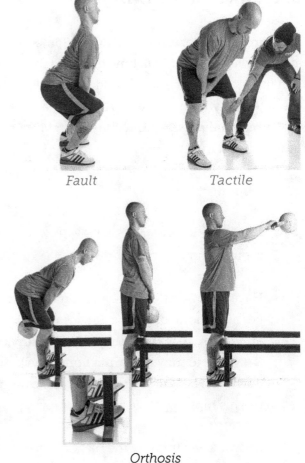

Fault   *Tactile*

Orthosis

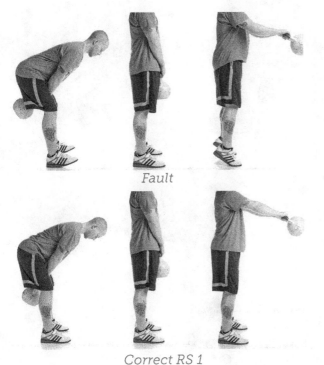

Fault

Correct RS 1

7. Foot rocking.

RS 1 violation. On the back swing into RS 1, the weight transfers back onto the heels, and the toes rise off the ground. In RS 2, the weight shifts forward onto the balls of the feet, and the heels lift. Feet should remain flat on the floor, with weight planted just in front of the heel.

 "Feet flat!" or "Grip the floor with your toes!"

 Demonstrate a correct transition from RS 2 to RS 1 to RS 2.

Kettlebell Swing Common Faults and Fixes, cont.

8. Frankenstein swing.

Russian Swing Position 2 violation. Sometimes an athlete will have a difficult time grasping the idea that the hips drive the swing, and insist on lifting the kettlebell with his arms, maintaining a consistent arms-straight-out-from-the-body stance as he hinges and stands.

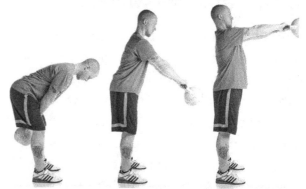

Frankenstein swing sequence

 "Hips first!"

Demonstrate correct RS 1, RS 2, RS 3 sequencing.

Have the athlete execute a swing with the upper arms tight to the ribs. If necessary, tie the arms in place with a lifting belt or skinny band! Only able to move his arms from the elbows down, the athlete will quickly figure out how to use his hips to get the kettlebell moving.

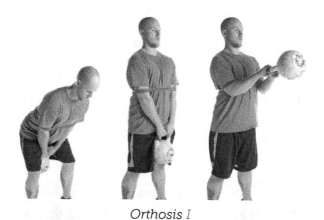

Orthosis I

Loop a towel through the handle of the kettlebell. Have the athlete grasp the ends of the towel close to the kettlebell handle. Then have him practice the Russian swing. He'll quickly realize that if he tries to lift the 'bell with his arms, it will hang straight down. Allow him to experiment until he figures out how to get the 'bell to float.

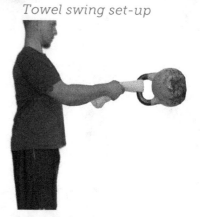

Towel swing set-up

Orthosis 2: Towel swing

Kettlebell Swing Common Faults and Fixes, cont.

9. Kettlebell does not go overhead.

American Swing Position 4 violation. While getting the kettlebell completely overhead is probably not necessary from a training perspective, it *is* necessary when we are establishing standards for CVFMHI as competition and sport. The "Three at the Top" positional drill can be very helpful here, as the athlete takes the time to familiarize himself with the correct overhead pose.

 "More hip!" or "Pull back at the top!"

 Demonstrate correct AM 4.

 Hold your hand over your athlete's head and tell him to hit it with the kettlebell.

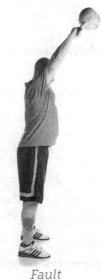

Fault

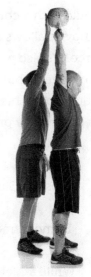

Tactile

10. Bent arms.

American Swing Position 4 violation. Athlete holds 'bell overhead with soft elbows. As the kettlebell swings overhead, elbows should be fully extended. The "Three at the top" Positional Drill is an effective correction.

 "Straight arms!"

 Demonstrate a correct AM 4.

 While athlete holds in AM 4 adjust his position.

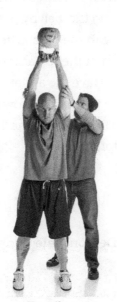

Fault

Tactile

Kettlebell Swing Common Faults and Fixes, cont.

11. Ship's figurehead.

American Swing Position 4 violation. As the bell rises, the athlete throws his torso into a forward lean, exaggerating the extension of his spine until he looks like the figurehead on the prow of a ship. This fault allows the athlete to put more weight overhead than he could with a correct swing; the extra distance the hips travels allows a longer period for the production of force. It's also way of cheating ROM; the 'bell is not fully overhead, but by throwing himself forward, he manages to get his arms behind his ears, thus fulfilling a commonly prescribed point of performance.

 "Abs on! Glutes on!" or "Stand up straight!"

 Demonstrate a correct AM 4.

 While athlete holds in AM 4 adjust his position.

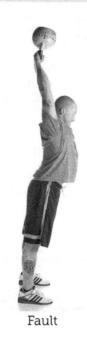

Fault

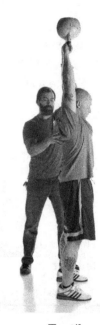

Tactile

12. Kettlebell droops.

American Swing Postion 4 violation. During the swing, the 'bell should align with the extended arms. If the kettlebell hangs toward the ground, the athlete is elevating the 'bell by pulling with the arms rather driving with the hips. Often this happens because the extension of the hip as it travels from AM 1 to AM 2 is too slow. Have the athlete work through AM 1 and AM 2 until he figures out how to "snap" the hips to create power. The "Three at the Top" positional drill can be very helpful here.

 "Straight bell!" or "Bell points away!"

 Demonstrate a correct AM 4

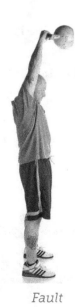

Fault

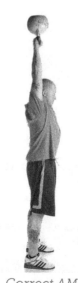

Correct AM 4

Now three weeks into our idealized intro program, our trainees have begun to accrue some of the tools required for some more technically challenging workouts. We're going to keep it relatively simple for one more week, though. Did I say simple? What I meant was, *Simply brutal*. This week, our crew is going to take on "Streisand".

"Streisand" consists of intervals of 19 pull-ups, 29 push-ups, 39 sit-ups, and 49 squats alternating with three minute rests. This sequence repeats for four more cycles, yielding a total volume of 95 pull-ups, 145 push-ups, 195 sit-ups, and 245 squats. Ideally, each round should take three minutes or less to complete, yielding a roughly 1:1 work/rest ratio.

Customizing "Streisand" for Athletes of Varying Ability Levels

Prescribing Correct Movement Complexity

This week I had the opportunity to take our trainees through a formal progression toward the kipping pull-up. Harry, who already had kipping pull-ups, if of a wild and ad hoc variety, very readily picked up our more compact and efficient technique. It remains to be seen, though, if he'll be able to keep moving well as he heads into the later rounds of "Streisand" and fatigue challenges his form. Push-ups, sit-ups, and squats will be no problem, although I'll keep a bumper plate ready in case his feet start turning out.

Amy surprised us all (including herself!) by getting her first strict pull-up last week. Today she has the option of doing band-assisted pull-ups or piked ring rows. She decides to go with the band-assisted pull-ups. I give her a 1" band and set her up with a box tall enough that she can put her foot in the loop without too much trouble. As a back-up, I set up a pair of rings. If she tires to the point she can do less than ten pull-ups in the allotted interval, I'll have her default down the hierarchy to the next most complex movement: the piked ring row. Push-ups necessitate another decision: fewer push-ups with less assistance (12" box) or more push-ups with a 20" box? As long as she can crank out at least 10 push-ups per effort, she can work off the shorter box. For sit-ups and squats, she's good to go.

I think Tim is ready for an upgrade or two. Today he'll be doing ring rows, push-ups on the floor, feet-anchored sit-ups, and air squats.

Prescribing Correct Volume

The reality is that most of your athletes will not be able to accomplish a round of "Streisand" in three minutes, at least not consistently. Someone like Harry may complete the first round in less than 3 minutes, but you can pretty much count on his last rounds being closer to five. And less experienced athletes may needs 5-6 minutes just to complete the first round! As commonly practiced, "Streisand" can take forty minutes or more.

That's not the intended stimulus of this workout. But when faced with group of athletes of varying abilities, how do figure out, in a timely fashion, a volume of exercise that will take them about three minutes? The solution is structuring "Straisand" like this:

"By the Numbers Testing 'Streisand'"

AMRAP :30 of pull-ups. If you get to 19 pull-ups before time is up, move on to...
AMRAP :40 of push-ups. If you get to 29 push-ups before time is up, move on to...
AMRAP :50 of sit-ups. If you get to 39 sit-ups before time is up, move on to...
AMRAP :60 of squats. If you get to 49 squats before time is up, rest.
Rest for three minutes, and then complete for a total of five cycles.

If an athlete can complete his first round in under three minutes, he rests for three, and then starts his next, always trying to stay ahead of the clock. For example, if he finishes his first round in 2:31, he starts his next at 5:31, etc. An athlete who can consistently stay ahead of the clock and complete every round will record a time to completion somewhere under 27:00—a very good score for "Streisand".

The average athlete will end up accruing W pull-ups before the call for "Push-ups!" comes at the 30 second mark, X push-ups before it's time to move on to sit-ups, Y sit-ups in the allotted time, and Z squats before three minutes is up. He'll record how many reps of each movement he got within the time allotted, and after three minutes rest, he'll go again.

Harry and Amy will both do this version.

Tim is not at a point where he needs to be thinking about the clock. He's still working on con-sistently demonstrating sound mechanics. But after three weeks, I'm ready to start upping the volume a bit. I assign him five rounds of 6 ring rows, 8 push-ups, 10 sit-ups, and 12 squats. He's to take his time and perform his reps as perfectly as he can. When he finishes his squats, he'll rest exactly 3 minutes, and then start again.

"3...2...1...GO!"

Harry

Harry finished his first round of "Streisand" in 2:51. That's super impressive! He started his next round at 5:51, and this time, his form on the kipping pull-ups deteriorated, and he started having trouble stringing them together. At 6:30, the cut-off point for pull-ups, he had just dropped off the bar after completing his last rep. He finished round two just under the wire at 8:58. In round three, which he started at 11:58, he continued to struggle with the kip, and was only at 13 pull-ups the clock hit 12:30—oh well, time to shift to push-ups. Because he failed to complete all the assigned work for the round, after his squats, I brought him back to starting with the group, and asked him to switch back to strict pull-ups. Why? Because his kipping pull-ups looked terrible! He had totally reverted to his prior bad habits. Following BtN, because he was messing up a complex movement, I had him default to a simpler movement he could do well, one that preserved the desired stimulus—in this case, "Pull to Object (vertical)".

When time was called at 27:00, he had a score of 74 pull-ups, 140 push-ups, 200 sit-ups, and 237 squats. With a little more time and seasoning, this kid will CRUSH this workout, of that I'm sure.

Amy

Amy was able to stay with band-assisted pull-ups all the way through the workout. After round two I had her switch from the 12" box to the 20" box for her push-ups. When the smoke cleared she had racked up 61 pull-ups, 85 push-ups, 140 sit-ups, and 182 squats.

The skeptic might ask, "61 pull-ups? That's it?" Well, what of it? What makes 95 a magic number? 95 pull-ups is not a necessary or appropriate amount of volume for the average trainee anyway. Working at her highest intensity on band-assisted pull-ups, the reps Amy totaled in five sets of thirty seconds is exactly the right volume for her...today. She hit red line intensity in a carefully circumscribed manner. Next time she'll get more—*because she'll be ready for it.*

Tim

As expected, Tim was able to complete his work in the assigned time. He seemed surprised and gratified when the rest of the group included him in their congratulatory fist bumps, given that he had been taking his time with the workout, but Amy and Harry recognized that Tim was working at what was, for today, exactly the right intensity for him. He put out, just the way they did. Still, later he pulled me aside and said, "That was very good. But next time, I want to go against the clock, too."

And therein lies the magic of MMGPP.

Category: Push Object (vertical)

Movement screen: N/a (no formal movement screen, but if your trainee is lacking shoulder flexion, approach the push press with care)

Ability screen: Press x 5

By turning the press into a core-to-extremity (that is, force generated by a powerful extension of the hips before amplified by the actions of the limbs) movement, the push press allows the athlete to put more weight overhead by harnessing the power of the explosively extending hip. It's a great developer of "finishing" strength, as the triceps must work to fully lock out the elbow under a greater load than the strict press imposes, and it's a necessary step toward learning the push jerk.

Teach the barbell push press only to those trainees who've demonstrated competence with the strict press. If the trainee doesn't have the flexibility to finish the press in a correct overhead support position, it doesn't make any sense to ballistically load that limited range of motion with a barbell. With that in mind, Amy should have no problems with the push press. Harry can lock out a press correctly, but his so-so flexibility makes it difficult; I'll keep an eye on him today. Tim, who cannot yet hit a good overhead support position, will keep strict pressing his dumbbells.

Push Press Teaching Script

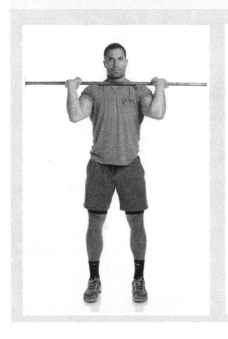
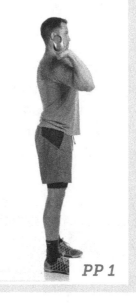

PP 1

"With a light barbell, begin in your press set-up position: feet under the hips, midline braced, bar held with a full-fist grip just outside the shoulders. Raise your elbows until your upper arms are about at about 45 degrees relative to the ground. Push your shoulders up; ideally, the bar is sitting on top of your deltoids, rather than on the sternum. This is **Push Press Position 1 (PP 1)**.

"The push press is a 'core to extremity' exercise, in which hip extension provides the initial impetus. This requires the shoulders provide a stable platform for the bar, so that the force generated by the hip can be efficiently transmitted. The problem here is that the way we've learned to close the hip—hinging back—inclines the torso forward, potentially causing the bar to slide off.

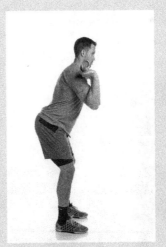

Hinging back causes the bar to slide off shoulders.

"To flex the hips without changing back angle, stand with the weight in the heels, squeeze your glutes tightly, and push your knees out so that your pelvis drops 2-4" directly over the heels. Imagine you are standing with your glutes and shoulder blades against a wall, maintaining continuous contact as you descend. The bar should be lined up over the front of the heel. This is **Push Press Position 2 (PP 2)**.

"Pushing through the heels, return to **PP 1**.

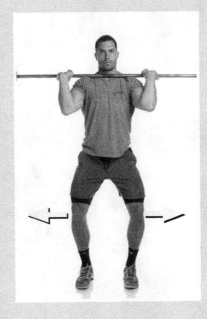

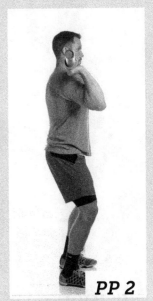

PP 2

"Now, pull your head back (sexy double chin!) and push the bar up in front of your nose. You may remember this as Press Position 2, but for our purposes now, this is **Push Press Position 3 (PP 3)**.

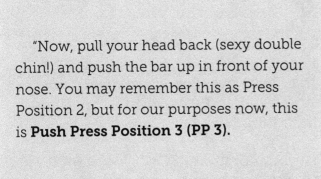

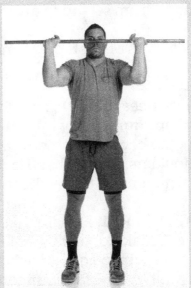

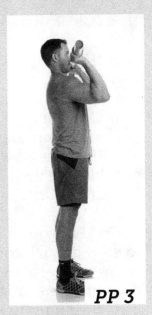

PP 3

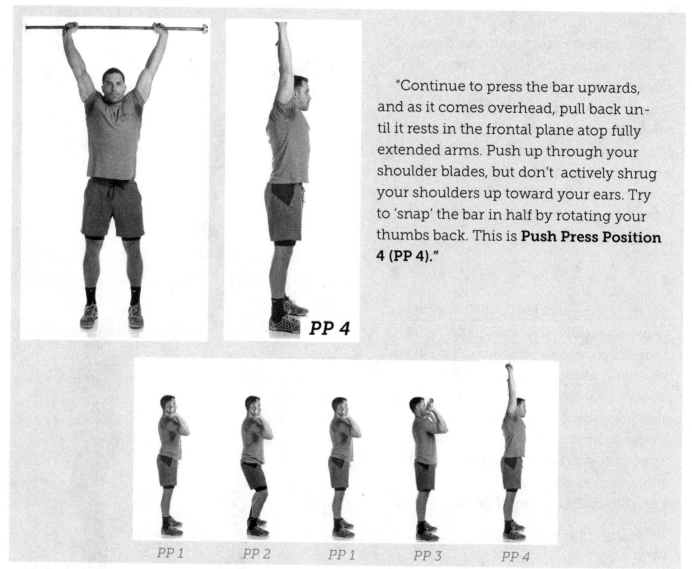

"Continue to press the bar upwards, and as it comes overhead, pull back until it rests in the frontal plane atop fully extended arms. Push up through your shoulder blades, but don't actively shrug your shoulders up toward your ears. Try to 'snap' the bar in half by rotating your thumbs back. This is **Push Press Position 4 (PP 4)**."

PP 4

PP 1   PP 2   PP 1   PP 3   PP 4

Positional Drills

"1! 2! 1! 2!" Drill transition from set-up to dip, emphasizing vertical torso in PP 2.

"1! 2! 1! 3! 4! 1!" Drill positions of push press one at a time, making corrections as necessary.

"1! 2! Go!" Bring your trainees from **PP 1** to **PP 2**. Explain that on your command "Go!", you want them stand up aggressively into **PP 1** and then immediately execute **PP 3** and **PP 4**. They are not to begin pressing until they have stood up completely. They should drive their shoulders into the bar! Have them wait in **PP 4** for your command "Reset!" or "One!", at which point they will return to **PP 1**.

"1! Go!" Put your trainees in **PP 1**. Explain that on your command "Go!", you want them to draw down into **PP 2**, making the descent into the dip smooth and controlled. As soon as they hit **PP 2** they are to aggressively rebound through **PP 1** into **PP 3** and **PP 4**, where there are to wait in **PP 4** for your command "Reset!" or "One!", at which point they will return to **PP 1**.

As trainees progress with the push press, they will eventually put loads overhead that are too heavy for them to lower under control. If you wish, you can begin now to train them how to receive heavy loads on the shoulders safely.

How to Reset a Heavy Push Press

"Eventually the push press will allow you to put overhead loads in excess of 120% of your strict press max. This makes coming back to **Push Press Position 1** problematic, as the weight will be too heavy to lower under strict control. Instead, you'll do a controlled drop onto the shoulders, with your hips and knees absorbing the impact.

"Start in **Push Press Position 4**: bar overhead, lined up in the frontal plane, elbows locked, shoulders torqued, glutes and abs locked.

"Lower the bar to **Push Press Position 3**: bar halfway down to the shoulders, head back, and continuing to try to 'snap' the bar in half.

"Receive the bar on the shoulders and immediately sit down into a 1/4 front squat: elbows high, hips hinged back, knees out, midline braced. The squat decelerates the bar and eventually (in the space of a second) brings it to a halt. Stand to reset."

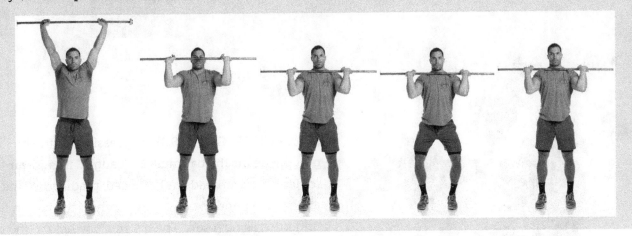

Dumbbell Push Press Teaching Script

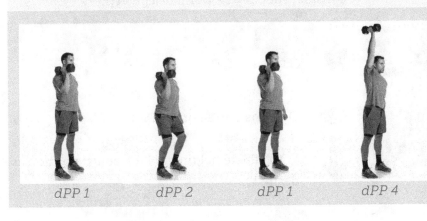

dPP 1   dPP 2   dPP 1   dPP 4

"The db push press is a dumbbell press powered by the dip and drive of Positions 1 and 2 and finishes in **dPP 4**. **dPP 3** is omitted because there's no need to pull the head back out of the way."

Push Press Faults and Fixes

1. Bad rack position

Push Press Position 1 violation. It's common for athletes to mistakenly set up for the push press as they would for the press (full fist, elbows low) or the front squat (bar back on fingertips).

A. LOW ELBOWS. The elbows should be elevated until the forearms are at about 45 degrees.

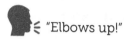 "Elbows up!"

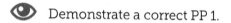 Demonstrate a correct PP 1.

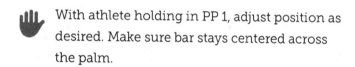 With athlete holding in PP 1, adjust position as desired. Make sure bar stays centered across the palm.

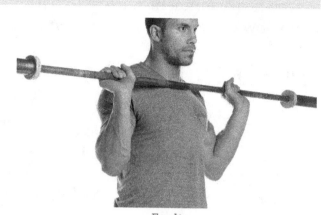

Fault

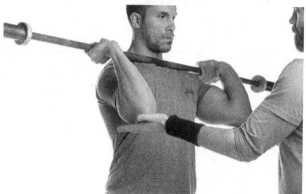

Tactile

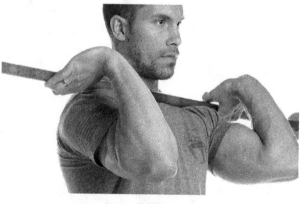

Fault

B. BAR ON FINGERTIPS. Push pressing off the fingertips means the bar must be "caught" in mid-air for lockout overhead, and at speed, predisposes the athlete to a hand sprain as he "catches" the bar on his fingertips as he resets. The bar must be held in the fist as much as possible. If the athlete can't hold the bar in his palms and elevate his elbows at the same time, consider subbing the dumbbell push press.

 "Full fist grip!"

 Demonstrate a correct PP 1.

 With athlete holding in PP 1, adjust position as desired.

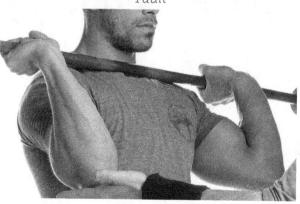

Corrrect PP 1

Push Press Faults and Fixes, cont.

2. Hinge back/forward lean during dip.

Push Press Position 2 violation. Athlete inclines torso forward in dip. May be caused by sitting back rather than pushing knees out; also, descending too low, so that the dip turns into a partial squat.

 "Knees out!" or "Butt tight!" "or "Slide down the wall!" or "Too low!" as appropriate.

 Demonstrate a proper PP 2.

 With athlete holding in PP 2, adjust position as desired.

Place a piece of PVC against the trainee's back, making contact with shoulder blade and butt. Have him dip down 2-4", making sure to maintain contact at both points. Another alternative is to have him practice his dip/drive with his back against a wall (see **Fault #4, "Leaning Back."**

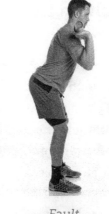
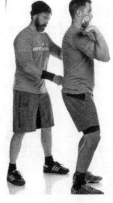

Fault *Tactile 1*

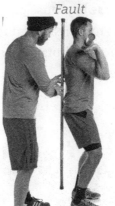
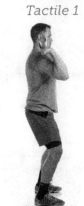

Tactile 2 *Correct PP 2*

3. Hyperextended lumbar during dip.

Push Press Position 2 violation. Very flexible athletes can maintain a vertical thoracic spine while still hinging back at the hip, which causes the lumbar spine to overextend. These athletes must be reminded to not only squeeze the glutes but to lock rib cage down toward the pelvis by contracting the abs as well.

 "Abs on!" or "Six pack!"

 Demonstrate a proper PP 2.

 With athlete holding in PP 2, karate chop him in the gut to remind him to keep his abs tight. That'll show him! I kid, I kid. Just give him a tap, with the verbal command, "Abs on!"

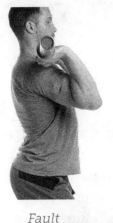
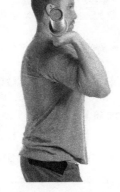

Fault *Correct PP 2*

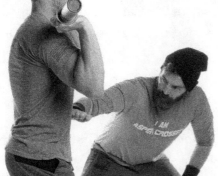

Tactile

Push Press Faults and Fixes

4. Leaning back, pushing from toes (muted hip function).

Push Press Position 2 violation. Some athletes have a difficult time maintaining a neutral pelvic position as they descend in the dip—the pelvis stays in line with the femurs instead of the spine. This often results in the weight shifting forward onto the balls of the feet. This is problematic for a couple of reasons: 1) it means relying on the quads extending the knee to produce force, rather than the big muscles of the posterior chain extending the hip, greatly reducing potential force production, and 2) it puts unnecessary compressive strain on the lower back.

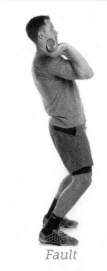
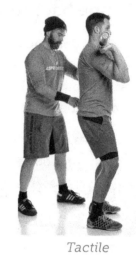

Fault　　　　*Tactile*

 "Compress on heels!" or just "Heels!"

 Demonstrate a correct PP 2

 With athlete holding in PP 2, adjust position as desired.

 Have athlete stand with shoulder blades and butt to the wall and practice transition from PP 1 to PP 2 and back by sliding down and up the wall.

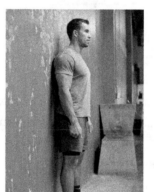
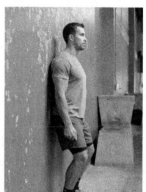

Orthosis

5. Pressing too soon.

Push Press Position 1 violation. Accelerating into PP 1 from PP 2 transfers to the bar the force generated by the extending hip. If the bar is not seated directly on the shoulders, efficiency is compromised; holding the bar off the body essentially turns the arms into a spring system that dampens the energy transfer. In this instance, the "1! 2! Go!" Positional Drill is very helpful.

 "Drive your shoulders into the bar!"

 Demonstrate proper transition from PP 2 to PP 1.

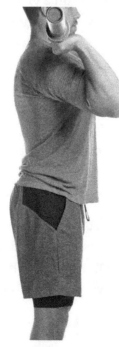

Fault　　　　*Correct PP 1*

Push Press Faults and Fixes, cont.

6. Ship's figurehead.

Push Press Position 4 violation. The cue "Head through!" is problematic. If the trainee thrusts his head "through the window", he will often end up on the hyperextended position pictured here. The athlete needs to be stacked in a straight line: load over shoulders over hips over knees over the front of the heel.

 "Abs and glutes lock in!" or "Stand straight!"

 Demonstrate a proper PP 4

 With athlete holding in PP 4, adjust position as desired.

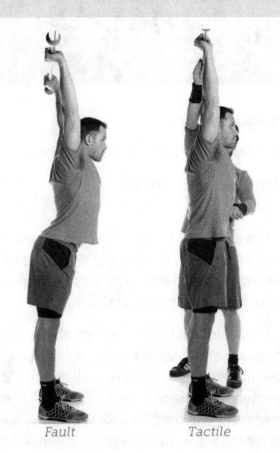

Fault   *Tactile*

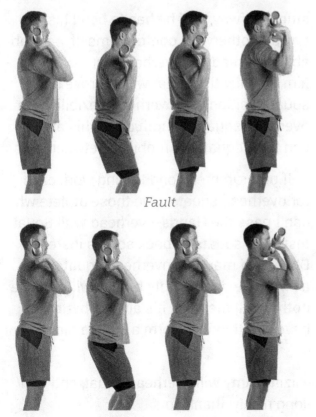

Fault

Correct PP 2 to PP 1 transition

7. Elbow droop in drive.

Push Press Position 1 violation. As athlete drives up out of PP 2, his elbows drop to point straight at the floor. This decreases the stability of the bar sitting on the shoulder. He must maintain upper back tension to keep elbows high, and use Valsalva to ensure stiffness of the torso. The "2! Go!" Positional Drill is useful here.

 "Tight back!" or "Elbows high!" or "Big breath!" as appropriate.

 Demonstrate a proper PP 2 to PP1 transition.

 With athlete holding in PP 2, adjust position as desired.

OVERHEAD SQUATS

Category: Squat

Movement screen: Hands-overhead Wall Squat Test

Ability screen: Front squat x 5

The overhead squat increases the challenge of the front squat by elevating the load to arm's length overhead. It is a great developer of midline strength, and is the foundation movement for the snatch. It requires a flawless air squat with a very upright torso, as well as a great deal of shoulder flexibility and stability.

Those unable to keep an upright torso while squatting, or who may have a good squat but lack adequate shoulder flexion, should not be forced to overhead squat. Here's a simple test: have your athlete stand facing a wall about 1" away from his toes. Have him put his arms straight overhead, one hand over the other, with thumbs turned back slightly. If he can squat below parallel without crashing into the wall, he is good to go. If he can't, let him back up a few inches and try again (some athletes' anthropometry will forbid a toes-to-wall squat, anyway). If he gets stuck halfway, or if he has to bend his elbows or otherwise contort himself, he probably isn't ready to overhead squat. Teach him mobilizations that will improve his squat position and overhead flexibility. On overhead squat strength days, this athlete can front squat and mobilize between sets.

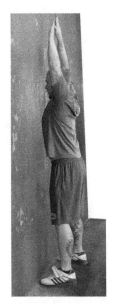 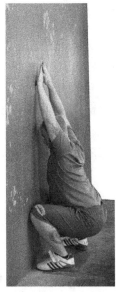 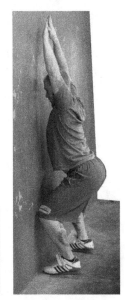

Start here   *Good to go*   *Stuck? Uh oh!*

If programmed conditioning work calls for overhead squats, give those athlete who can't pass the Hands-overhead Wall Squat test front squats or back squats instead. Dozens of mangled overhead squats with a PVC pipe or an empty barbell will achieve nothing. Remember, it's always better to have an athlete perform a simple movement well than a more complex movement badly.

That means today Harry is front squatting and mobilizing, Amy will overhead squat, and Tim will work on his dumbbell squats, which are coming along nicely, thank you.

Overhead Squat Teaching Script

"Start with PVC dislocates. With a wide grip, raise the pipe with straight arms, shrugging your shoulders as it passes overhead. Without bending your elbows, touch the small of your back with the bar, then return to starting position. Each time you successfully pass through, move the hands a little closer. The 'sticking point' you can just barely get through without bending your elbows is the grip width you should use for the overhead squat. A wider grip would inhibit stability in the shoulders. A narrower grip would make it difficult to 'bail out' forward in the event of a missed lift.

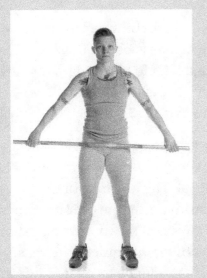 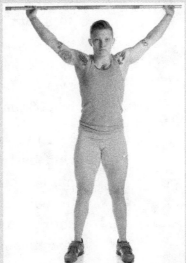 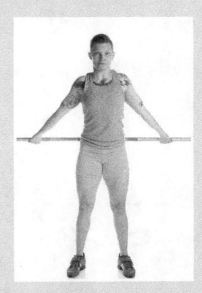

The "sticking point" is a good indicator of optimal OHS grip width.

"With your grip established, place the bar behind your neck, on top of the traps. Push it straight up to arms' length. The bar is now in the frontal plane, congruent with the line of gravity. Let the bar fall back slightly on your wrists, and try to 'snap' it in half by rotating your thumbs back. Brace your midline by locking in your glutes and abs, and with your feet in your normal squat stance, screw them into the floor. This is **Overhead Squat Position 1 (OS 1),** the start and finish of every repetition.

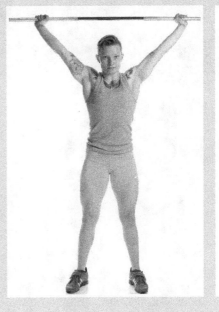 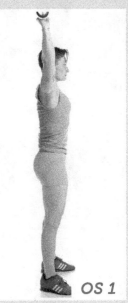

OS 1

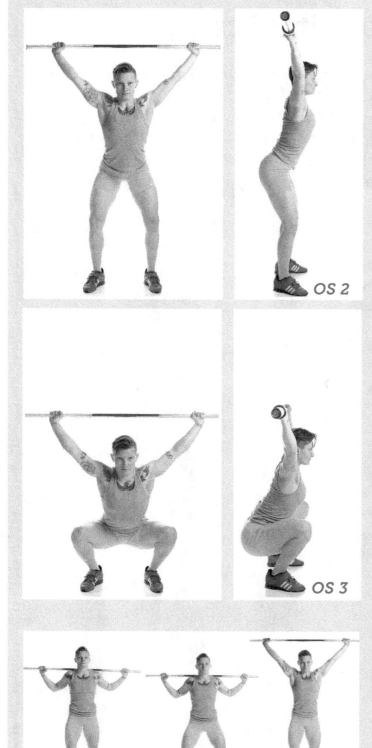

OS 2

OS 3

Snatch Push Press sequence. To set up for the overhead squat, take the bar out of the rack and snatch push press it into OS 1.

"Unlock your knees. Sit your hips back, but keep your torso as vertical as possible. Push your knees out. This is **Overhead Squat Position 2 (OS 2).**

"Sit straight down between your heels, until the hip crease is below the knee. The overhead load should be lined up directly over the front of the heel. This is **Overhead Squat Position 3 (OS 3).**

"In the overhead squat, moving the load with 'best leverage' and 'best efficiency' is mission critical. The distance of the load from its fulcrum point (the ground under your center of mass) means any deviation from the line of gravity quickly increases 'moment', or a tendency to rotate toward the ground. The bar must move straight down and straight up, remaining in or just behind the frontal plane, for the lift to be successful.

"When overhead squatting out of the rack, the set-up procedure is similar to setting up for the back squat. Take a wide grip on the bar. Try to 'snap it in half'. Duck underneath the bar and position it securely on the traps as you get in a well-organized partial squat. Step the bar up out of the rack. Once the bar has been walked out, it must be snatch push pressed or snatch push jerked (from behind the neck) into place. Run your standard set-up checklist (feet screwed into the ground, glutes and abs on 100%, big breath, employ Valsalva technique) and then squat."

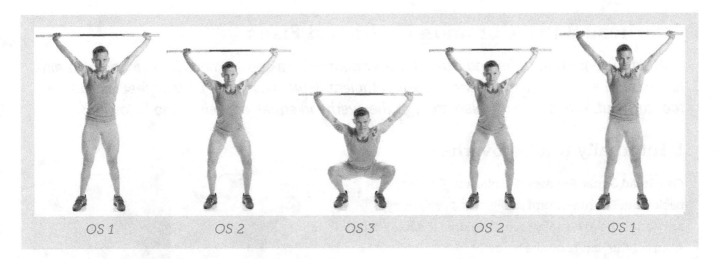

OS 1   OS 2   OS 3   OS 2   OS 1

Positional Drills

"1! 2! 3! 2! 1!" Take athletes through each position of the overhead squat. Have them hold each position while you make necessary adjustments.

"1! 2! 3! Go!" Bring athletes into bottom position and make necessary corrections; when they look good, on your command "Go!", they return to OS 1.

"Five in the hole." This is "1! 2! 3! Go!" with a five second hold in the bottom position.

Bailing Out of the Overhead Squat

"Occasionally excessive load or a lack of concentration can result in a missed lift. For bailing out of an overhead squat, the rule is: DON'T ARGUE WITH THE BAR. If it wants to go forward, by all means, let it fall forward, and step back out of its way. If the bar starts going back, simply allow it to, basically performing a dislocate as we practiced at the beginning of instruction, and rapidly stepping or hopping forward to get out of danger. DO NOT USE SPOTTERS!"

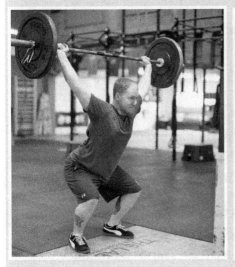
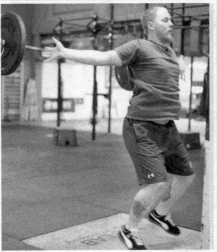
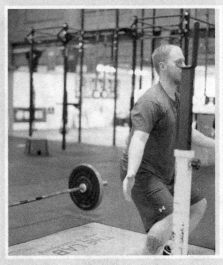

Overhead Squat Common Faults and Fixes

All of the common faults and fixes of the air squat—breaking at knees first, unable to maintain neutral spine, spinal overextension, insufficient depth, weight on balls of feet, excessive foot turn out, knees cave in—also apply to the overhead squat, as well as the following:

1. Internally rotated overhead.

Overhead Squat Position 1 violation. Elbows point backward. For maximum stability and efficiency, arms must be externally rotated against the fixed position of the hands on the barbell.

 "Show armpits!" or "Break the bar in half!"

 Demonstrate a correct OS 1.

 With athlete holding in OH 1, turn her arms so that the point of her elbows are facing forward.

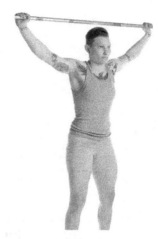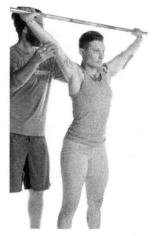

Fault   *Tactile*

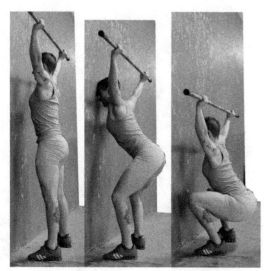

Fault   *Tactile*

2. Excessive forward lean

Overhead Squat Position 3 violation. A squat with a torso angle that might be acceptable for a low bar back squat will put the shoulders in an unstable and possibly unsafe position in the overhead squat. I included this as it *is* a common fault, but if your athlete can pass the OH wall squat test, it's unlikely she'll display it.

 "Chest up!" or "Pull the hips in!"

 Demonstrate a correct OS 3.

 While athlete holds in OS 3 adjust her position, pushing down on hip and bringing the bar forward. Block hips with your knee to provide stable fulcrum.

 Have athlete practice squatting with nose to the wall and pipe overhead. Sticking point hold applies as in the Hands Overhead Wall Squat Test.

Start.   *Stuck.*   *Good.*

304

Overhead Squat Common Faults and Fixes, cont.

3. Bar too far forward.

Overhead Squat Position 3 violation. For maximum stability and efficiency, the barbell must located as close as possible to the line of gravity throughout the action of the squat.

 ""Pull back on the bar!"

 Demonstrate a correct OS 3.

 While athlete holds in OS 3, adjust her position. Block hips with your knee to provide stable fulcrum.

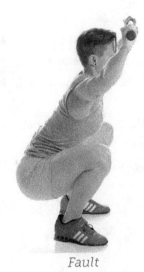

Fault

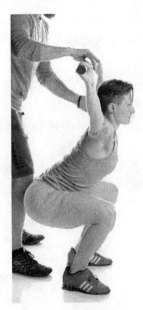

Tactile

4. Bar too far back.

Overhead Squat Position 1 violation. If the trainee has some forward lean in the bottom of her overhead squat, she'll need to pull back on the bar to keep it in the line of gravity. If she continues pulling back on the bar as she stands back up, she'll finish with the bar too far behind her. Remind her that in OS 1, the bar in her hands should be stacked over the shoulders over the hips over the front of her heels.

 "Bar forward!"   Demonstrate a correct OS 1   While athlete holds in OS 1 adjust her position.

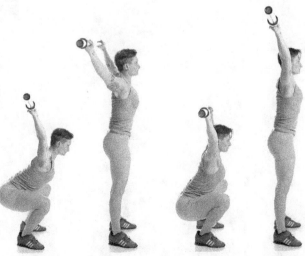

Bad: bar is returned behind line of gravity. Good: bar returned in line of gravity.

Overhead Squat Common Faults and Fixes, cont.

5. Soft elbows.

Global positional variation. Bar must be held over-head with arms locked straight. Under any but the most minimal load, bent elbows will mean a missed lift.

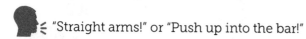 "Straight arms!" or "Push up into the bar!"

👁 Demonstrate a correct OS 1, 2, or 3.

✋ With athlete holding in OS 1, 2, or 3, push elbows in and up to straighten them.

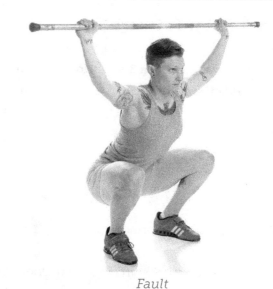

Fault

Tactile

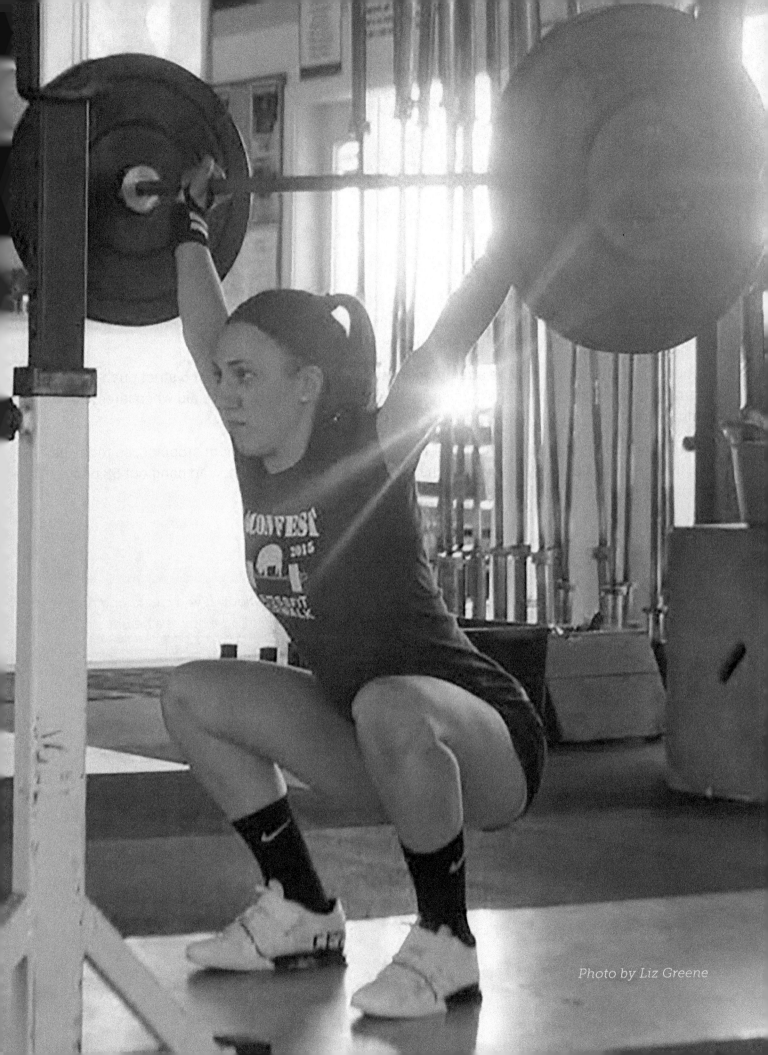

Photo by Liz Greene

Category: Push Away from Object (horizontal)

Movement screen: N/a

Ability screen: Push-up x 5

The ring push-up adds challenge to the traditional push-up by forcing the athlete to stabilize his body while supporting himself in a frictionless plane.

Ring push-ups should only be attempted by athletes who can do at least 5 strict push-ups. Learning to stabilize on the rings in push-up position will be an invaluable aid when later attempting ring dips.

Tim has turned out to have a talent for push-ups! He can do 18 without stopping, so today he can try ring push-ups. Amy will work on her strict push-ups. Harry, who can bang out 58 push-ups in one minute, is good to go.

Ring Push-up Teaching Script

Begin with a pair of rings set about 18-20" apart and 2-4" off the floor. If you can't hang rings that low due to strap length limitations, have your athlete set his feet on a box at a height sufficient to bring his body to standard push-up body angle when he is set up.

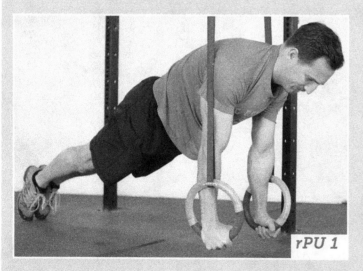

"Take a thumbs-around grip with arms inside the rings and assume a strong plank position. Hands should be slightly turned out, the right to about 1 o'clock, the left to 11. Rather than curl your toes under, with your feet firmly together, balance on your pointed toes with the insteps of your feet facing the floor. Glutes and abs should be strongly engaged to create a hollow body position. This is **Ring Push-up Position 1 (rPU 1)**.

"Lower yourself until your elbows are higher than your shoulders. Your forearms should be vertical. Your body should still be in a straight line from toe to shoulder. This is **Ring Push-up Position 2 (rPU 2).**

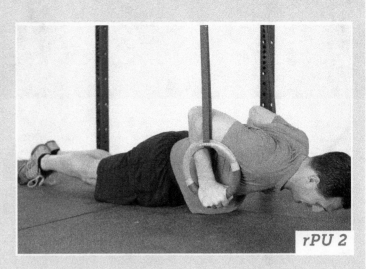

rPU 2

"Still screwing your hands into the rings, push to return to **rPU 1.**"

Ring Push-up Common Faults and Fixes

All of the common faults and fixes of the push-up—insufficient depth, incomplete lockout, sagging or piking at the hips, elbows flaring out or collapsing in—also apply to the ring push-up, as well as the following:

1. Rings turn in.

Ring Push-up Position 1 and 2 violation. The athlete must work continually to maintain a stable shoulder position. As soon as the rings begin to turn in toward the body, the elbows begin to flare out and the shoulders to internally rotate, causing inefficiency due to loss of torque and eventual injury due to impingement.

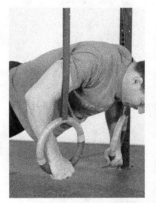
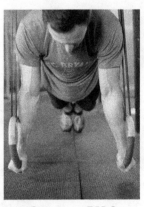

Fault   Correct rPU 2

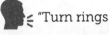 "Turn rings out!"   Demo correct rPU 1.

2. Rings come away from body

Ring Push-up Position 1 violation. Rings must remain directly under the shoulders. Pectoral tension is required to keep them in position.

 "Squeeze your chest!"

 Demo correct rPU 1.

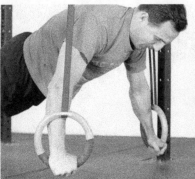

Fault   Correct rPU 1

HIP EXTENSIONS

Category: Hip and Trunk Extension

Movement screen: N/a

Ability screen: Good morning x 5 with 20/15kg barbell

The hip extension develops the athlete's ability to extend the hips while maintaining a neutral spine. Loaded up, this exercise is an excellent developer of posterior chain strength.

The ability screen for hip extensions is being able to do 5 good mornings to parallel with the floor using an empty barbell. Harry and Amy pass it without a problem. Tim is not able to bend that far without starting to round to his back, so today he'll keep working on good mornings.

Hip Extension Teaching Script

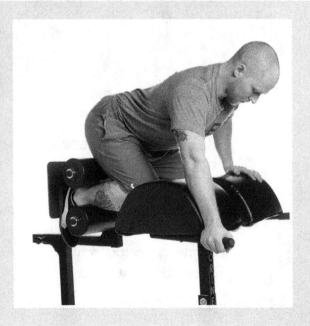

"Climb up onto the GHD bench. Facing the floor, fit your lower legs legs between the foot anchor pads and press your feet against the back plate.

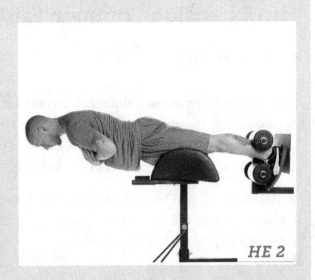

"The foot anchor assembly of the GHD bench should be set at a length that puts your thighs atop the pad, with your hips out in front, as you set up with your body prone and parallel to the floor. Your midline should be strongly braced. Hands can crossed at the chest, touching the temples, or held behind the head. This is **Hip Extension Position 2 (HE 2).**

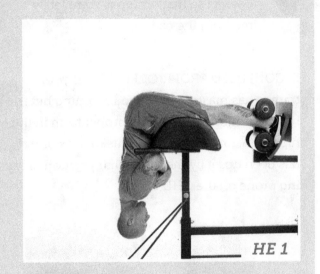

"Maintaining a neutral spine, bend the hips to lower your torso until the top of your head is pointing at the floor. Free of the restriction of the pad, the pelvis moves in line with the spine. This is **Hip Extension Position 1 (HE 1).**

"To return to **HE 2**, squeeze your glutes, pressing your thighs hard into the pad. Make sure you keep your abs as engaged as possible to support your back."

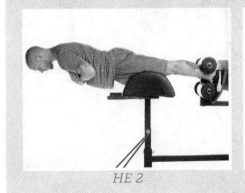

HE 2

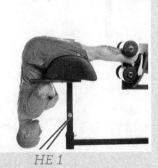

HE 1

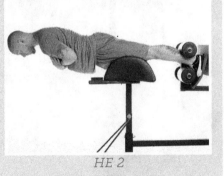

HE 2

Positional Drills

"1! 2! 1!" Practice the positions of the hip extension one at a time, with your trainees holding the pose while you make necessary corrections. Make sure your athletes maintain a neutral midline.

Hip Extension Common Faults and Fixes

1. Back rounds

Hip Extension Position 1 violation. To perform the hip extension, the athlete must keep his back straight throughout the movement. There are a couple possible causes preventing correct execution.

A. INCORRECT SET-UP. If the foot-anchor is set too far back, the pad will block his torso as he attempts to pike, causing his back to round.

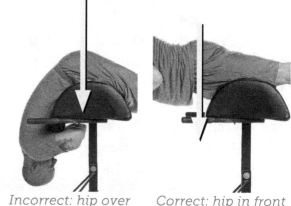

Incorrect: hip over bench　　*Correct: hip in front*

 Make sure the athlete has set up the foot rest so that his hip is completely free from the pad.

B. CONFUSED PROPRIOCEPTION. If your trainee has mastered the good morning but is having trouble maintaining proper form in the hip extension, it's likely that his motor control has been upset by the unfamiliar position of lying prone on the GHD bench.

 "Chest up!" or "Shoulders back and down!"

 Use Good Morning Positions 1 and 2 to demonstrate hip flexion and extension with a neutral spine.

 With the athlete in HE 2, adjust his back. Don't let him surrender back tension as he lowers into HE 1.

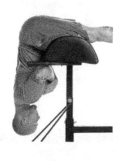 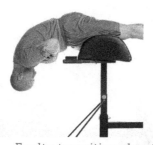 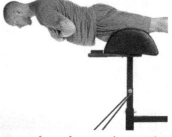 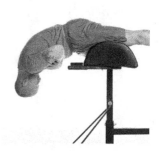

Faulty transition due to confused proprioception

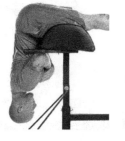 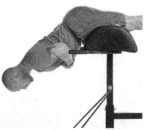 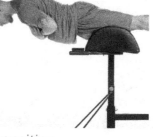 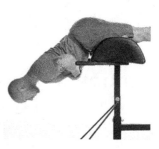

Correct transition

MUSCLE CLEANS

Category: Pull Object (ground to shoulder)

Movement screen: Front rack test

Ability screen: Deadlift x 5

We initiate our new trainees into the movements of weightlifting—the clean and the snatch—with the muscle clean. Pedagogically, the muscle clean is simply the best way to introduce the clean. If a trainee hasn't mastered the front squat, is dropping under the bar to catch it in a partial or full front squat going to end well? (Short answer: no.) Make it easy on your new athletes, and let them concentrate on the mechanics of the first and second pulls, and the upper body mechanics of the third pull, before adding complexity.

As an athlete gradually masters the muscle clean, he'll concurrently be improving his front squats, and eventually can begin receiving the bar lower and lower (the height of the catch being a function of the load relative to his power), in efficient, aesthetically pleasing positions. This may fly in the face of traditional weightlifting pedagogy, but that's okay. Our goal is not to create weightlifters, but MMGPP athletes who can clean and snatch competently.

Even seasoned athletes can benefit from learning the muscle clean. At lower weights it reinforces sound upper body mechanics in the turnover (third pull). At heavier weights it strengthens the turnover.

While the muscle clean is not formally prescribed in any benchmark workouts, it can be seamlessly substituted for the sumo deadlift high pull. In terms of the "It's all about progression" philosophy of BtN, the muscle clean is preferred because it has direct transferability to the power and full clean, whereas the SDHP, with its extra-wide stance and narrow grip, has no logical successor.

For those with sufficient strength, the muscle clean is also a good choice for a workout that calls for power cleans. In their efforts to get the fastest possible cycle time, strong athletes often end up performing power cleans with no foot movement and only a perfunctory knee bend in the catch—what amounts to a sloppy muscle clean. Why not *consciously* perform muscle cleans, and sharpen up the execution?

Harry and Amy both have creditable front squats, so they are cleared for the muscle clean. Tim's squat is improving, as is his deadlift set-up, but he can't front rack a barbell. Today he can learn the basics of the muscle clean with dumbbells.

Muscle Clean Teaching Script

"Let's start by reviewing front rack position, because that's where you're going to catch the bar at the end of the muscle clean.

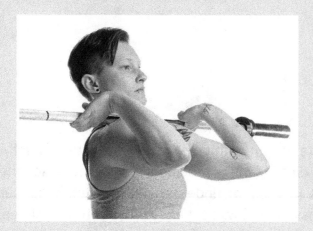

"Take a clean-width grip on the bar (about thumb's length from the edge where the gnurling meets the smooth central section of the bar) and curl it up onto your shoulders. Elevate your shoulders and lift your elbows until they are pointing straight ahead. Let your fists relax and the bar to roll back on your fingertips. Ideally, the elbows and wrists should be in line. Remember, the bar should be resting on your shoulders, not in your hands.

"Following our principles of best leverage and best efficiency, in the muscle clean the barbell travels in a straight line up the torso before coming to rest on the shoulders. We're going to rehearse that bar path.

"Lower the bar to waist height.

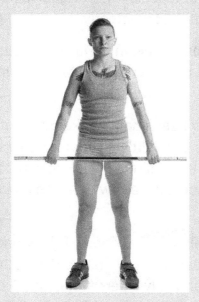

"At this point let's establish what we'll call 'reset' position: feet under the hips (6-9" apart), midline braced, shoulders back, arms internally rotated so that the elbows point outward, and wrists curled under. When 'reset' is called, return to this position.

"Reset."

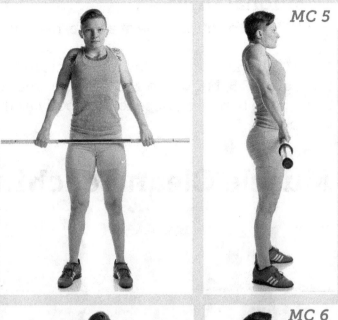

MC 5

"Shrug your shoulders up and back, elevating the bar but keeping it close to the body. This is **Muscle Clean Position 5 (MC 5)**, otherwise known as 'finish.'

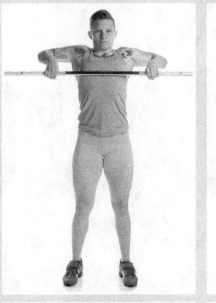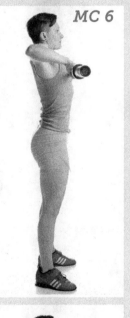

MC 6

"Now lift the bar by pulling your elbows high. The bar should remain within an inch of the chest. This is **Muscle Clean 6 (MC 6),** also known as 'scarecrow.'

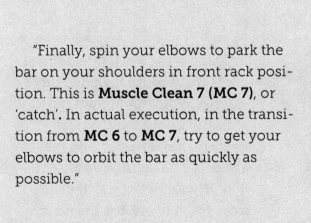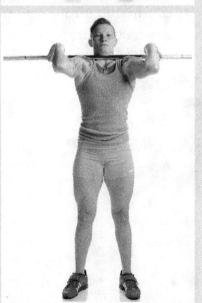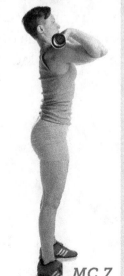

"Finally, spin your elbows to park the bar on your shoulders in front rack position. This is **Muscle Clean 7 (MC 7)**, or 'catch'. In actual execution, in the transition from **MC 6** to **MC 7**, try to get your elbows to orbit the bar as quickly as possible."

MC 7

Positional Drills

"5! 6! 7!" Drill positions one at a time, making corrections as necessary.

"5! Go!" Also known as a "tall muscle clean." At the command "Go!", trainees move through **MC 5**, **MC 6**, and **MC 7** in one smooth and aggressive motion. Remind them to keep the barbell as close to their body as they can. It should ruffle their t-shirts on its way up.

Muscle Clean Teaching Script, cont.

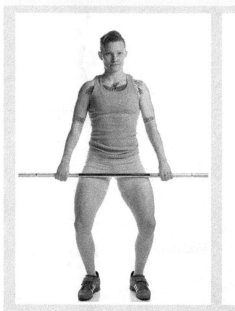
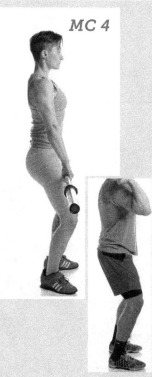

MC 4

"Reset. Now, squeeze your butt tight, and flare your knees out so that you sit down about two or three inches. Weight is centered on the foot with a slight emphasis on the heel. The bar rests about three-quarters of the way up your thighs, right where the pockets of your jeans would be. This is **Muscle Clean Position 4 (MC 4)**, also known as 'high hang' or 'pockets.'

"Notice the strong resemblance between **MC 4** and Push Press Position 2. Except for the placement of the bar, they're the same!

"On my command "GO!", driving through your heels, stand explosively and shrug simultaneously into **MC 5**. It's essentially a jump, except your feet don't leave the floor. Accelerate the bar with a pull of the arms (**MC 6**), then flash the elbows around to receive the bar on the shoulders—that's **MC 7**. Ready? GO!

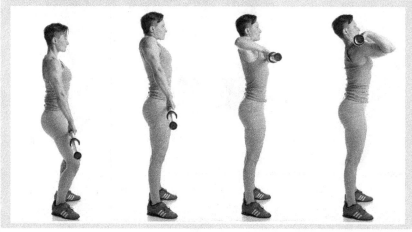

"Did the bar feel lighter that time? It's because the powerful extension of your hip put momentum on the bar that effectively makes it lighter, and thus easier to pull up onto your shoulders. This aggressive extension from **MC 4** to **MC 5** is the heart of the clean."

Positional Drills

"4! Go!" Also known as the "high hang muscle clean." Point out to the trainees that the violent extension of the hip should make the bar feel noticeably lighter as they pull it up to **MC 7**. Emphasize the necessary of moving the elbows quickly around the bar.

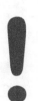

The transition from MC 4 and MC 5 (and later, PC 4 to PC 5) often creates such force that the athlete is carried up onto his toes. At this point, knees, ankles, and hips are all in extension, so this position is commonly referred to as "triple extension". Do NOT teach your athletes to try to get into this position! If it happens as a natural consequence of a super-aggressive drive from the heels, that's fine. But if an athlete intentionally tries to stand up on her toes, she'll often put an anterior-direction impetus on the bar and will have to jump forward to catch it. Simply teach her to explode off the heels, and concentrate on landing with her weight

"We're now going to work on pulling from the floor. Understand that each new stage we'll look at it is only setting you up for that explosion at **MC 4.**

"We'll practice as if we have bumpers on our bar. The bumpers we use have a diameter of approximately eighteen inches. This is standard. An eighteen-inch diameter means the bumpers have a radius of nine inches. Squat down behind the bar until it's about nine inches off the floor.

"Unlike the set-up for the deadlift, when setting up for the clean, allow the bar to travel out from the shin until it's over the point at which your big toe meets your foot. That's about where the laces of your shoes begin. The weight is distributed across the foot, with a slight emphasis on the forefoot. Knees flare out. Wrists are curled under. The arms are straight, internally rotated, and from the side, vertical, with the leading edge of the shoulder slightly in front of the bar. The spine in 'absolute' extension, gaze forward. This is **Muscle Clean Position 1 (MC 1)**, or 'floor.'

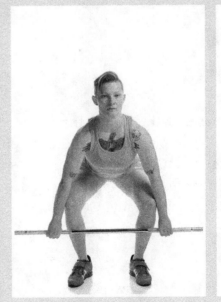
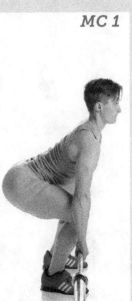

MC 1

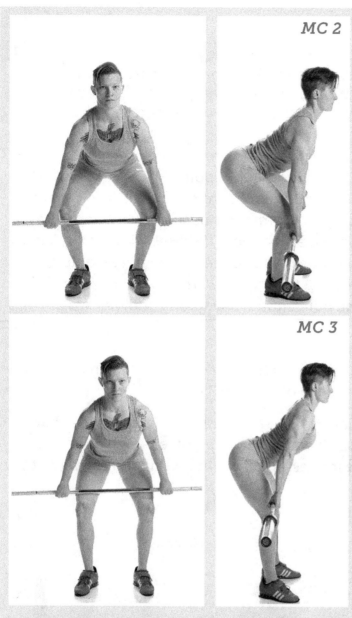

MC 2

MC 3

"Next: stand until the bar is just touching the bottom of the knee cap. This is **Muscle Clean Position 2 (MC 2)**, 'low hang' or 'hang below the knees.' The back angle should be maintained from **MC 1**. Flaring the knees out wide as the bar rises, instead of pulling them back, helps. Be patient!

"From **MC 2,** push with the legs while simultaneously sweeping the bar back into the body. Your hips will rise, and your shoulders will come out slightly in front of the bar as your shins go vertical. The bar is now an inch or two above the knee. This is **Muscle Clean Position 3 (MC 3)**, sometimes referred to as 'hang'. **MC 3** puts tension on the hamstring, which is vital for the explosive hip extension to come.

"As the bar reaches mid-thigh, shift the torso to vertical *while simultaneously sitting straight down over the heels.* This preserves the tension created in the hamstrings as the knees extended and hips rose in **MC 3**. That's important—you'll use that tension to help launch the bar into the air. The bar continues traveling up the leg. This returns us to **MC 4.** When I say 'GO!', you know what to do, right? Ready? GO!

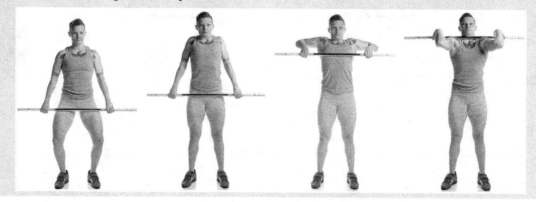

"Notice that in **MC 7** you are standing tall. No rebend of the knees is necessary (or desirable) in the muscle clean, as you are not trying to get under the bar; instead, you are pulling the bar to you. Later, with the power clean and clean, we'll learn how to retreat under the bar."

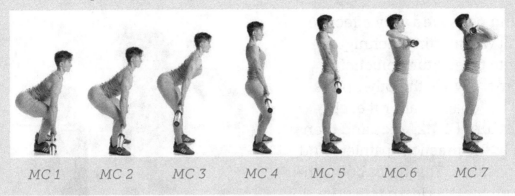

MC 1   MC 2   MC 3   MC 4   MC 5   MC 6   MC 7

Positional Drills

"1! 2! 3! 4! 5! 6! 7!" Drills positions of the muscle clean one at a time, making corrections as necessary. Do not call next position until you are satisfied that all trainees are performing the current position correctly.

"1! 2! 3! 4! Go!" Take the trainees from floor to pockets, and at "Go!" they execute a high hang muscle clean.

"1! 2! 3! Go!" Take the trainees from floor to mid-hang, and at "Go!" they execute a hang muscle clean.

"1! 2! Go!" Take the trainees from floor to low hang, and at "Go!" they execute a hang-below-knees muscle clean.

"1! Go!" At "Go!", trainees execute a full muscle clean.

A Word About Timing

"Although you are being taught the muscle clean in a slow, segmented, and rather mechanical fashion, the way the clean and its more complex variants are actually performed is very smooth, although the timing changes from position to position. Moving from **MC 1** to **MC 2** is relatively slow. There is an acceleration as you move from **MC 2** through **MC 3** to **MC 4**. At **MC 4** the acceleration becomes an explosion. In the full clean, the transition from **Position 4** to **5** to **6** to **7** is one of the fastest movements in all sports.

"But moving with precision—and weightlifting is a sport where the divide between success and failure can be measured in millimeters—at speed requires endless slow, methodical practice. Drill moving through all seven positions of the muscle clean until you simply can't do it any way but correctly."

Coaching Pairs

Coaching pairs are a very effective way to drill weighlifting technique. Each athlete takes a turn practicing the movement while the other plays "coach". The "coach" calls off each position in turn ("1." "2," etc), and then tries to help the practicing athlete find the right position. This helps both athletes. If your athletes learn to recognize what is good or bad in the movement of others, they have a better chance of executing correctly themselves. You can aid them by sketching stick figure diagrams of the movement they can use as visual reference. Posi-

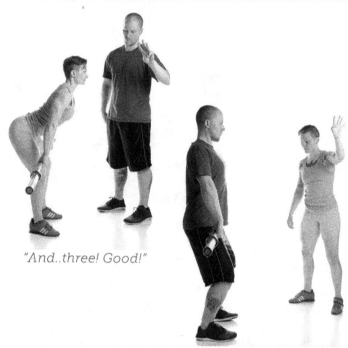

"And..three! Good!"

"Four. Find your heels! Good!"

Teaching the Hook Grip

"Weightlifters use a hook grip on the barbell. While the standard grip is fingers closed around the bar, and thumbs over the fingers, the hook grip reverses the order: with palms pronated, thumbs wrap around the bar first, and then fingers lock the thumb in place.

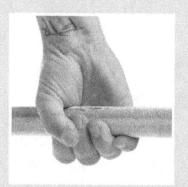 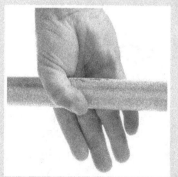 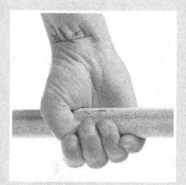

"The hook grip allows you to pick up heavy weights without maximally contracting the forearm flexors. A combination of tight back and relatively relaxed arms provides for the most efficient transmission of force from the hips to the bar.

"After the elbows come high during the third pull (**MC 6**), allow your fists to relax and your thumbs to pop out as you spin your elbows around the bar. This increases your speed, and allows you to get the elbows higher as you receive the bar on your shoulders."

Setting Up From the Floor

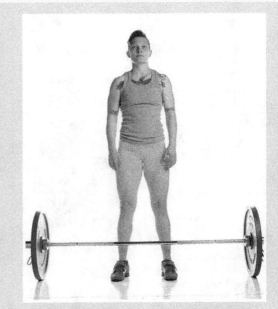

"To set up to muscle clean a bar from the floor, start by standing with your feet hip-width apart. Run your standard set-up: screw your feet in, brace your midline, pack your shoulders.

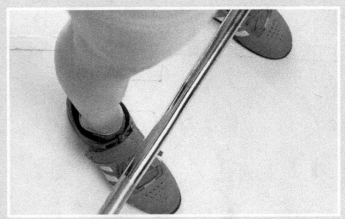

"The bar should be slightly away from the leg, over where the bones of your feet meet the phalanges of the toes (about where your shoelaces start).

"Squat down and get your hook grip on the bar. Sit on your heels and retract your shoulder blades as strongly as you can while still keeping your arms loose and relaxed.

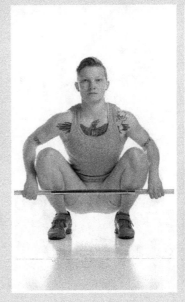
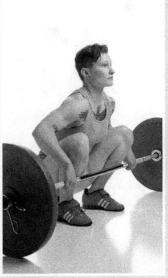

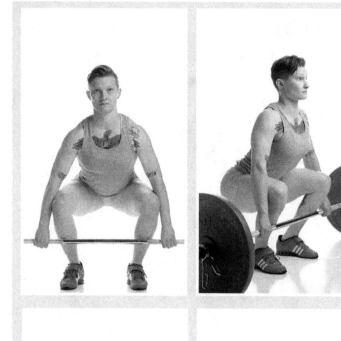

"Depress your shoulder blades and lift your chest, setting your back into 'absolute' extension. Then internally rotate your arms so that the points of your elbows are facing out. Curl your wrists unders.

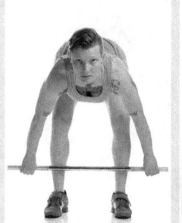 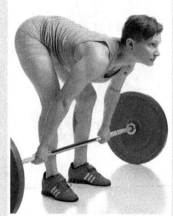

"Maintaining this absolute spinal extension, push your hips up.

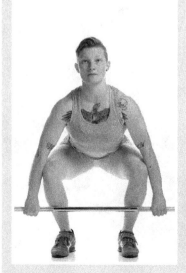 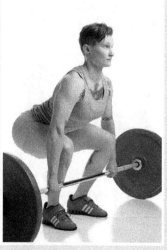

"Then, by strongly engaging your hamstrings, pull your hips back down until your shoulders are directly over the bar. At this point your whole body is set in tension and and you're ready to lift."

Muscle Clean Faults and Fixes

1. Deadlift set-up.

Muscle Clean Position 1 violation. New trainees will often set up for their clean as if for the deadlift. While not totally terrible (at least they won't hurt themselves), it will make it more difficult for them to get into a proper position to jump the bar into the air. Get the trainee to let the bar come out over her foot, and to sit until her shoulders are directly over the bar.

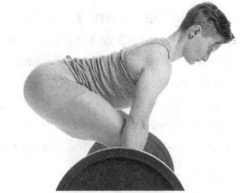

Fault

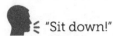 "Sit down!"

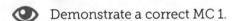 Demonstrate a correct MC 1.

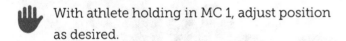 With athlete holding in MC 1, adjust position as desired.

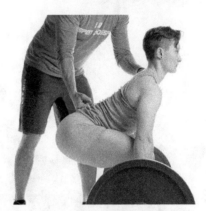

Tactile

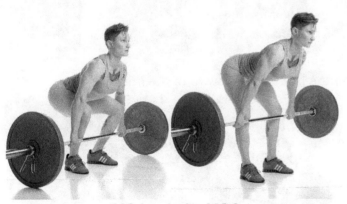

MC 1 to faulty MC 2

2. Hips rise too soon.

Muscle Clean Position 2 violation. Athlete's butt shoots into the air as she pulls from MC 1 to MC 2. Back angle must be maintained, with shoulders staying vertical over the bar. Care must be taken to set the hamstrings in tension before lift is initiated. Review set-up as necessary.

 "Squat it off the floor!"

 Demonstrate proper transition from MC 1 o MC 2.

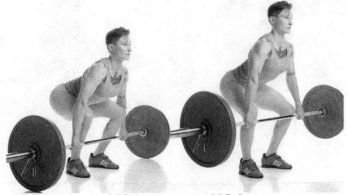

MC 1 to correct MC 2

Muscle Clean Faults and Fixes, cont.

3. Jumping bar from in front of knees.

Muscle Clean Position 3 and Muscle Clean Position 4 violation. Another very common error is rushing the movement and simply ripping the bar from the floor. Listen for the characteristic clang of the bar bumping the knees as the trainee jumps too soon. With light weights it doesn't make that much difference (indeed, some lifters practice the muscle clean just like that), but it doesn't reinforce positions that will be critical when the weights get heavier. Maximum acceleration should be reached when the back is vertical AND the bar is in the line of gravity.

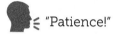 "Patience!"

 Demonstrate a proper transition from MC2 to MC 4.

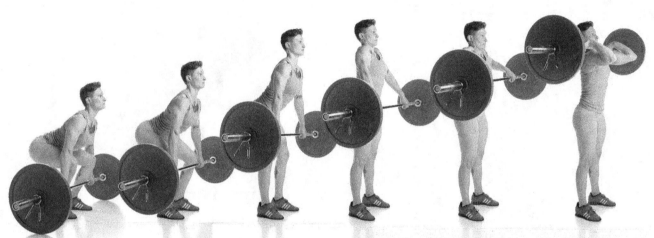

Jumping too soon puts the bar away from the body and forward of the line of gravity

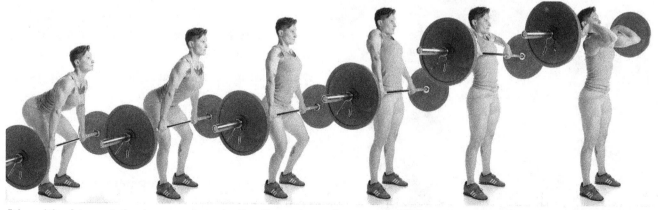

It's critical to get the bar as close to the line of gravity as possible to create optimal leverage. The bar brushes along the leg and then travels vertically so close to the body that it "ruffles the t-shirt".

Muscle Clean Faults and Fixes, cont.

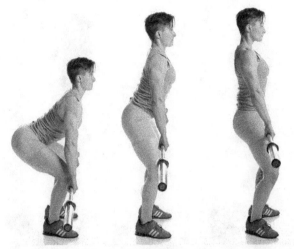

MC 2, no sweep, MC 4

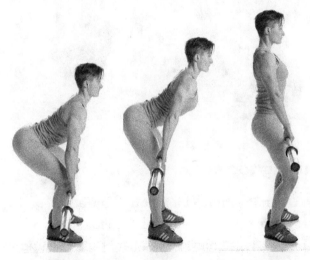

Proper transition: MC 2, MC 3, MC 4

4. Not getting over the bar.

Muscle Clean Position 3 violation. As the athlete transitions from MC 2 to MC 3 she must set up MC 4 by extending her knees and actively sweeping the bar back toward her body. If she opens the hips instead, no tension is set in the hamstrings in MC 3, reducing the muscles' potential contribution of force in the explosion from MC 4 to MC 5.

 "Stay over the bar!" or "Push with your legs!" or "Sweep the bar in!"

Demonstrate a proper transition from MC2 to MC 4.

Tie a skinny resistance band around the center of the bar and run the athlete through positional drills. As she shifts from MC 2 to MC 3, put tension on the band to try to pull the bar away from her. The athlete will be forced to engage her lats and actively sweep the bar in to keep it in position.

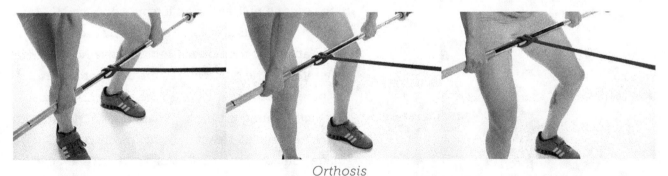

Orthosis

Muscle Clean Faults and Fixes, cont.

5. Reverse curling bar.

Muscle Clean Position 6 violation. In the initiation of the third pull, the bar must be kept close to the body.

 "Elbows up and back!" or "Keep the bar close!"

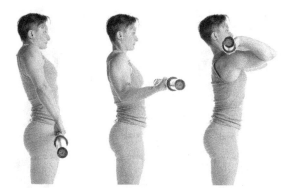

Fault

Demonstrate a correct transition from MC 5 to MC 7.

Position the athlete directly in front of a wall. Have her execute the positional drill "4! Go!" If she tries to curl the bar, her knuckles will collide with the wall. That'll learn 'er!

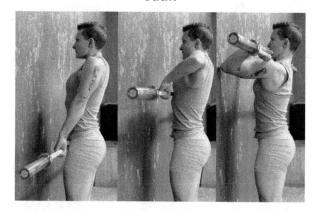

Orthosis

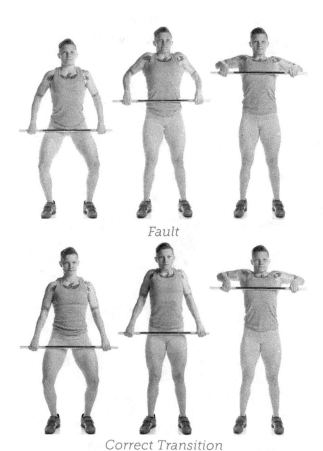

Fault

Correct Transition

6. Pulling too soon.

Muscle Clean Position 5 violation. Some athletes, especially older, stronger athletes used to relying on their upper body strength, have a hard time resisting the urge to row the barbell into position. Explain that in the second pull, as the athlete moves from MC 4 to MC 5 , the arms are like straps, or tow cables: not doing any work themselves, but transferring the force generated by the hips. Only as the bar approaches the top of its ballistic trajectory do the arms come into play, accelerating the bar's upward travel (and later, in the power and full clean, the athlete's descent). One image you could offer is that of a cartoon character with his arms stretching long as he jumps, only to snap back.

 "Long arms!" or "Stretch and snap!"

 Demonstrate a correct transition from MC4 to MC5.

326

Muscle Clean Faults and Fixes, cont.

7. Not getting it.

Muscle Clean Position 5 violation. Some trainees will have a difficult time grasping the core concept of the clean—that it is the violent extension of the hip, from MC 4 ("pockets") to MC 5 ("finish"), that puts the initial momentum and elevation on the bar. Instead they will carefully move through all positions up to pockets, stand up straight, and then laboriously use their arms to haul the bar up onto their shoulders.

The solution is to put them in MC 4, and then tell them to jump as hard as they can, without worrying about racking the bar.

If you're lucky, the bar will float up. If not, if it barely moves, it's likely that the trainee is locking her elbows as she jumps. Get her to relax her arms, and then repeat until the bar floats. Once she's got a handle on that, then instruct her to jump just as she has been, but add MC 6 and MC 7. The bar will rocket into the air (probably nearly knocking her out), and the light of understanding will come on in her eyes. Then have her repeat the action, except this time, her feet are not to leave the ground.

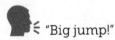 "Big jump!"

👁 Demonstrate a proper transition from MC 4 to MC 5.

✋ Ask the trainee to stand tall. Hold your hand 2" above her head. Ask her to execute a muscle clean and jump to drive the top of her head into your palm as she hits MC 5. This will force her to explosively extend her hips. If her arms are relaxed, inertia will cause the bar to rise.

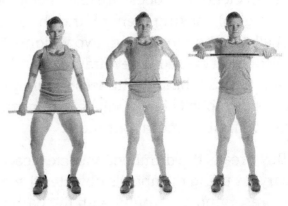

Fault

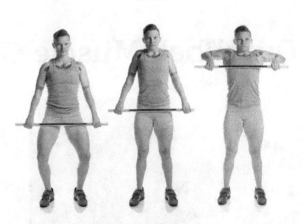

Correct

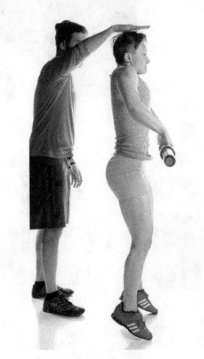

Tactile

Some trainees, due to lack of flexibility, will be unable to use the barbell to clean. Teach them to clean dumbbells instead. Because the 'bells can be held with a neutral (palm-facing grip), racking them on the shoulders can be a lot less painful than trying to rack a barbell. On the other hand, two weights flying about are inherently more challenging to control than one, and new trainees, who are often not especially coordinated, can have a hard time keeping dumbbells moving in one (saggital) plane. This relative instability means dumbbell cleans will be better utilized for relatively low weight high rep sets, instead of limit strength training.

BtN breaks the dumbbell muscle clean down into seven positions. This isn't really necessary, as using dumbbells obviates the need to move the knees around the load as it rises. But preserving continuity with the barbell muscle clean will make running positional

Dumbbell Muscle Clean Teaching Script

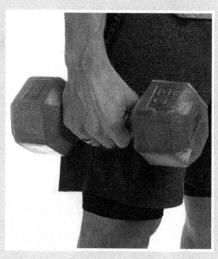

"Grab a pair of dumbbells. Make sure the pinky side of your hand is closer to the dumbbell head than your thumb side. This will help balance the dumbbell in your hand, and make it easier to seat on your shoulder.

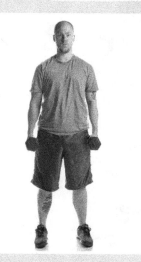 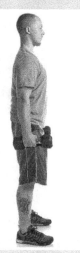

"Reset position is feet under your hips and screwed into the ground, glutes on, abs locked down, shoulders back and down, arms at your sides.

"With your palms facing in toward your center line, park the thumbside end of your dumbbells on top of your shoulders. Keep your elbows in tight to your ribs. This **Dumbbell Muscle Clean Position 7 (dMC 7)**—where we'll land.

"Reset.

"In the dumbbell muscle clean, we're going to approximate the seven positions of the barbell muscle clean. Instead of being in front of the body, the load will be on either side of the body, moving in a straight path congruent with the line of gravity.

"**Dumbbell Muscle Clean Position 1 (dMC 1)** looks like this: Feet are hip width, weight slightly forward on the feet, spine is neutral. Hips are hinged back with knees bent. The wrists are tilted slightly forward to allow the front (thumb side) plate of the dumbbell to touch the floor.

"Maintaining the same back angle, stand up until the dumbbells are beside your knees. This is **Dumbbell Muscle Clean Position 2 (dMC 2).**

"Continue your upward travel by pushing with your knees. Sweep the dumbbells slightly back as the hips rise. This is **Dumbbell Muscle Clean Position 3 (dMC 3).**

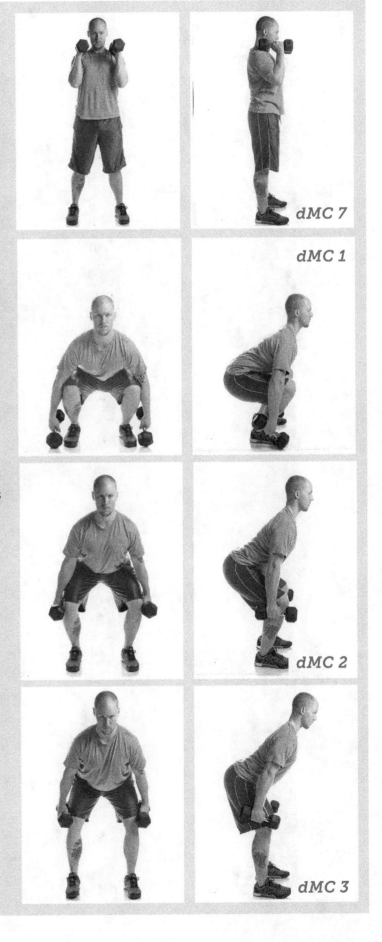

dMC 7

dMC 1

dMC 2

dMC 3

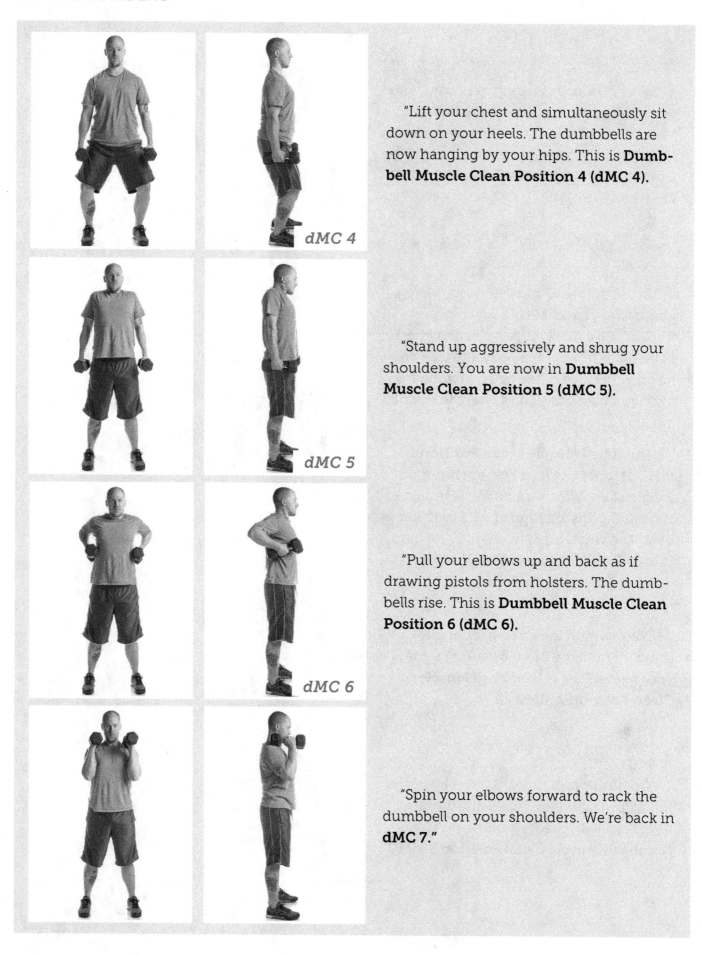

dMC 4

"Lift your chest and simultaneously sit down on your heels. The dumbbells are now hanging by your hips. This is **Dumbbell Muscle Clean Position 4 (dMC 4).**

dMC 5

"Stand up aggressively and shrug your shoulders. You are now in **Dumbbell Muscle Clean Position 5 (dMC 5).**

dMC 6

"Pull your elbows up and back as if drawing pistols from holsters. The dumbbells rise. This is **Dumbbell Muscle Clean Position 6 (dMC 6).**

"Spin your elbows forward to rack the dumbbell on your shoulders. We're back in **dMC 7."**

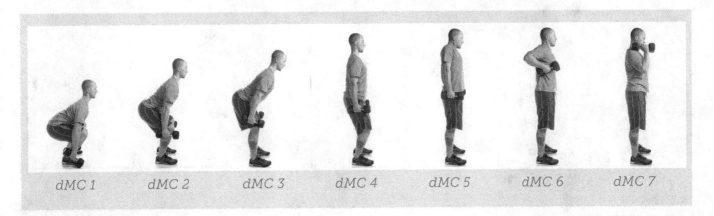

dMC 1   dMC 2   dMC 3   dMC 4   dMC 5   dMC 6   dMC 7

Positional Drills

"1! 2! 3! 4! 5! 6! 7!" Rehearse the path of the dumbbells in the db muscle clean. Drill positions one at a time, making corrections as necessary.

"1! 2! 3! 4! Go!" Take dumbbells from floor to high hang, then practice aggressive hip extension and arm pull.

"1! Go!" Full movement.

Dumbbell Muscle Clean Faults and Fixes

Positional faults of the barbell muscle clean apply, as well as...

1. Curling the dumbbells.

Dumbbell Clean Position 6 violation. Athlete hammer curls dumbbells into place. The dumbbells should rise in a straight line along the sides before being racked on the shoulders. A comparison can be made between this action and the drawing of imaginary pistols.

 "Elbows high!" or "Draw your pistols!"

 Demonstrate a correct transition from DbMC 4 to DbMC 7.

 Have athlete stand facing a wall and practice. If he tries to curl the dumbbells out, they will hit the wall.

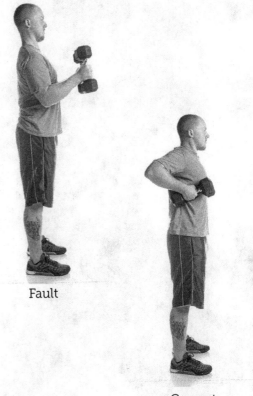

Fault

Correct

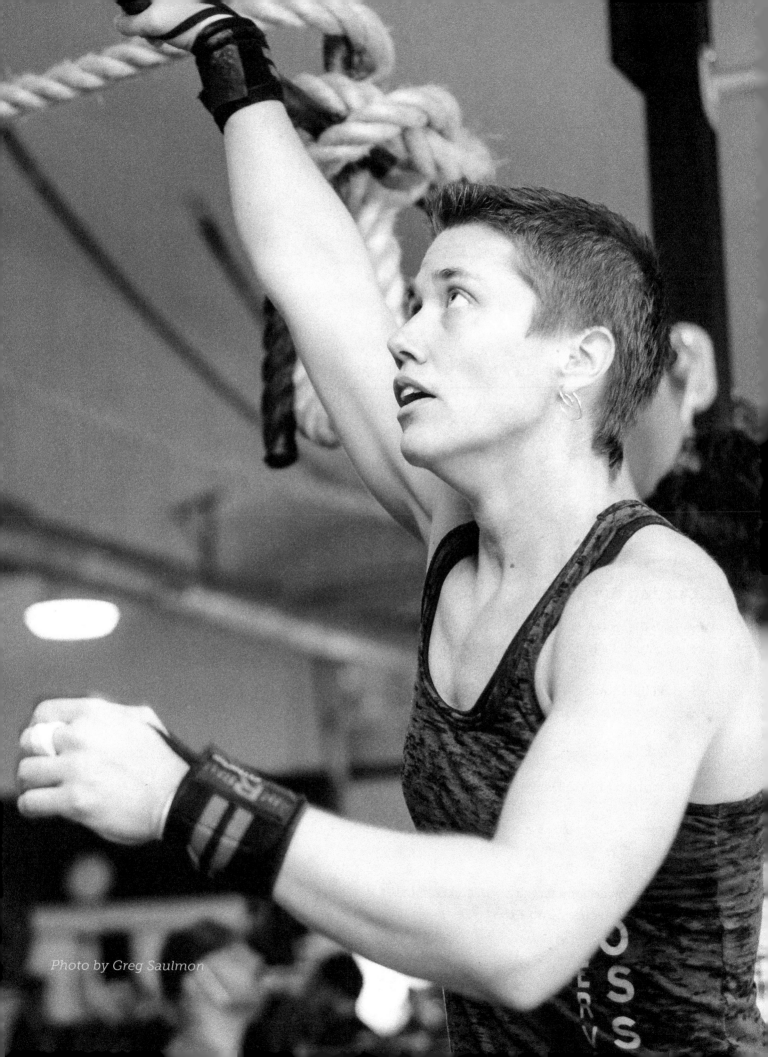

WEIGHTED PULL-UPS

Category: Pull to Object (strict, vertical)

Movement screen: N/a

Ability screen: Pull-up x 5

Once an athlete has a certain number of strict pull-ups (we set the floor at five), it becomes possible to begin using the principle of progressive resistance to increase vertical pulling strength. The weighted pull-up uses the same positions as the strict pull-up (or chin-up), and the same common faults and fixes apply.

Team Space Monkey assignments: Harry will do weighted pull-ups, Amy will continue to develop her strict pull-ups, and Tim will do five sets of three jumping pull-ups with slow eccentrics.

Weighted Pull-up Techniques

"Unless you're inordinately tall, you're probably going to begin standing on a box. (Jumping up to the bar with weights hanging from a belt is impractical at best, dangerous to your procreative capacity at worst). Make sure your gear of choice is secure (vest straps fixed, dip belt fitted correctly, kettlebell or dumbbell between your feet), then get your grip and hang next to the box. When you've finished your set, move back to the box. Don't drop off the bar! If you've got weight strapped to you it'll greatly increase your impact on landing, unnecessarily stressing your knees, and even if you drop the kettlebell or dumbbell first, you may inadvertently land on it, breaking an ankle. Go back to the box, then step down.

"WEIGHT VEST. Convenient, but not useful for limit strength tests for stronger athletes; many weight vests are a fixed weight, and even those that are adjustable are usually limited to 40lbs or so.

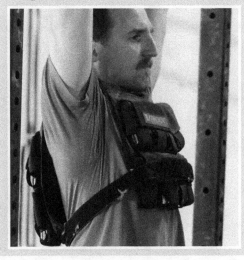

"DIP BELT. Dip belts are necessary for stronger athletes attempting to test max efforts in the weighted pull-up. Wear the belt just above the hips. Pull the carabiner through the opposite side U-ring, thread it through the handle of a kettlebell or hole in the center of a plate, then attach on the original side.

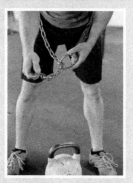 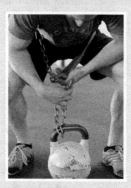 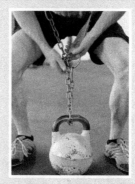 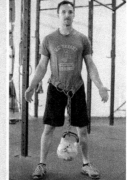

"KETTLEBELL. Hook the toe of one foot through the handle of a kettlebell. Bring your other foot in front and press the heel of that foot back into the toe of the hooking foot, holding the 'bell in place.

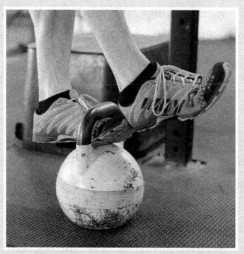 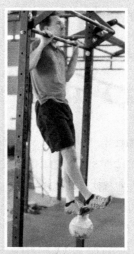

"DUMBBELL. With the dumbbell resting on the floor or on a box, trap the handle between your feet, so that one head of the dumbbell rests on your insteps."

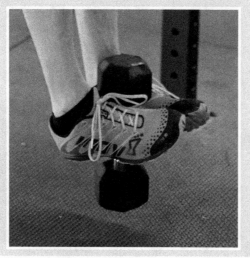 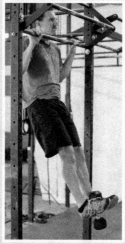

THE L-SIT

Category: Hip and Trunk Flexion (static)

Movement screen: N/a

Ability screen: N/a (tuck sit), tuck sit x 10 sec (half-tuck sit), half-tuck sit x 10 sec (L-sit knee extensions), L-sit knee extensions x 10 (L-sit)

In the L-sit, the athlete supports her weight atop a pair of parallettes set shoulder width. The legs are held out straight in front, hips piked to 90 degrees, while the torso is held vertical. It's a great developer of lower abdominal strength, and helps progress the athlete toward tough exercises like the L pull-up and strict toes-to-bar.

Although a three minute L-sit has been suggested as the gold standard of performance, it's probably a little bit more realistic to set a goal for your athletes of holding a one minute L-sit. The best way to train for this is to work 4 x :15 or 3 x :20 efforts.

I'm pretty sure Harry and Amy will be able to progress all the way to a full L-sit today. Tim doesn't have the hamstring flexibility for an L-sit, but he'll derive much training benefit from one of its simpler variants.

L-Sit Teaching Script

"We'll start with the simplest variation of the L-sit: the tuck sit.

"Set up a pair of parallettes about shoulder-width apart. Check the spacing by placing your lower arm, elbows to straight fingertips, between them. You should just about touch on both sides.

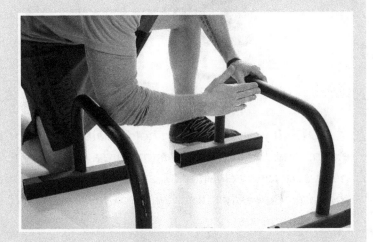

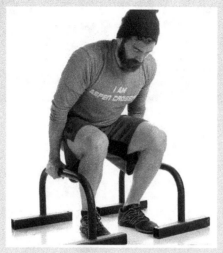

"Crouch down between the parallettes and grip them at their centers. Set your shoulders back and down. Screw your hands (right: clockwise, left: counter-clockwise) into the bars.

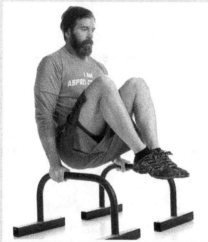

"Push down into the parallettes while simultaneously tucking your knees up into your chest. Keep your shoulders back and down. Resist the urge to cross your ankles. This is a **Tuck Sit.** If this is too challenging, put one foot down, and keep the other knee high.

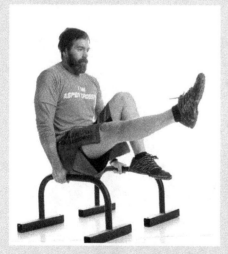

"But if you can manage that easily, try this: keeping the knees high, extend one leg. Hips remain flexed, shoulders back and down, fists twisting into the bars. This is a **Half-tuck Sit.**

NOTE: If your athlete can hold a half-tuck sit for 10 seconds, he's ready to try L-sit knee extensions. L-sit knee extensions are a great way to start building the strength and flexibility necessary for an extended L-sit hold. By virtue of the fact they are performed for repetitions, they are also easily integrated into the standard WOD format, giving you another weapon for your training arsenal.

"We'll work towards a full L-sit with L-sit Knee Extensions. L-sit knee extensions are a great sub for L-sit holds programmed in a WOD. Use a 1:2 rep/seconds ratio, e.g., a 20 sec L sit equals 10 L-sit knee extensions.

"Return to your Tuck Sit. We'll now refer to it as **L-sit Knee Extension Position 1 (kLS 1).**

"Keeping both knees high, contract your quads to extend your knees. Keep your legs straight, knees and feet together, toes pointed. Keep screwing your hands into the bars and pulling your hips forward. Feet must remain at least hip height to count. This is **L-sit Knee Extension Position 2 (kLS 2).**

"Flex your knees to return to **kLS 1**.

"Once you can do ten repetitions of L-sit Knee Extensions, begin working on your L-sit hold. **L-sit Knee Extension Position 2** is now a full **L-sit (LS 1)**. Point your toes to keep legs tight."

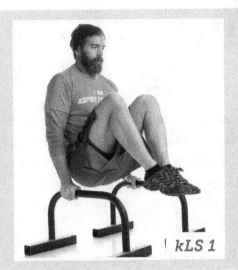

kLS 1

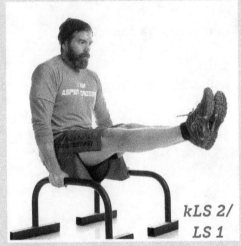

kLS 2/ LS 1

L-sit Faults and Fixes

1. "W" sit.

L-sit Position 1 violation. If athlete's hamstrings are too tight, his quads will not be strong enough to fully extend the knees while he is attempting to L-sit. If cues don't fix it, have him default to the most complex variation he can perform well.

 "Knees straight!"

 Demonstrate a correct LS 1.

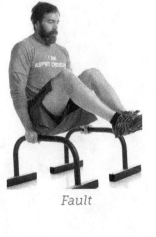

Fault

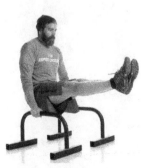

Correct LS 1

L-sit Faults and Fixes, cont.

2. Tilt.

L-sit Position 1 violation. An athlete may be able to hold his legs out straight in front of him, but if he lacks upper back strength he'll tilt forward until his hips are behind his hands and his feet are pointing at the floor.

 "Pull your hips foward!"

 Demonstrate a correct LS 1.

 With athlete holding in LS 1, adjust position as desired.

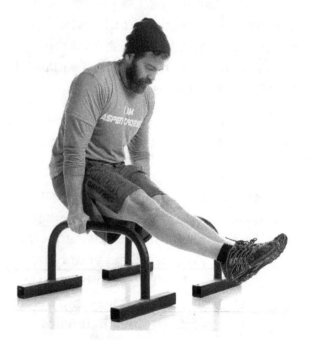

Fault

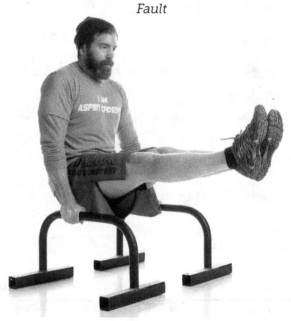

Correct LS 1

Category: Hybrid (hip and trunk flexion, push object away [horizontal], single-leg squat)

Movement screen: N/a

Ability screen: Butterfly sit-up x 5, bench press x 5, forward lunge x 5

The Turkish get-up is a whole body exercise that starts with the athlete lying on the floor, then has him one-arm floor press an object to full extension, stand to support the object overhead, then return to supine. The TGU builds shoulder stability and flexibility, hip mobility, stability in the lunge position, and overall body coordination, balance, and strength. There are many methods to teach the TGU; this one is mine. I've omitted certain traditional elements in favor of a simpler version more accessible to a broad population.

Like all complex exercises, the best way to learn the Turkish get-up is by breaking it down into a series of discrete positions, each with its own energy, rhythm, and balance. Instead of thinking of it as one gross motor pattern—standing up from a supine position with a weight pressed overhead—encourage your athletes to think of the TGU as a sequence of poses. As they practice, they should pause briefly at each point to self-assess and improve their position before proceeding to the next pose.

Harry and Amy should do well with the TGU, although Harry's tight shoulders may be an issue. I anticipate a very challenging time for Tim; he won't be using any weights today. Just working on the positions of the TGU will have a huge benefit for him, though.

Turkish Get-up Teaching Script

"Initially, the best way to learn the Turkish Get-up is with no weight at all. You'll carefully work through each successive position as you hold aloft an imaginary kettlebell. (*However, the photos all feature an athlete holding a 'bell, just so we don't have to print them twice—Ed.*)

"Have a seat on the floor, then lie back, with legs out straight and feet together. An imaginary kettlebell is by your right hip. Slip your right hand through the handle, palm up, and grasp it toward the corner to which your thumb points. Now reach across your body to clasp your left hand over your right.

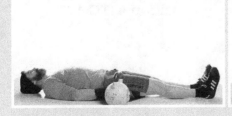
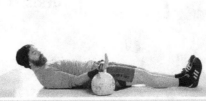
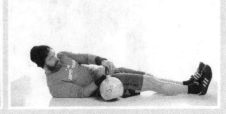

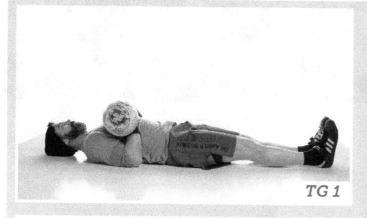

TG 1

"With the help of the left hand, do an assisted bicep curl to get the bell into a racked position: wrist straight, bell resting on forearm and biceps, arm resting on your ribs. This is **Turkish Get-up Position 1 (TG 1)**.

TG 2

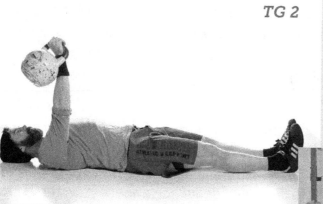

"Set your shoulders back and down. Then floor press the kettlebell straight towards the ceiling. Maintain this orientation throughout the rest of the movement. Keep one eye on the kettlebell at all times. This is **Turkish Get-up Position 2 (TG 2)**.

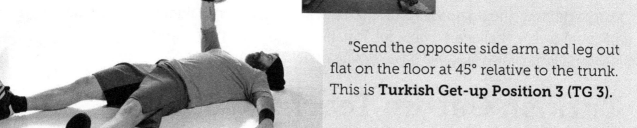

"Note the similarity to the first position of the bench press.

"Send the opposite side arm and leg out flat on the floor at 45° relative to the trunk. This is **Turkish Get-up Position 3 (TG 3)**.

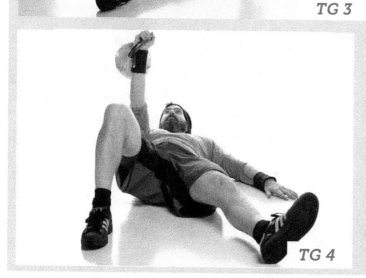

TG 3

"Draw the foot on the same side as the kettlebell up by your buttocks. This is **Turkish Get-up Position 4 (TG 4)**.

TG 4

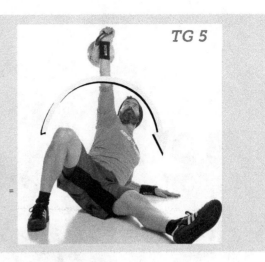

TG 5

"Pushing through the right heel, roll yourself onto your side to sit up onto your opposite elbow. This is **Turkish Get-up Position 5 (TG 5).**

Positional Drills

Depending on your trainees, it can be helpful to build the Turkish get-up one pose at a time, only adding a new position once all the preceding poses have been mastered.

"1! 2! 1!'
"1! 2! 3! 2! 1!"
"1! 2! 3! 4! 3! 2! 1!"
"1! 2! 3! 4! 5! 4! 3! 2! 1!"

Use a brief description of each new position to help your trainees stay organized, as follows:

"1! Seat the weight on your chest and set your shoulder blades back and down.
"2! Press the weight toward the ceiling.
"3! Opposite side arm and leg out to 45 degrees.
"4! Draw same side foot up by your butt.
"5! Pushing through the heel of the same side foot, roll onto your side to sit up on the opposite elbow."

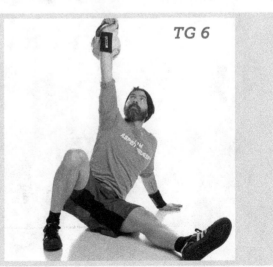

TG 6

"Plant your palm and extend your arm to lift your torso. This is **Turkish Get-up Position 6 (TG 6).**

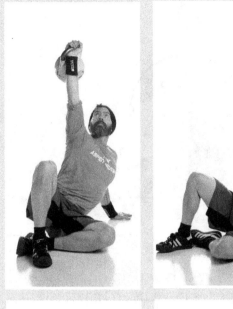
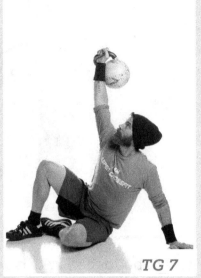

TG 7

"Now switch your feet by flexing the left knee to draw the left heel towards the right toe. As the left foot approaches, lift the right foot and allow the left leg to pass underneath. Then replace your right foot on the ground. This is **Turkish Get-up Position 7 (TG 7).** *(Note! Due to a childhood injury, my left elbow doesn't straighten all the way. Floor support arm should be locked straight.—Ed.)*

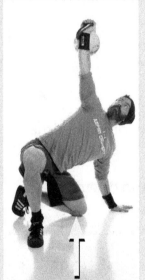
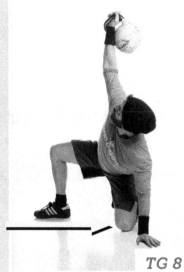

TG 8

"Bracing your weight on your left hand, lift your hip and draw the left knee straight back until it is straight up-and-down under your body. Keep the lower leg perpendicular relative toward your facing direction. Ideally, the foot, knee, and hand are in a straight line. This is **Turkish Get-up Position 8 (TG 8).**

TG 9

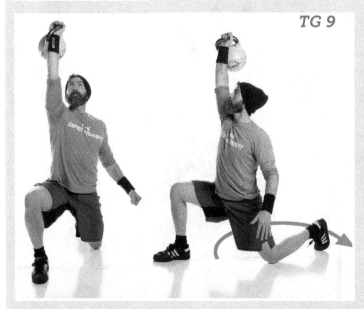

"Shift your torso vertical, simultaneously pivoting your rear foot around the planted knee to bring your lower left leg around behind you. At this point, you should be in an ideal lunge position, with your knees slightly outside your hips, and your front knee lined up over the ankle. Curl your left toe under. This is **Turkish Get-up Position 9 (TG 9).**

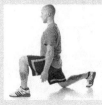

"Note the similarity of **TG 9** to Walking Lunge Position 2.

"Pushing through the rear toe and through the front heel, stand up. Make sure feet are set shoulder-width apart. This is **Turkish Get-up Position 10 (TG 10)**. Savor your momentary triumph over gravity!

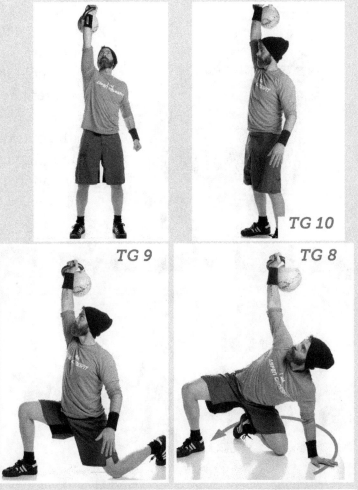

TG 10

TG 9

TG 8

"To return to the starting position, reverse the process.

"Take a big step straight back with the left foot. Sink the knee to the floor, returning to **TG 9**. Externally rotate the rear (left leg) 90 degrees, then draw the hip to the right to bring the left hand to the floor just outside the knee. You're back in **TG 8**.

"Bracing your weight on your left hand, omit **TG 7** to simply pull your left leg all the way through and sit down, returning you to **TG 6**.

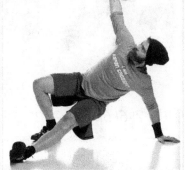
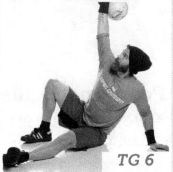

TG 6

"Alternately, you can lower your hip to the ground, then slide your left leg forward until it is behind your right foot. We're back in **TG 7**. Switch your feet and extend your left leg to **TG 6**.

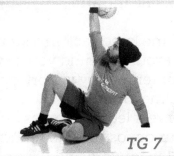
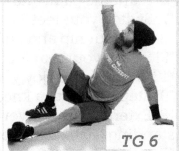

TG 7

TG 6

"Sink to your elbow (**TG 5**) and then lie flat on your back (**TG 4**). Extend the bent leg (**TG 3**), draw the opposite arm and leg in to the side (**TG 2**) and then lower the weight to your chest (**TG 1**). Take your time and hit each pose cleanly.

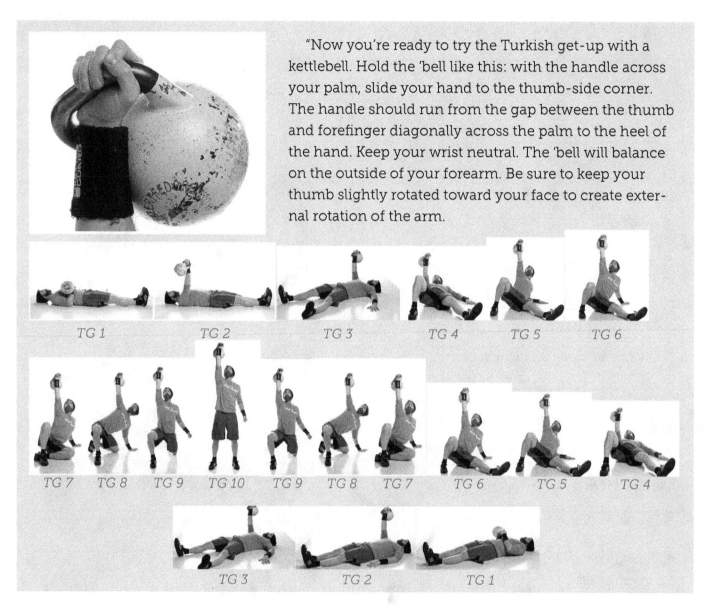

"Now you're ready to try the Turkish get-up with a kettlebell. Hold the 'bell like this: with the handle across your palm, slide your hand to the thumb-side corner. The handle should run from the gap between the thumb and forefinger diagonally across the palm to the heel of the hand. Keep your wrist neutral. The 'bell will balance on the outside of your forearm. Be sure to keep your thumb slightly rotated toward your face to create external rotation of the arm.

TG 1   TG 2   TG 3   TG 4   TG 5   TG 6

TG 7   TG 8   TG 9   TG 10   TG 9   TG 8   TG 7   TG 6   TG 5   TG 4

TG 3   TG 2   TG 1

Positional Drills

"1! 2! 3! 4! 5! 6! 7! 8! 9! 10! 9! 8! 7! 6! 5! 4! 3! 2! 1!" Use all the pose descriptions mentioned earlier, plus:

"6! Plant the palm and extend the arm.
"7! Switch your feet.
"8! Lift your hip and pull the knee back in a straight line.
"9! Swing your rear foot around behind you as you pivot into a kneeling lunge.
"10! Stand and enjoy your temporary victory over gravity.
"9! Step back into a kneeling lunge.
"8! Externally rotate your rear leg 90 degrees, then pull your hip to the side of the standing leg to draw your opposite hand to the floor.
"7 and 6! Slide your rear leg forward and have a seat.
"5! Down on your elbow.
"4! Flat on your back.
"3! Extend your bent knee.

"2! Opposite side arm and leg in.
"1! Lower the weight to your chest."

Turkish Get-up Common Faults and Fixes

Poor execution of the TGU is best fixed via positional drills. Talk the trainee through each position in sequence, and address mistakes as they arise. The athlete's supine starting position, and the stresses of unfamiliar positions, will make it difficult for him to respond to cues. Take your time and put him in the right shapes.

1. Incorrect kettlebell position.

Turkish Get-up Position 1 violation. The 'bell should be held near the corner of the handle closest to the thumb, with the handle diagonal across the palm and the bell resting against the back of the forearm. Arm should be externally rotated, with thumb turned toward face. Wrist should be neutral.

 "Thumb knuckle points to nose!"

 Demonstrate correct kettlebell grip.

 Position arm and wrist so kettlebell is at correct angle.

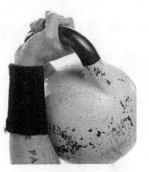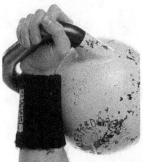

Fault   *Correct grip*

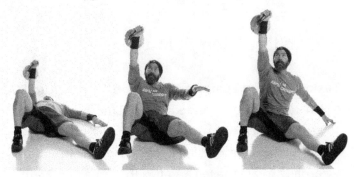

Faulty sequence

2. Sit-up, not roll-up

Turkish Get-up Positions 4 and 5 violation. The initial move off the floor isn't a sit-up, per se, or if it is, it's a rotating, lateral sit-up. The athlete must push with the bent leg to roll himself onto his side.

 "Push through the heel!" or "Roll up on opposite elbow!"

 Demonstrate proper transition from TG 4 to TG 5.

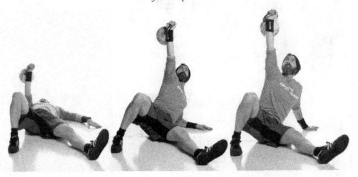

Correct sequence

Turkish Get-up Common Faults and Fixes, cont.

3. Drawing to knee to centerline.

Turkish Get-up Position 8 or 9 violation. Once the feet have switched and the hip is raised, the knee of the leg on the floor should be drawn straight back, rather than in toward the centerline. In TG 8, the upper legs should be at a 90 degree angle. This keeps the knees outside the hips, promoting lateral stability.

A similar error can fault can occur as athlete steps down into TG 9, committing a walking lunge "tightrope walk" error.

 "Knee straight back!" or "Step straight back!"

 Place a foot or small object in front of trainee, and instruct him to draw his knee or step back in a straight line with it.

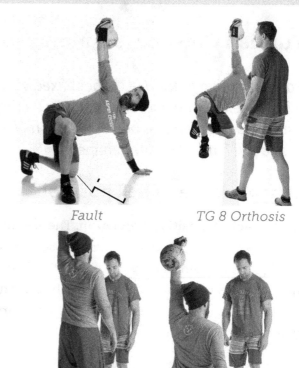

Fault   *TG 8 Orthosis*

TG 9 (descending) Orthosis

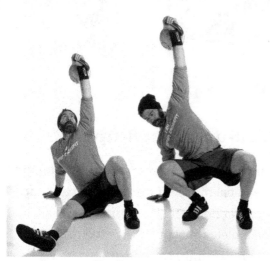

Faulty sequence

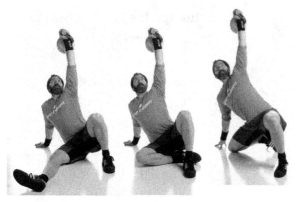

Correct sequence

4. Can't pull leg through.

Turkish get-up Position 7 violation. To get from TG 6 (seated with leg extended) to TG 8 (half kneeling, supported by one arm), it's necessary to lift the hip and drag the extended leg back. If the athlete fails to externally rotate the leg and flex the knee first, he'll find this prohibitively difficult, if not impossible.

 Explain the problem.

 Demonstrate how to get into TG 7: turn knee of extended leg toward the floor, draw heel toward toe of other leg and switch.

Turkish Get-up Common Faults and Fixes, cont.

5. Short lunge.

Turkish Get-up Position 9 violation. When the athlete pivots into a kneeling lunge, the knee of the forward leg should be over the ankle. When he stands up, this will keep shear force off the knee. This fault is caused by not sliding the bent knee far enough back in the transition to from TG 7 to TG 8.

 "Rear knee further back!"

 Demonstrate proper transition from TG 8 to TG 9. Emphasize the quality of the lunge.

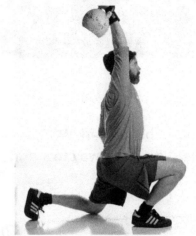

Fault

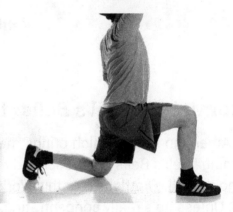

Correct TGU 9

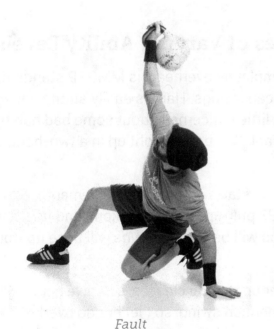

Fault

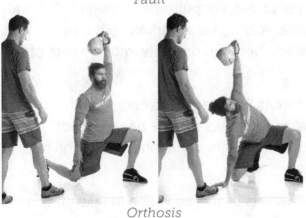

Orthosis

6. Reaching back.

Turkish Get-up Position 8 violation. Once the athlete has stepped back into a reverse lunge, his next move should be to reach for the ground beside his rear knee as that leg externally rotates 90 degrees. A common mistake is reaching way back and sitting his haunch down on the heel, without pivoting the leg.

 "Reach beside your knee!"

 Demonstrate proper TG 8.

 Place a foot or small object in line with athlete's rear knee, indicating where you want him to place his hand.

For our fourth benchmark WOD, I selected "Hell's Bells". A mix of running, kettlebell swings, and pull-ups, it's a great way to introduce implement training into our workouts.

"Hell's Bells"

Three rounds for time of
Run 400m
20 Kettlebell swings @ 24/16kg
11 pull-ups

Customizing "Hell's Bells" for Athletes of Varying Ability Levels

The American swing, which brings the kettlebell completely overhead, is MMGPP standard, so performing "Hell's Bells" as prescribed requires American swings. Harry's easily strong enough to swing the 24kg kettlebell for this workout, but I'm a little concerned about some bad habits he has. Unless he's really concentrating, he tends to yank the 'bell straight up in a two-handed snatch and then throw his head forward.

I agree he can do American swings, but warn him if he starts committing movement faults I'll have him revert to Russian swings. There are only 33 pull-ups in this workout, and he's had another week to practice, so I think his kipping pull-ups will be fine. The runs will pose no trouble for him at all.

Amy has had some experience with kettlebells in her bootcamp classes, so I give her a 25lbs kettlebell. She's also demonstrated a knack for the American swing, so I let her go overhead but, to provide a safety buffer, limit her to 15 swings per round. For pull-ups, I assign 1/2" band-assisted pull-ups. 33 pull-ups is not at all unreasonable volume for a workout, but I tell her to expect to break her second round of 11 into two sets, and her third possibly into two sets of four, then a set of three.

It's fair to say that Tim is not a runner, and I have doubts he'll be able to complete the first 400m run in 2 minutes or less. To be on the safe side, and to make sure he has plenty of time to think about his positioning in the other exercises, I tell him to run one lap around our building—200m.

Despite my best efforts, Tim has a tendency to "squat" his swing, so I set him up with two benches blocking his knees. Now he'll *have* to hinge back into RS 1, rather than squat down. I limit him to 12 Russian swings per round—2 sets of 6, with a brief reset between sets—and then 10 ring rows, 2 x 5.

Prescribing Correct Volume

Without a time cap, "Hell's Bells" can easily stretch out to 15 plodding minutes. But this workouts is supposed to be a sprint, not a grind; that requires a consistent pace on the runs, sets that go close to unbroken, and transition time between exercises kept to a minimum.

The trick is to impose a structure on "Hell's Bells" that facilitates that experience. Here's what I came up with:

"By the Numbers Testing 'Hell's Bells'"

Three cycles of
AMRAP 2: Run 400m. If you complete the run <2:00, move immediately to...
AMRAP 1: Kettlebell swings. If you get to 20 before one minute is up, move on to...
AMRAP :30 Pull-ups. If, during the first two cycles, you get to 11 before thirty seconds is up,
move immediately back to the 400m run. If, during the last cycle, you get to 11 before
time is up, you're done.

This version of "Hell's Bells" is constrained to 10:30. One could just as easily train for a 12:00 "Hell's Bells" with three rounds of a 2:00 run, 1:15 to get 20 kbell swings, and :45 to get 11 pull-ups, or a 9 minute "Hell's Bells" with 1:30 run, 50 seconds for swings and 40 seconds for pull-ups. Adjust as necessary for your group.

"3...2...1...GO!"

Harry

Harry blasted through his first 400m run in 1:15. Fast! And then, just like he promised me he wouldn't do, he proceeded to do "overhead" swings with his hands at about 1 o'clock and the 'bell pointing to 4 o'clock—a sure sign he was pulling with his arms, not powering the swing with his hips. Verbal and tactile cues didn't work, so after he finished his pull-ups (at 2: 30) and went out for his next run, he returned to find a red, 32kg kettlebell waiting for him. I told him to finish with Russian swings, knowing the heavier bell would mollify him. He called time at 8:51. Pretty blazing! But not an "as Rx'd" score. Next time.

Now, I *could* have let it go. Harry's swings weren't the very worst I've ever seen, and would've passed muster at many gyms. But my clients pay for coaching specifically because they want to know what to improve. Had I turned a blind eye to Harry's not-to-standard movement, he wouldn't have been getting his money's worth. And it's not just that. If I let him skate by, I would've been doing a disservice not only to him, but my gym, and the greater MMGPP community, too.

Amy

Amy, slower on the runs, finished up at 10:15. Next time she'll do the full volume of swings, and probably at the rx'd weight of 16kg, as well. Maybe kipping pull-ups, too? We'll see!

Tim

Tim finished his assigned work just before the ten minute mark, and surprised me by asking if he could go out and run for the remaining time. He was sweating hard, but seemed to feel energized by the exertion, not beaten down, so I told him, "Hell yeah, man!" And he went back out. I tried to wave him down after his first 200m lap, but he kept going for the full 400m.

When he got back, Amy and Harry were waiting for him at the garage door, and there were high fives all around. Great way to finish the week!

BOX JUMPS

Category: Jump and Land

Movement screen: N/a

Ability screen: Jump and land x 5 (tuck jump), tuck jump x 1 (box jump)

The box jump involves taking off from the ground, pulling the knees high, then landing in a well-organized partial squat atop a box. It builds explosive strength, and at high reps demands stamina and endurance.

Because MMGPP training prioritizes power output, many athletes will rebound their box jumps to complete the assigned work as quickly as possible. However, unless an athlete has specific competitive goals, you should discourage rebounding. Rebounding increases the risk of Achilles tendon injury, and for the general trainee, it's not worth it.

Harry and Amy will do fine with box jumps. Tim's jumping mechanics have improved to the point I'm willing to let him try jumping to stacked plates, or even the 12" box. Let's see what happens!

Box Jump Teaching Script

"We begin instruction of the box jump with the box step-up. The box step-up is a walking lunge onto a raised platform. We use the step-up as an introduction to the box jump because it teaches the proper way to descend from the box. Those with knee and ankle issues that make jumping up onto an object unsafe can use the step-up as a substitute exercise.

"Begin with your feet shoulder-width and screwed into the deck, butt tight, ribs locked down, shoulders packed. This is **Box Step-up Position 1 (bST 1).**

bST 1

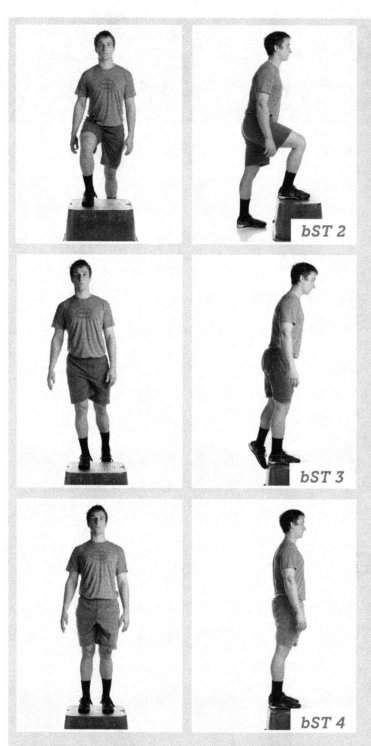

bST 2

bST 3

bST 4

"Lift your right knee and plant your foot atop the box. Make sure the entire sole of your foot is in contact. Immediately create torque by screwing your foot into the box clockwise. **Box Step-up Position 2 (bST 2).**

"Rock your center of gravity slightly toward your right foot. Then, pushing through the heel, extend the right knee and hip. **Box Step-up Position 3 (bST 3).** Try to avoid pushing off the toe of the trailing leg.

"When your right knee and hip are fully extended, bring your left foot forward and set it firmly on the box, screwing it in counterclockwise. Stand tall. This is **Box Step-up Position 4 (BU 4).**

"To return to the floor, shift your weight back onto your right foot, and step back and down with the left—**bST 2.** Once your left foot is on the floor, shift your weight to the left and bring your right foot down to return to **Box Step-up Position 1.**

"Now try it on the other side: step-up left, step-up right; step-down right, step-down left. Always step down first with the foot that came up second."

"The box jump isn't a measure of your vertical leap, but instead your ability to explode off the ground, rapidly flex your hips to pull your knees high, then land safely.

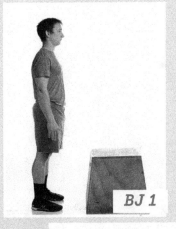

BJ 1

"Set your feet under your hips, screw in your feet, brace your midline, set your shoulders. This is the set-up, **Box Jump Position 1 (BJ 1)**.

"Jumping and landing can be broken down into two familiar positions: the hip hinge and the squat. Your take-off is based on the hinge. Landing is based on the squat.

"To hinge, push your hips back, loading your hamstrings. Keep your shins as vertical as possible! Simultaneously draw back and internally rotate your arms. Gaze should remain forward. This is the wind-up, **Box Jump Position 2 (BJ 2)**.

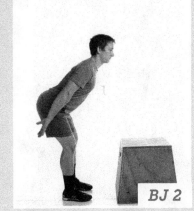

BJ 2

"To jump, launch yourself from your heels, and throw your hands forward as you externally rotate your arms. Because the vector of force is up, not forward, before you leave the ground your torso will shift to vertical, which will cause a forward translation of the knees. This very quick passing position is **Box Jump Position 3 (BJ 3)**. Notice how this 'rhymes' with **Muscle Clean Position 4.**

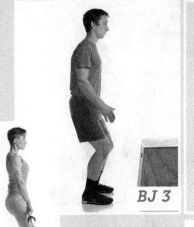

BJ 3

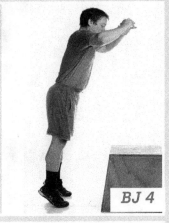

BJ 4

"As you leave the ground, your knees, hips, and ankles should be fully extended. This is the take-off, **Box Jump Position 4 (BJ 4).**

"Once you've left the ground, pull your knees high and outside. At maximum efforts, this will look as if you're sitting at the bottom of a squat while in midair. This is the tuck, **Box Jump Position 5 (BJ 5).**

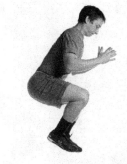

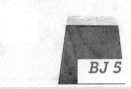

BJ 5

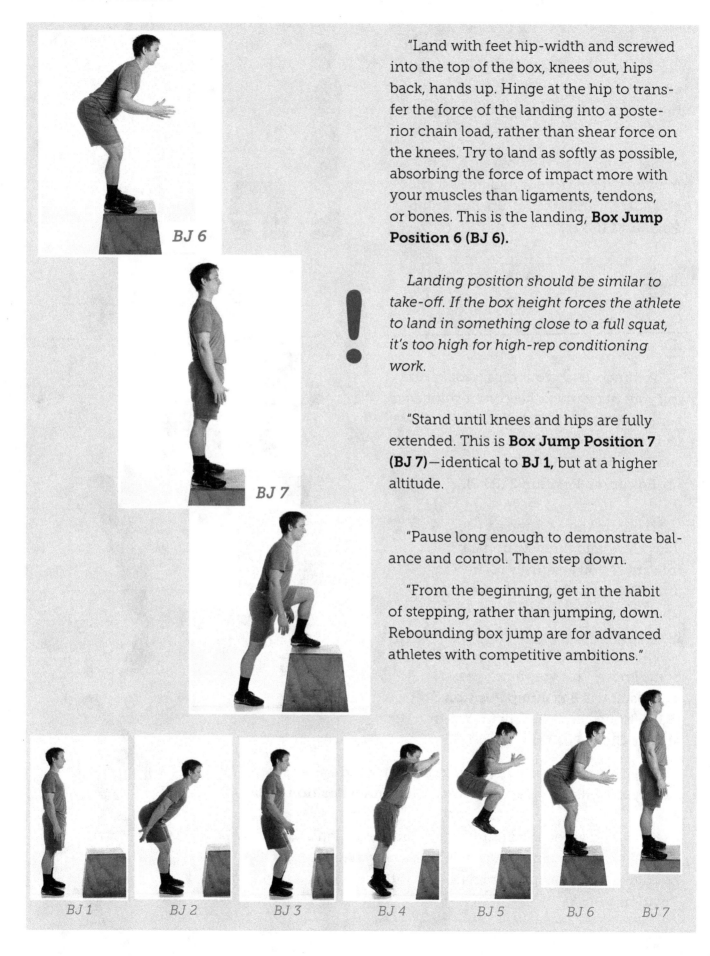

BJ 6

BJ 7

"Land with feet hip-width and screwed into the top of the box, knees out, hips back, hands up. Hinge at the hip to transfer the force of the landing into a posterior chain load, rather than shear force on the knees. Try to land as softly as possible, absorbing the force of impact more with your muscles than ligaments, tendons, or bones. This is the landing, **Box Jump Position 6 (BJ 6).**

Landing position should be similar to take-off. If the box height forces the athlete to land in something close to a full squat, it's too high for high-rep conditioning work.

"Stand until knees and hips are fully extended. This is **Box Jump Position 7 (BJ 7)**—identical to **BJ 1,** but at a higher altitude.

"Pause long enough to demonstrate balance and control. Then step down.

"From the beginning, get in the habit of stepping, rather than jumping, down. Rebounding box jump are for advanced athletes with competitive ambitions."

BJ 1   BJ 2   BJ 3   BJ 4   BJ 5   BJ 6   BJ 7

Positional Drills

"1! 2! 1! 2!" Drill athletes on the hip hinge and stand. Make sure their shins stay vertical and that they are internally rotating their arms as they draw them back.

Tuck jump. Before letting athletes attempt to jump onto the box, drill positions 1, 2, 3, 4, 5—which basically constitute a "tuck jump" (historically, a sub for double-unders). This will give you the opportunity to make some corrections in terms of mechanics before adding the challenge of actually jumping up onto an object. Make sure the knees come high and outside in BJ 5.

Box Jump Common Faults and Fixes

All faults and fixes common to jumping mechanics apply, including knees forward on wind-up, knees collapse on wind-up, no internal rotation of arms during wind-up, knees collapse on landing, as well as...

1. Landing with less than whole foot on box.

Box Jump Position 6 violation. Landing on the box with less than the full surface of the sole of the foot is just asking for trouble. A miss can lead to a painful shin abrasion, or worse.

 "Whole foot on box!"   Demonstrate a correct landing on top of the box.

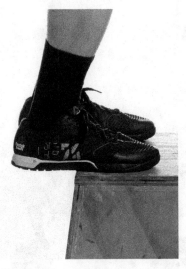

Fault

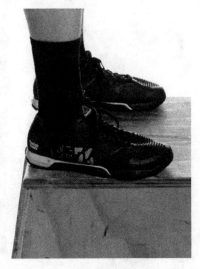

Correct BJ 5

Box Jump Common Faults and Fixes, cont.

2. Failure to come to full extension on top of the box.

Box Jump Position 7 violation. Athlete does not come to a full stand before stepping down. Remind athlete that knees and hips must straighten completely for rep to count.

"Stand up!"　　　　　　　　　　Demonstrate a proper Box Jump Position 6.

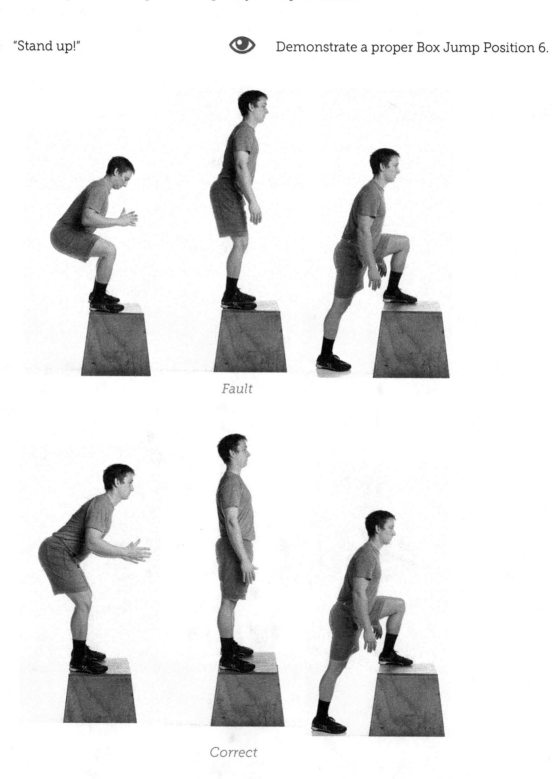

Fault

Correct

THRUSTERS

Category: Hybrid (squat, push object [vertical])

Movement screen: Front squat with push press grip

Ability screen: Dumbbell squat x 3 and dumbbell push press x 3 (dumbbell thruster), Front squat x 3 and push press x 3 (thruster)

"Thruster" is the popular name for an old-time physical culture exercise called the squat press. To do a thruster, the athlete front squats to full depth and then stands up aggressively to press the bar overhead.

Moving a large load a long distance very quickly with a fast cycle time, the thruster might be the quintessential MMGPP movement...if it's done well. Otherwise, it's exactly the sort of thing that haters make image macros about.

Not everyone can (or should) thruster with a barbell! It requires a good deal of wrist and shoulder flexibility to execute correctly. If a new athlete cannot set up properly for a barbell push press, or if he can't front squat with the bar held in the fists while holding elbows high, he should NOT do thrusters with the barbell. Substitute dumbbells instead. Otherwise you are setting him up for injury, or humiliation on the Internet.

Case in point: Tim. His dumbbell squat is improving rapidly, and he should be back squatting soon, but it'll be a long time, if ever, before he can safely front squat a barbell. No problem! Today he can superset dumbbell squats and dumbbell presses. He won't be doing dumbbell thrusters, per se; he's still too stiff to safely try to dumbbell push press. But the dumbbell squat/press combination will preserve much of the desired stimulus of the thruster.

Although Harry and Amy should both be fine with barbell thrusters, as with the dumbbell squat and back squat, we're going to start everyone with the dumbbell thruster. Let's get to work!

Dumbbell Thruster Teaching Script

"Not everyone will be able to thruster with a barbell, but everyone should learn the dumbbell thruster. The dumbbell thruster is the classical sub for wallballs if no medicine ball was available, and it's part of fun dumbbell complexes like the 'man-maker.'

"Set up as you would for a dumbbell squat: feet shoulder-width and screwed into the floor, midline braced, shoulders packed. Holding dumbbells with the knife edges of your hands next to the loading plate, set one end of the dumbbell on each shoulder. Your elbows should be tucked into your ribs, the dumbbells parallel to the floor. This is **Dumbbell Thruster Position 1 (dTH 1).**

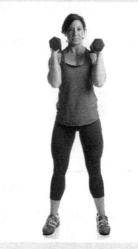 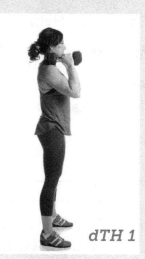

dTH 1

"Unlock your knees and sit your hips back. Push your knees out. Keep your chest up. This is **Dumbbell Thruster Position 2 (dTH 2).**

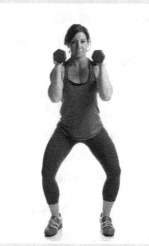 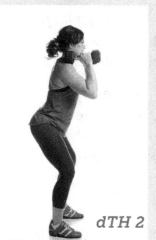

dTH 2

"Sit straight down under the crease of your hip is below the top of your knee. Keep your elbows close to the ribs. This is **Dumbbell Thruster Position 3 (dTH 3).**

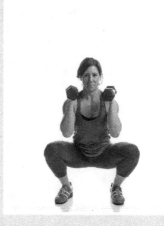 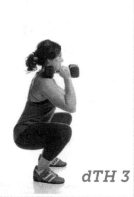

dTH 3

"Drive back up through **dTH2** into **dTH 1**.

"Just as in the barbell thruster, drive your shoulders into the dumbbell to transfer the force produced by the legs and hips.

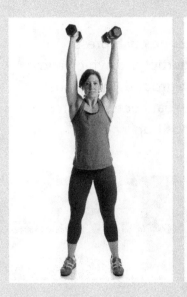
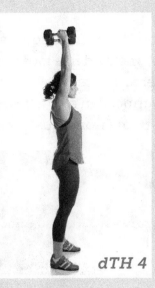

dTH 4

"Push the dumbbells up until elbows are straight. Palms should be facing in. This is **Dumbbell Thruster Position 4 (dTH 4).**

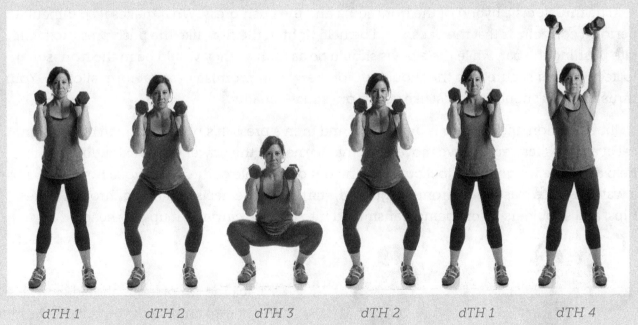

dTH 1   dTH 2   dTH 3   dTH 2   dTH 1   dTH 4

Thruster Teaching Script

"Pick up your barbells and execute three front squats.

"Now do three push presses.

"What's the difference between rack position for the front squat and the push press? In the front squat, the bar is seated on the shoulders, and held in a loose fingertip grip, which allows one to keep the elbows high enough the upper arms are parallel to the ground. In the push press, the bar is seated on the shoulder but is gripped in a tight fist, the bar centered across the palm. The elbows are high, but not as high as in the front squat rack position.

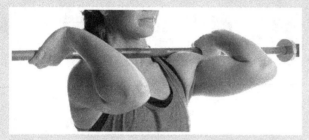
Front squat rack position

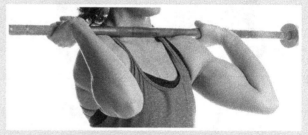
Push press rack position

"The thruster is a hybrid of the front squat and the push press. What makes it so difficult to perform correctly is that the bar should be held tight in the fists, like the push press, to facilitate pushing the bar, while the elbows should be as high as they would be in the front squat, to keep the bar secure atop the shoulder. Nor is any compromise in squat form allowed. Your thruster squat should look just like your front squat—quality.

"In execution, the thruster is not a squat and then a press. It's not segmented or mechanical at all. It's a fast, aggressive movement that harnesses the power of the extending hip to help drive the weight up to lockout. Coming out of the hole of the squat, you should visualize a wave of force blasting up from the ground, starting in the heels and rising through knees, hips, and shoulders before being transmitted into the bar, carrying it up overhead.

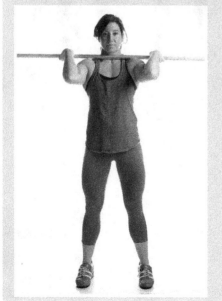

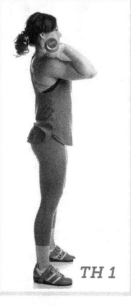
TH 1

"Rack the bar on your shoulders with a full-fist grip and crank your elbows as high as possible. Set your feet shoulder-width, create torque in your hips, brace your midline. This is **Thruster Position 1 (TH 1).** (Note: if your athlete can't do this, stick with dumbbell thrusters.)

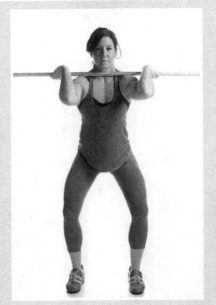
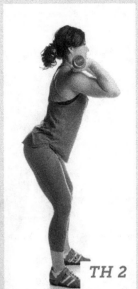

"Keeping your elbows as high as you can, unlock your knees, hinge your hips back, and push your knees out. This is **Thruster Position 2 (TH 2).**

TH 2

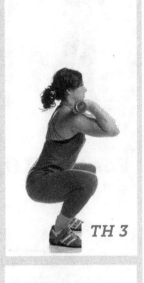

"Sit down into a full squat, keeping the elbows high as possible. This is **Thruster Position 3 (TH 3).**

TH 3

"Stand up to **Thruster Position 2**—elbows high, hips hinged back, shins vertical.

"Hips forward to **Thruster Position 1.**

"Now pull your head back and push the bar up in front of your nose. This is **Thruster Position 4 (TH 4).** If it seems familiar, it's because it's the same pose as **Push Press Position 3** (except for the stance, which is squat-width in **TH 4**).

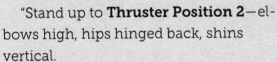

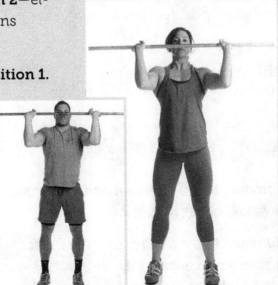

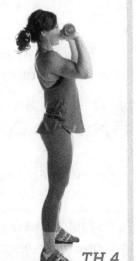

TH 4

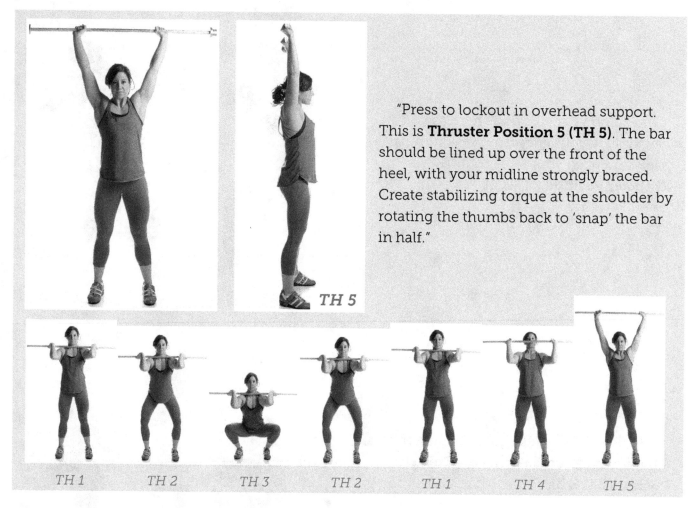

"Press to lockout in overhead support. This is **Thruster Position 5 (TH 5)**. The bar should be lined up over the front of the heel, with your midline strongly braced. Create stabilizing torque at the shoulder by rotating the thumbs back to 'snap' the bar in half."

TH 5

TH 1   *TH 2*   *TH 3*   *TH 2*   *TH 1*   *TH 4*   *TH 5*

Positional Drills

"1! 2! 3! 2! 1! 4! 5!" Drill positions of the thruster one at a time, making corrections as necessary.

"1! 2! 3! 2! Go!" Bring trainees through positions of squat back up to **TH 2**. On the command "Go!" they aggressively drive their shoulders into the bar to push press it overhead.

"1! 2! 3! Go!" Bring athletes into the bottom of the squat. Then, on the command "Go!", they accelerate out of the "hole" to drive the bar overhead.

Thruster Common Faults and Fixes

All faults and fixes common to the air squat and front squat: weight on toes, knees cave in, insufficient depth, elbows low, chest wilts, etc.

All faults and fixes common to the push press: bar in crooks of fingers, not fist; elbows too low; pressing too soon, ship's figurehead, etc. The exception is the push press's emphasis on vertical body position; the hip hinge of a Front Squat Position 2 applies.

Category: Push away from object (vertical)

Movement screen: N/a

Ability screen: Bar dip x 10

Similar to bar dips, ring dips require the athlete to support herself with extended arms, descend until her elbows are higher than her shoulders, then push back up to support. The critical difference is that the unlike the bars, which have a fixed position, the rings are in a "completely frictionless plane", which means the athlete must work much harder to create the stability necessary for the productive application of force.

Explain to your trainees that often an athlete's first attempts at support on the rings will cause his arms to shake violently as his brain figures out how to stabilize on the rings. At first this lack of stability will make ring dips much more difficult than bar dips. Later, once your athletes are familiar with the apparatus, that difference will lessen.

It's pointless to put on the rings, even just to practice support, athletes who lack the strength to do full bar dips without assistance. Keep trainees on the bars until they can do at least five full dips. There's no need to rush.

With that in mind, only Harry will do ring dips today. Amy will stay on the bars, and Tim, the parallettes.

Ring Dip Teaching Script

"A spotter will hold the rings still. Grasp the rings and hop up to support position— same as on the stationary bars. Once you are stable, ask the spotter to let go.

"Generally speaking, your arms will begin to shake, your muscles firing wildly as your brain tries to figure out which are required for stabilization.

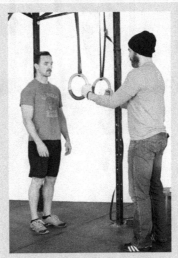
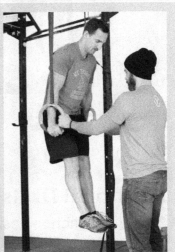

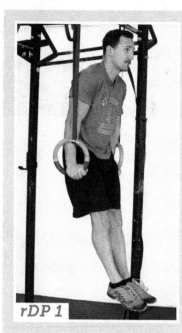

rDP 1

"Keep your thumbs facing forward, and keep the rings close to your body. Holding a strong hollowed-out position (feet together, toes pointed, midline stable, shoulders packed), you are in **Ring Dip Position 1 (rDP 1)**. Hold **rDP 1** for ten seconds. More advanced athletes can try externally rotating their arms to turn the rings out.

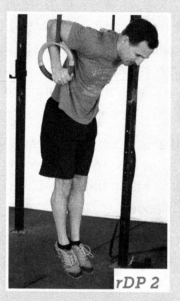

rDP 2

"If you can hold a reasonably stable support, try a ring dip. Lower yourself until you can feel the rings touch your biceps, then push back up to full elbow extension. Keep the rings close to your body; the action mimics drawing a pistol from its holster. At the bottom of the movement, the toes are pointed at the floor as the torso leans forward slightly. This is **Ring Dip Position 2 (rDP 2)**."

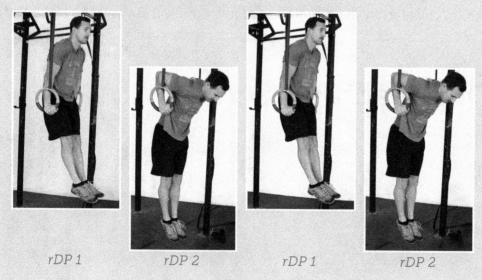

rDP 1   rDP 2   rDP 1   rDP 2

Positional Drills

"1! 2! 1! 2!" Practice positions of the ring dip one at a time, making corrections as necessary.

Ring Dip Common Faults and Fixes

All faults and fixes common to the dip apply, including partial ROM, shoulder dump, and spinal overextension, as well as...

1. Rings coming away from body/elbows flare out.

Ring Dip Position 2 transition to rDP 1 violation. Rings must be kept close to the sides, with thumbs facing forward.

 "Thumbs forward!" or "Rings close!"

 Demonstrate a correct transition from rDP 2 to rDP 1.

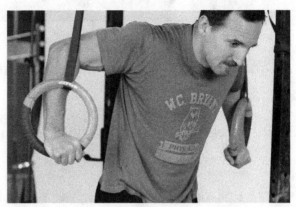

Fault: rings move away from body, turn in

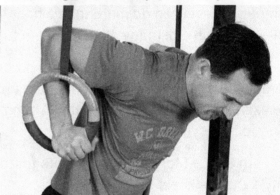

Correct: rings are kept close and parallel to body

2. Triceps extensions.

Ring Dip Position 2 violation. Rather than lower and raise his COG, the athlete bends from the hips and then straightens up. With the body straight, its center of gravity must travel up and down, somewhere between 8-10", while the elbows travel back and the shoulders stay just in front of the rings. Discourage the athlete from hinging forward from the elbow and piking at the hips.

 "Stay vertical!" or "Draw pistols!"

 Demonstrate a correction rDP 2.

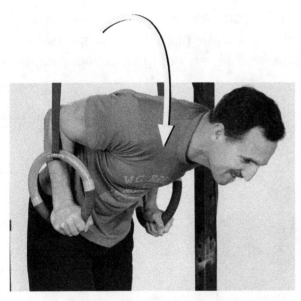

Fault: hip remains at same height

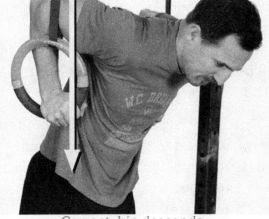

Correct: hip descends

Category: Hybrid (Pull to object [strict, vertical], hip and trunk flexion [static])

Movement screen: N/a

Ability screen: Pull-up x 5 and L-hang knee extensions x 10 (L Pull-up)

The L Pull-up is a challenging variation of the dead hang pull-up. It seems to have fallen out of fashion these days, perhaps because its positions are so demanding that few athletes not at competitor level can do more than a handful in any recognizable form. It can be performed as a pull-up or chin-up; many athletes seem to find the chin-up variation easier on the shoulders.

If you do include L pull-ups in your programming, when it comes time to choose a variation for developing athletes, prioritize either the upper body pull or the static hip flexion component of the exercise, i.e., the pull-up or the L-hang, depending on what else is going on in your programming for the cycle.

Team Space Monkey assignments for this movement will shake out like this: Harry, L pull-ups; Amy, L-hangs knee; Tim, tuck hangs.

L-Hang Teaching Script

"Climb up on a box under the pull-up bar. Grasp the bar with a full, thumbs-around grip. Make sure your pinky knuckles point toward the ceiling; this helps create external rotation at the shoulder.

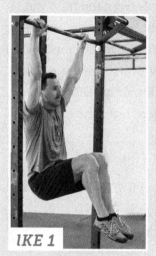

lKE 1

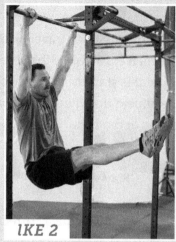

lKE 2

"Step off of the box into a static hang with active shoulders. Pull your knees as high as you can, keeping knees and feet together. This is a **tuck hang**, what we'll call **L-hang Knee Extension Position 1 (lKE 1)**.

"Then, keeping the knees high, contract the quads to extend your knees. When your legs are straight, you're in **L-hang Knee Extension Position 2 (lKE 2)**, otherwise known as an L-hang.

"These two positions can be cycled to build up strength for the L-hang static hold.

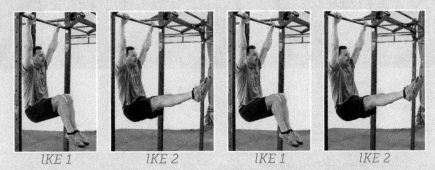

lKE 1   lKE 2   lKE 1   lKE 2

"The L-hang is an L-sit executed while hanging from the pull-up bar. It's a necessary first step toward the L Pull-up. Don't give up anything else about your position! Hips remain flexed, shoulders back and down, fists twisting into the bars.

"If you can hold **L-hang Knee Extension Position 2** for at least 20 seconds, and you've got at least five strict pull-ups, try an L pull-up. **L-hang Knee Extension Position 2** is now **L Pull-up Position 1 (lPL 1)**. Hanging from the bar, feet together, legs straight, hips piked, shoulders active, drive the elbows down until your chin is clearly over the bar. This is **L Pull-up Position 2 (lPL 2)**. Straighten your arms to return to **L Pull-up Position 1**. Make sure your feet remain higher than your hips."

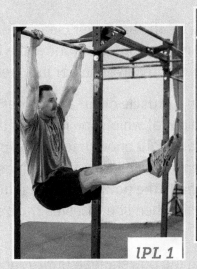
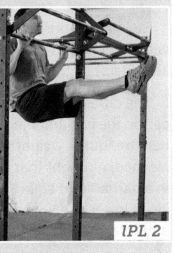

lPL 1   lPL 2

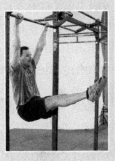
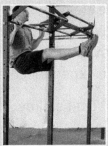
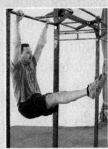
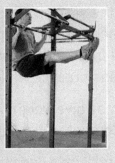

lPL 1   lPL 2   lPL 1   lPL 2

L Pull-up Common Faults and Fixes

All faults and fixes common to the pull-up apply, including midline breaks, chin fails to clean bar, and arms don't come to full extension.

All faults and fixes common to the L-sit apply, including W-sit and tilting.

POWER CLEANS

Category: Pull Object (ground to shoulder)

Movement screen: Front squat Position 2 test

Ability screen: Muscle clean x 5

Building on the muscle clean, the power clean adds a pull-accelerated drop toward the floor, with feet shifting from "jumping" position (under the hips) to "receiving" position (under the shoulders) so the athlete may receive the bar in a well-organized partial front squat.

The difference between a muscle clean and power clean is the height at which the athlete receives the bar, and the height at which she receives the bar is a function of the weight relative to her strength. A weight that's light enough for her to pull easily to shoulder height can be muscle cleaned. A weight that can be pulled about as high as the sternum, but no further, can be caught in a partial front squat. That's the power clean. As the weights get heavier, she'll catch the power clean lower and lower, until, when she receives the bar in the bottom of a front squat, she's doing a full clean.

DO NOT begin teaching the power clean until your trainee has mastered the muscle clean! If moving through the seven positions of the muscle clean has not yet become a matter of unconscious competence, further complexifying the movement by requiring a drop into an instantly organized partial front squat is not going to improve matters. Let those athletes still developing their muscle cleans practice while you teach more experienced athletes the power clean.

This method may give weightlifting purists fits. That's okay. My goal is to get the general trainee moving competently as quickly as possible.

Fast, strong, and with a decent front squat, Harry will excel at power cleans. Amy's slowly getting over a fear of fast-moving barbells, but her positions are so good, I know she'll do well, too. Tim still can't use a barbell for squatting, but his dumbbell squats and jumping mechanics are are sufficiently developed that I can teach him the dumbbell power clean.

Power Clean Teaching Script

"The power clean has five positions in common with the muscle clean: **Power Clean Position 1**, **Power Clean Position 2**, **Power Clean Position 3**, **Power Clean Position 4**, and **Power Clean Position 5** are all identical to their muscle clean equivalents. The arm pull of **Power Clean 6** is the same as in MC 6, but you'll be in free fall, with your feet off the ground. More on that in a bit.

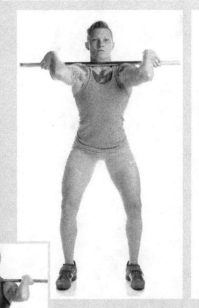
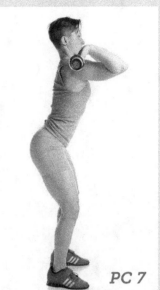

PC 7

"Unlike the full stand of MC 7, **Power Clean Position 7 (PC 7)** is a partial front squat—exactly like Front Squat Position 2 (FS 2). If your trainee cannot hit this position, DO NOT attempt to teach her the power clean.

"This partial front squat of **PC 7** is the result of a rapid reversal of direction from the upward impetus created by exploding from **PC 4** into **PC 5**. As the arms pull into **PC 6**, the feet shift from under the hips to under the shoulders. In that transition, the lifter is in free fall for a split second, which allows her to work against the inertia of the bar to accelerate herself toward the floor. The load is received as her shoulder pass below the bar.

"Let's practice that footwork.

"Stand tall with your feet under your hips. Now, move your feet out from your center line, about 2-4", until they are under your shoulders. Hinge back at the hips. With your weight toward the heels and kneels pushed out, you should be in a well-organized partial squat.

"Move your feet back under your hips. On my command 'Go!', drop into that partial squat, and freeze. Ready? Go!

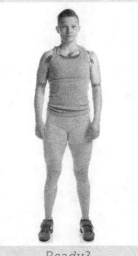
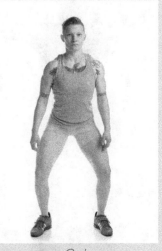

Ready?   *Go!*

369

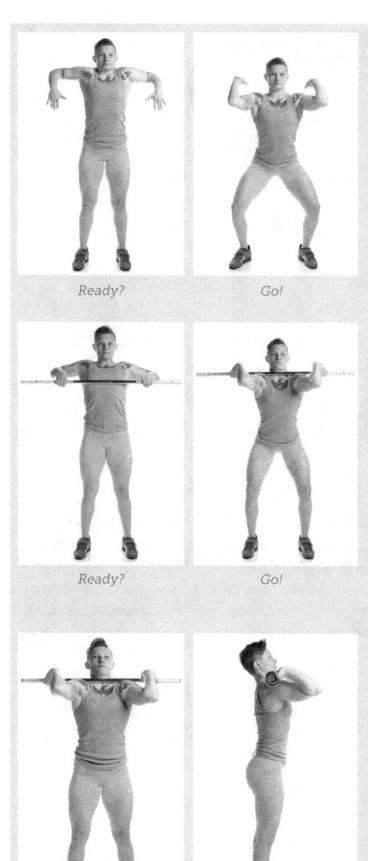

Ready? Go!

Ready? Go!

PC 8

"Stand and reset. Let's try that again, this time miming the action of the third pull. Set-up in **PC 6** with an imaginary barbell—feet under the hips, elbows high. On my command 'GO!', execute a drop squat while simultaneously whipping your elbows around to bring your thumbs to your shoulders.

"Good! Now, pick up your barbell (make sure it's lighter than what you usually work out with—unless you're unusually strong, doing this drill with a 20kg bar will be uncomfortable).

"Hit **PC 6** for me. On my command 'GO!' drop squat and spin your elbows around the bar to land in **PC 7.**

"I want you to stick the landing and freeze right where you are. Ready? GO!

"Self-assess. Are you in a good partial front squat? Weight back toward the heel, slight toe turnout, knees pushed out, hips hinged back, elbows high, gaze forward? If not, get organized.

"Then stand up into Front Squat Position 1—now **Power Clean Position 8 (PC 8)** or 'stand'. Drill as necessary until you've got a feel for it."

Positional Drills

"5! 6! 7! 8!" Practice positions one at a time, making corrections as necessary.

Power Clean Teaching Script, cont.

"Reset. Now we'll work from **Power Clean Position 4**. On my command 'Go!', stand up aggressively to get the bar moving (thus hitting **PC 5**). In action, **PC 6** sees you in mid-air, hauling on the bar while simultaneously hinging back and sliding your feet out to squat width. Instead of thinking 'pull the bar up,' think 'pull yourself under'. Your elbows will spin around the bar and should be pointing straight ahead when you come to rest in the partial front squat of **Power Clean Position 7**. I want you to freeze there, in your catch position. Ready? Go!

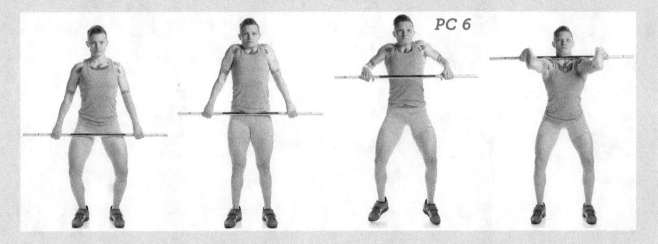

"Self-assess! Are you in a well-organized partial front squat? If so, stand up into **PC 8**. If not, make the necessary corrections to your position, and then stand to completion.

"Make sure you pause and self-assess in the catch. Each time you don't land perfectly, remind yourself how you should be landing, fix what's wrong, and then try again. This iterative process of execute, self-assess, self-correct will, over time, greatly improve the quality of your positions.

"The bar should join the body with little to no ballistic impact. If the bar is slamming into your body, or landing on your clavicles instead of your shoulders, calibrate your pull more carefully. Don't overpull. Pull the bar to you."

Positional Drills

"4! 5! 6! 7! 8!" Practice the positions of the high hang power clean one at a time, making corrections as necessary.

"4! Go!" Practice the high hang power clean. Make sure the athletes pause in **PC 7** to self-assess and correct before standing up the bar.

Power Clean Teaching Script, cont.

"Reset. The pull from the floor in the Power Clean uses exactly the same positions (except **PC 6**, as discussed) as the Muscle Clean."

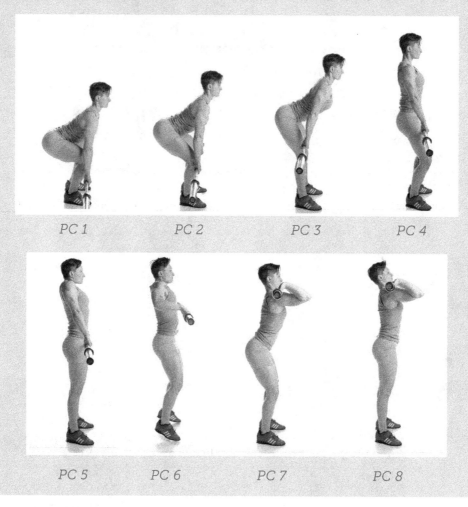

| PC 1 | PC 2 | PC 3 | PC 4 |

| PC 5 | PC 6 | PC 7 | PC 8 |

Positional Drills

"1! 2! 3! 4! Go!" Practice the positions of floor, hang, extend, pockets one at a time, making corrections as necessary, before exploding through the second half of the movement.

"1! 2! 3! Go!" Practice the positions of floor, hang, extend, pockets one at a time, making corrections as necessary, before exploding through the second half of the movement.

"1! 2! Go!" Practice the positions of floor, hang, extend, pockets one at a time, making corrections as necessary, before exploding through the second half of the movement.

"1! Go!" Practice the power clean. Pause in **PC 7** to self-assess and correct before standing up the bar.

Power Clean Common Faults and Fixes

All faults and fixes common to the muscle clean apply, including deadlift set-up, hips rise too soon, jumping from in front of knees, not sweeping bar in, reverse curling bar, pulling too soon, and not finishing, as well as...

1. Knees coming forward in catch ("limbo-ing under the bar").

Power Clean Position 7 violation. Trainee shoves knees forward and leans back to descend, as if in a limbo contest. The receiving position for the power clean should be exactly the same as the initial hinge of the front squat: hips back, knees out, shins nearly vertical. It can be compared to sitting on a barstool. Tell your trainee, "You can't see it, you know it's there; just keep sitting back until you find it."

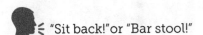 "Sit back!" or "Bar stool!"

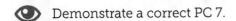 Demonstrate a correct PC 7.

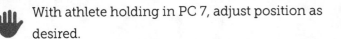 With athlete holding in PC 7, adjust position as desired.

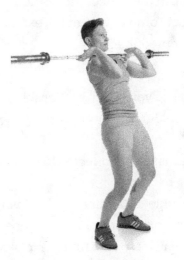

Fault

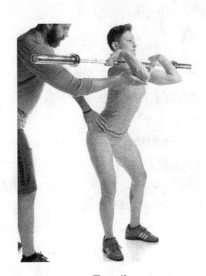

Tactile

Power Clean Common Faults and Fixes, cont.

2. Incomplete finish.

Power Clean Position 5 violation. Often in her rush to get down into receiving position, an athlete will neglect to finish the concentric portion of the lift. The hips must come to violent full extension in PC 5 for full power production.

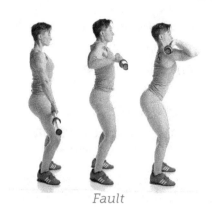

Fault

 "Squeeze your butt!" or "Finish!" or "Stand tall!" or "Jump! Fast elbows!"

 Demonstrate a correct PC 5.

 With athlete standing tall, hold your hand directly over her head. Have her execute a power clean, directing her to drive the top of her head into your palm as she explodes up into PC 5.

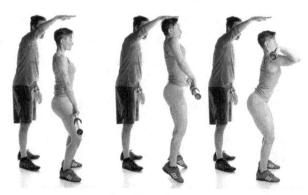

Tactile

3. Feet don't move.

Power Clean Position 7 violation. In transition from PC 5 to PC 7, feet must slide from under hips to under shoulders. Remember, a power clean is an abbreviated squat clean. PC 7 is synonymous with Front Squat Position 2.

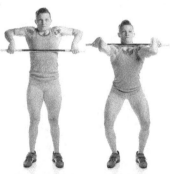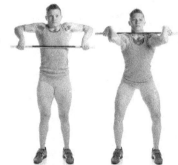

Fault   *Correct*

 "Feet slide out!"

 Demonstrate a correct PC 7.

 With athlete holding in PC 7, adjust position as desired.

 Draw desired foot position on ground with chalk.

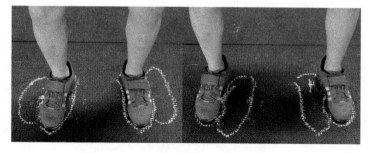

Orthosis

Power Clean Common Faults and Fixes, cont.

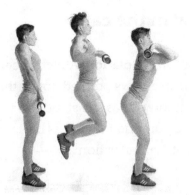

Faulty transition

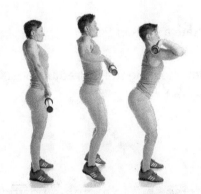

Correct PC 5 to PC 7 transition

4. Donkey kick.

Power Clean Position 6 to Power Clean Position 7 transition violation. Athlete kicks back and stamps down feet. Explain to athlete that the loud "crack" she often hears from weightlifters is a function of the speed with which their hard-soled shoes reset on the wooden platform, not an actual foot stomp.

🗣 "Don't move your feet!" often works wonders. You can also try "Heels to the ground fast!"

👁 Demonstrate a correct PC 6 to PC 7 transition.

5. Feet land too wide.

Power Clean Position 7 violation. If an athlete starts with her stance too wide, she'll often land too wide. This fault is also commonly caused by an unwilling-ness to sit down under bar; rather than bending the knees, the feet splay out. The bar should be received as if in FS 2.

🗣 "Squat stance!"

👁 Demonstrate a correct PC 7.

✋ With athlete holding in PC 7, adjust position as desired.

✚ Draw desired foot position on ground with chalk.

✚ Set two bumpers up to block feet at desired stance width.

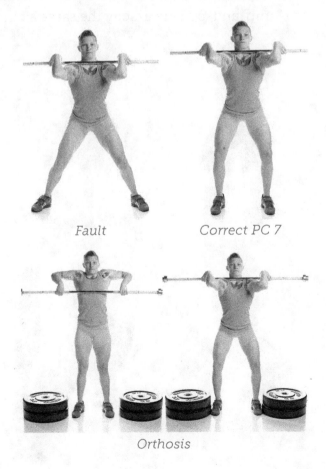

Fault   *Correct PC 7*

Orthosis

Power Clean Common Faults and Fixes, cont.

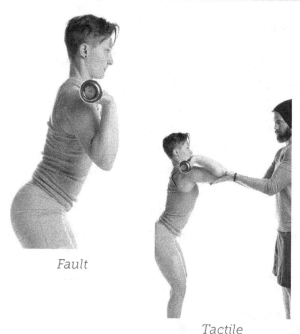

Fault

Tactile

6. Elbows low in the catch.

Power Clean Position 7 violation. Athlete receives bar on shoulders with elbows pointed down, then lifts elbows to point forward as she stands up to finish. Elbows must be pointing forward as bar lands on shoulders, *a la* Front Squat Position 2.

 "Elbows up!"

 Demonstrate a correct PC 7.

 With athlete holding in PC 7, adjust position as desired.

Dumbbell Power Clean

"In the dumbbell power clean the pull from the floor, the torso shift to jumping position, and the jump-and-pull are exactly the same as in the dumbbell muscle clean.

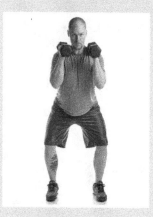

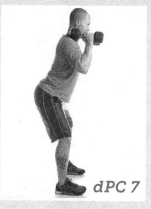

dPC 7

"The difference is that the dumbbells are caught in a partial squat. The dumbbells are racked on the shoulders, palms facing in, elbows in tight. This is **Dumbbell Power Clean Position 7 (dPC 7).** The dumbbells are then stood up to completion in **Dumbbell Power Clean Position 8.**"

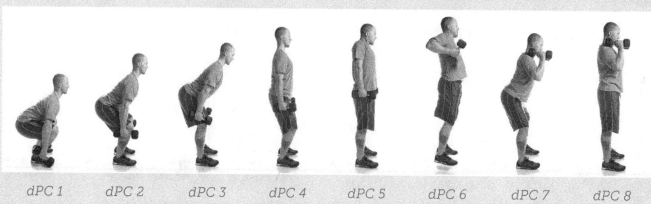

dPC 1   dPC 2   dPC 3   dPC 4   dPC 5   dPC 6   dPC 7   dPC 8

WALL HANDSTANDS

Category: Push Away from Object (vertical, inverted, static)

Movement screen: N/a

Ability screen: N/a (down dog hold), down dog hold x 20 sec (pike hold from box), pike hold from box x 20 sec (kick up to handstand), kick up to handstand (wall handstand)

Every MMGPP athlete should practice some version of the handstand. It strengthens the shoulder girdle and develops the athlete's proprioception in an unfamiliar and unsettling situation, i.e., being upside down. It's a necessary first step for more advanced movements like the handstand push-up, and later for the freestanding handstand, handstand walking, etc. BtN's progression begins with yoga's down dog pose. From there we increase the load by elevating the feet to bring the torso to vertical. If your athlete can handle a vertical torso piked hold from the box, he is strong enough to practice kicking up to handstand. We teach the kick up with hands planted, rather than a traditional gymnastic lunge into hand plant, because it reduces ballistic impact on the wrists and allows the athlete to set up with external rotation.

BtN teaches the back-to-the-wall HS first because it's easier to bail out should something go wrong. The nose-to-wall handstand is taught later, along with the wall walk.

Harry and Amy can handle this without problem. Tim will likely stay with the most basic pose.

Wall Handstand Teaching Script

"The positions utilized in the handstand progression series have much in common with those of the barbell press.

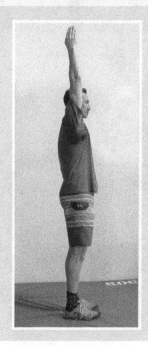

"Set up with feet together. Brace your midline by squeezing your glutes and locking your abs down. Push both hands overhead as if pressing a barbell. Unlike the barbell press, however, shrug your shoulders way up toward your ears. A small portion of your ears should be visible in front of your arms. A straight line could be drawn from your hands down through your shoulders and hips and ending at the front of your heel.

"Now let's turn that upside down. In the two handstand progression exercises that follow, we want to see straight arms in line with the spine, with the ears between the arms. We begin in a pose that will be familiar to those of you who've done some yoga: the downward-facing dog.

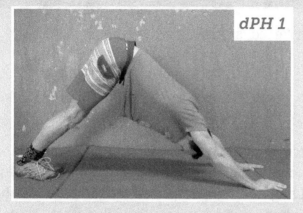

dPH 1

"Start in Push-up Position 1: feet together, butt and abs locked tight, shoulders back and down, hands planted just outside the shoulders and screwed into the ground. Keeping your legs and arms straight, draw your hips up and back until your head is between your arms. This is **Down Dog Pike Hold Position 1 (dPH 1).**

"If this is too easy, you can elevate your feet on a box, so that you are supporting more and more of your body's weight on your hands.

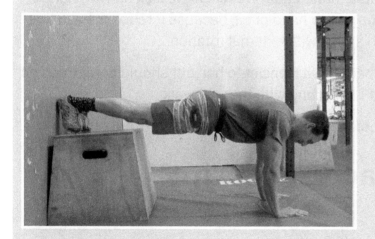

"Set a box against the wall. Start modestly, with a 12" box. Later you can use the 20", 24", or more. Get in a push-up position with your feet on the box. Set your feet against the wall.

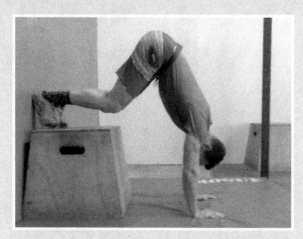

"Allowing your knees to bend, walk your hands back toward the box until the load starts to feel challenging.

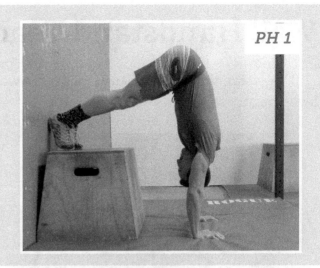

PH 1

"Pushing your heels into the wall, straighten your legs to load your hamstrings. Ideally, your torso is now perpendicular to the floor. This is **Pike Hold Position 1 (PH 1)**. To recover, walk your hands back out to push-up position and then step down."

Down Dog and Pike Hold Common Faults and Fixes

1. Looking at ground.

Down Dog Pike Hold and Pike Hold from Box Position 1 violation. Athlete cranes his neck to look at the floor. In the pike hold, the athlete should hold his head in a neutral position, with his gazed trained at his feet or on the box. The neck should be kept in line with the spine.

 "Head neutral!" or "Chin down!"

 Demonstrate a correct dPH 1.

 With athlete holding in dPH 1, adjust position as desired.

 Place a rolled up towel between chin and chest.

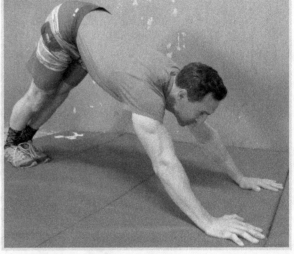

Fault

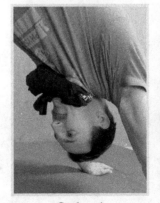

Orthosis

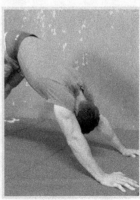

Correct DP 1

Wall Handstand Teaching Script, cont.

"Understand that the kick-up against the wall should be relatively effortless; it depends on leverage, not strength.

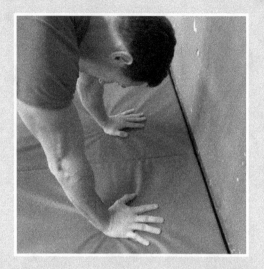

"Place your hands shoulder-width apart, 4-6" from the wall. Fingers should be splayed with middle fingers pointing to 12 o'clock. Screw your hands into the ground, right hand clockwise, left hand counter-clockwise, to create external rotation at the shoulder.

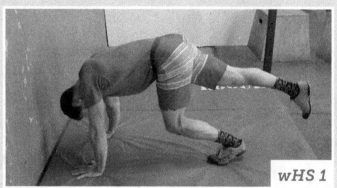

wHS 1

"Step back into a plank position. Then draw one foot up under you. The other leg should be kept straight. Squeeze the glute on that side to lift the leg about 6" off the ground. Throughout the kick-up, this leg should not touch the ground. Try to keep it in line with the torso. This is **Wall Handstand Position 1 (wHS 1).**

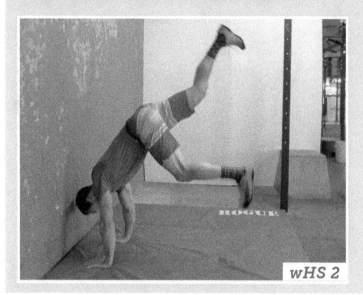

wHS 2

"Pushing with the cocked leg, swing the heel of your extended leg toward the wall. At the same time, actively engage the lats so that you are 'pulling' your shoulders over the fixed point of your hands. This is **Wall Handstand Position 2 (wHS 2).**

"Push off three times, trying to get the extended leg a little higher each time. Again, this is about leverage, not strength; bouncing off the floor, rather than throwing yourself at the wall.

"For some athletes, this will be enough to work on for awhile. Only when the athlete can, on the third push, easily tap the heel of his extended leg against the wall, is he ready to get completely upside down.

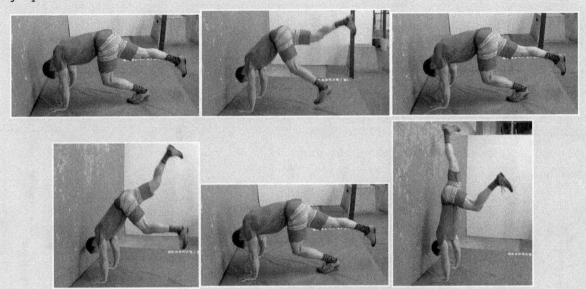

"On the third kick-up, look through your arms at the wall opposite you. This will bring your hips over your head, and both heels should make contact with the wall. Immediately push the ground away as strongly as you can, simultaneously bringing your feet together, pointing your toes, and contacting every muscle in the body.

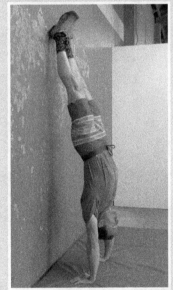

"Your goal is a straight body position: feet stacked over knees over hips over shoulders over hands. To defeat the natural tendency to arch into a backbend, hollow out as strongly as you can, drawing your pelvis toward your rib cage. In addition, push into the floor with your fingertips. Your heels should peel off the wall, putting you into a freestanding handstand (at least temporarily). This is **Wall Handstand Position 3 (wHS 3).**"

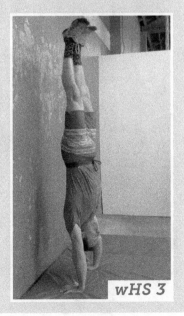

wHS 3

Wall Handstand Common Faults and Fixes

1. Knees bent/throws self at wall.

Wall Handstand Position 2 violation. Knee of extended leg is bent as the athlete tries to kick in toward the wall. Remind him that kicking up to handstand is a matter of leverage, not raw strength. He should strive to maintain a straight line from his hands through his midline down to the foot of his extended leg as he pushes off the leg cocked beneath him and pulls with his lats.

  "Straight leg!" or "Push off!"

Demonstrate proper kick-up technique.

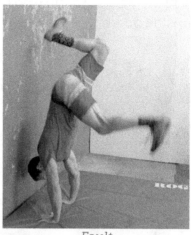

Fault

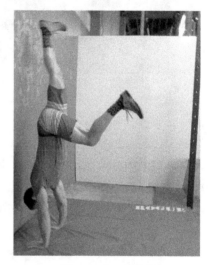

Correct wHS 2

2. Soft elbows.

Wall Handstand Position 3 violation. Elbows must be locked straight through kicking up and holding the handstand—otherwise, trainee risks falling on his head.

  "Straight arms!"

Demonstrate proper wHS 3.

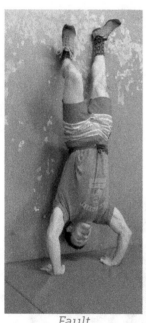

Fault

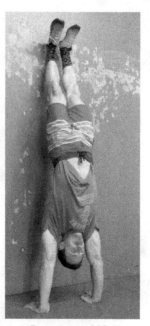

Correct wHS 3

Category: Hip and Trunk Extension

Movement screen: N/a

Ability screen: Hip extension x 5

The back extension develops strength and flexibility through the lumbar and thoracic spine. The athlete lays prone atop a GHD bench, hips fixed atop the pad, body parallel to the floor. He drapes himself forward, allowing his spine to flex, before slowly raising up one vertebra at a time until the lumbar and thoracic sections of the spine return to neutral.

The back extension is a more complex version of the hip extension. It requires a great deal more body awareness and control. So while Tim won't be doing back extensions today, his good mornings have improved to the point he can get on the GHD to learn the hip extension.

Harry and Amy will both practice back extensions.

Back Extension Teaching Script

"Climb up onto the GHD bench. Fit your legs between the foot anchor pads and press your feet against the back plate. Lay prone on the GHD pad. Your hips should be directly on top of the pad, trapped and unable to move. Adjust the length of the foot anchor assembly as necessary.

"Begin with your torso hanging over the pad, with the top of your head is pointing at the floor. Hands can be crossed at the chest, touching the temples, or held behind the head. This is **Back Extension Position 1 (BE 1).**

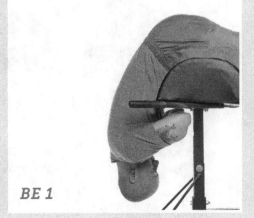

BE 1

BE 2

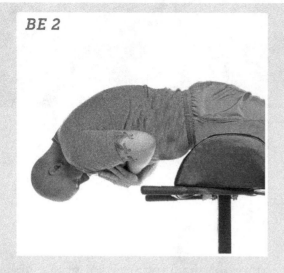

"Slowly raise up from your hips, vertebra by vertebra. Halfway up, your lower spine will be have returned to neutral, but your upper spine is still in flexion; we'll call this **Back Extension Position 2 (BE 2).**

BE 3

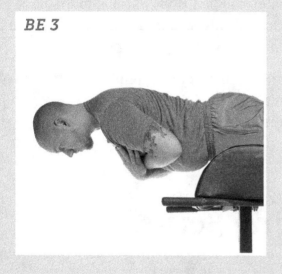

"Finish with knees, hips, and back in a line: body parallel to the floor, abs on, glutes on. This is **Back Extension Position 3 (BE 3).**

"Lower back to BE 1 and repeat. Slow and controlled is the way to go."

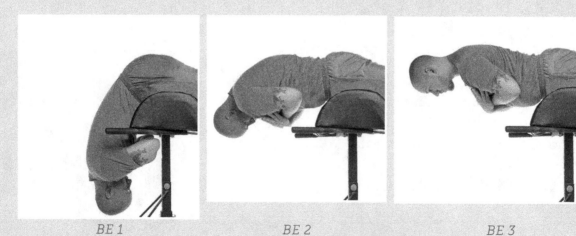

BE 1   BE 2   BE 3

Back Extension Common Faults and Fixes

1. Hip extension.

Back Extension Position 2 violation. Often an athlete will simply extend his hip to raise up, rather than carefully lift his spine one vertebra at a time. Explain to him that that the back extension is an uncurling of the spine, as if it is being lifted from below.

 "Snake up!"

 Demonstrate a proper transition from BE 1 to BE 2 to BE 3.

 Tap the athlete along the spine, ascending from the tailbone, to indicate from where the effort to extend should radiate.

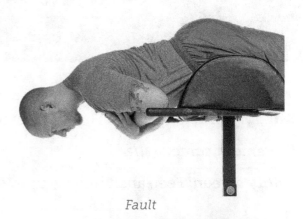

Fault

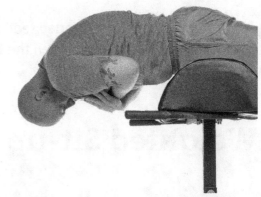

Correct BE 2

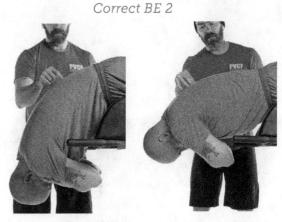

Tactile sequence: tap along the spine to give trainee positional feedback

WEIGHTED SIT-UPS

Category: Hip and Trunk Flexion (seated)

Movement screen: N/a

Ability screen: Feet-anchored sit-up x 20

The weighted sit-up is a loaded feet-anchored sit-up. It's included in By the Numbers as a necessary stepping stone between the feet-anchored sit-up and the challenging Roman chair sit-up.

Weighted Sit-up Teaching Script

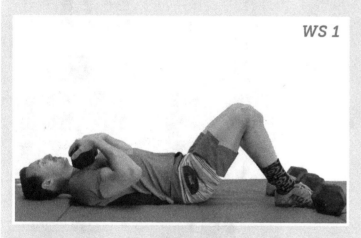

WS 1

"Set up two dumbbells and an Abmat, as when preparing for feet-anchored sit-ups. Have a seat and fit your feet under the handles of the dumbbells. Pick up the dumbbell of your choice (anywhere from 5-35lbs) and hold it by the ends against your upper chest. Lie back on the floor. This is **Weighted Sit-up Position 1 (WS 1).**

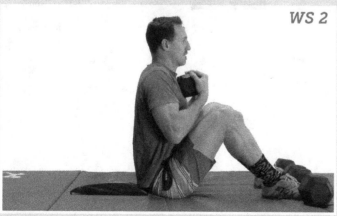

WS 2

"Contract your abdominal muscles to flex your trunk and push your lumbar vertebrae into the Abmat. Sit-up tall—your torso must incline slightly past vertical to the ground. This is **Weighted Sit-up Position 2 (WS 2).**

"Return to **WS 1** to begin your next rep."

Weighted Sit-up Common Faults and Fixes

1. Weight held out in front.

Weighted Sit-up Position 1 violation. The athlete holds the weight forward, over the fulcrum point of the movement. To get the maximum training benefit from this exercise, the weight must be carried as far out on the lever of the torso as possible. Behind the head would be most challenging, but might lead to neck strain. Keep weight on upper chest.

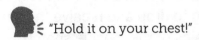 "Hold it on your chest!"

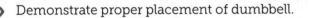 Demonstrate proper placement of dumbbell.

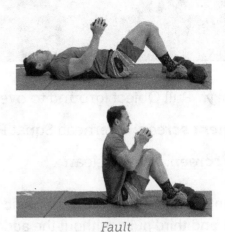

Fault

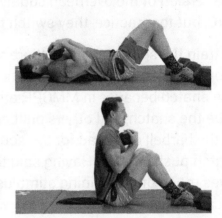

Correct

2. Weight held too low

Weighted Sit-up Position 1 violation. For the same reasons described above, holding the weight lower on the torso also decreases the challenge until the athlete is basically doing a regular feet-anchored sit-up. To get any extra training benefit, the athlete must hold the weight on his chest.

 "Hold it on your chest!"

 Demonstrate proper placement of dumbbell.

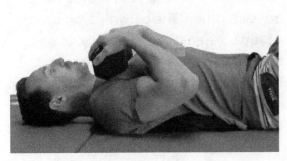

Fault

Correct WS 1

Category: Pull Object (ground to overhead)

Movement screen: Overhead Squat Position 1 test

Ability screen: Muscle clean x 5

The muscle snatch is the most basic version of the snatch. It teaches the positions of the first, second, and third pulls, without the added complexification of having to drop and receive the bar in some version of the overhead squat. In BtN, athletes learn the basics of the muscle snatch with PVC, but for practice, they switch to light barbells.

Why train the snatch at all? Is there a benefit for the average person in training the snatch over and above training the clean? The honest answer is that in a MMGPP training program athletes train the snatch because in MMGPP, athletes snatch. Some metabolic conditioning workouts prescribe the snatch, and others built around overhead squats certainly go quicker if you can snatch the barbell overhead for the squats, rather than clean, push press, lower behind the head, and snatch push press it. Having said that, when in doubt, confine your athletes to the clean. It preserves much of the training stimulus of the snatch without the extra risk to shoulders in their fifth decade of use, or tight from desk work.

The muscle snatch is appropriate for Harry and Amy, but not Tim, who lacks the overhead flexibility for ballistic work. He'll keep working on his dumbbell muscle cleans.

Muscle Snatch Teaching Script

"Let's start by reviewing overhead support position. Hold PVC at waist height, as far out toward the ends as you can manage.

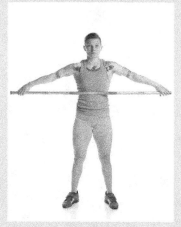
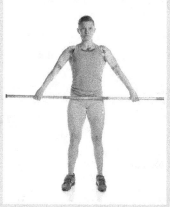

"Start slowly sliding your hands in toward each other. The bar will drop toward your hips; when it's in the crook of your hip (an inch or two below the crest of the pelvis, or the height at which you can raise one leg without jostling the bar), that's your snatch grip.

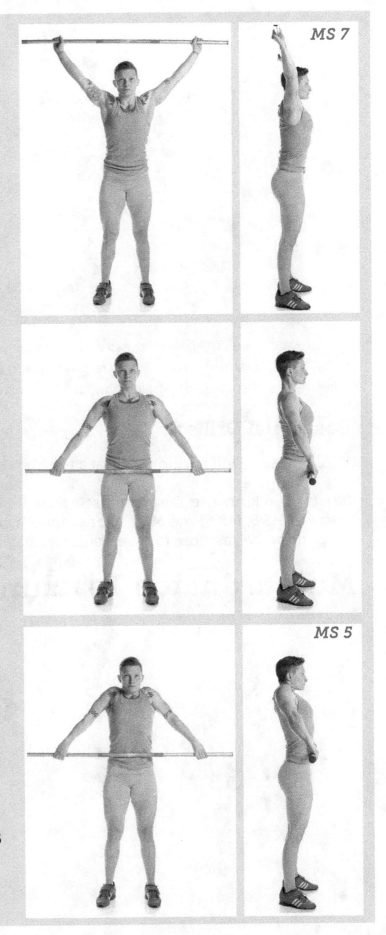

MS 7

MS 5

"With this snatch grip, press the bar from behind your neck straight up until your elbows lock out. Let it fall slightly back in your wrists. Attempt to 'snap' it in half externally rotating the arms. Brace your midline. However, instead of a shoulder-width stance, keep your feet hip width—about 6-9" apart. This is 'overhead', where you'll receive the barbell in the muscle snatch. We'll call it **Muscle Snatch Position 7 (MS 7)**, or 'catch'.

"Lower the bar in front of you to waist height.

"Reset position for these snatch progressions is the same as for the clean, except for grip width: feet under the hips, screwed into the floor to create external rotation at the hip, midline braced, shoulder blades retracted, arms internally rotated, wrists curled under. Whenever I call 'Reset', return to this position.

"Following our principles of best leverage and best efficiency, in the muscle snatch the barbell travels in a straight line up the torso before coming to rest overhead. We're going to rehearse that bar path.

"Shrug your shoulders, lifting the bar. This is 'finish'—**Muscle Snatch Position 5 (MS 5)**.

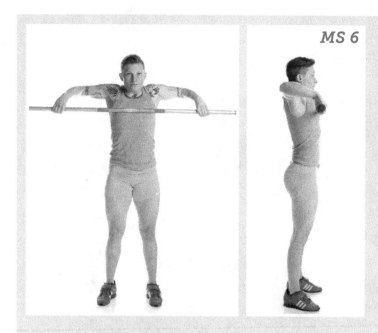

MS 6

"Now elevate the bar by pulling your elbows level with and behind the shoulders. The bar should remain within an inch of the chest. We'll refer to this as **Muscle Snatch Position 6 (MS 6)**, or 'scarecrow'.

"Continue to pull the bar overhead by extending the elbow and letting the bar roll over the wrists. As the forearms reach 135 degrees relative to the ground, the pull turns into a push to lockout—and we're back in **Muscle Snatch Position 7**."

Positional Drills

"5! 6! 7! Reset!" Drill positions one at a time, making corrections as necessary.

"5! Go!" Also known as the "tall muscle snatch." At the command "Go!", trainees move through **MS 5**, **MS 6**, and **MS 7** in one smooth and aggressive motion. Remind them to keep the barbell as close to their bodies as they can.

Muscle Snatch Teaching Script, cont.

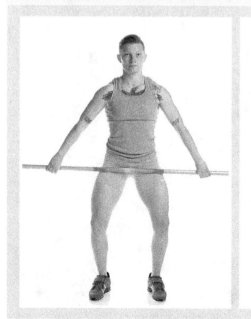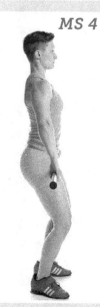

MS 4

"Reset.

"Now, with your weight in your heels, squeeze your butt tight and flare your knees out so that you sit down about 2-3". This is is **Muscle Snatch Position 4 (MS 4).**

"This position should be familiar to you. It's 'pockets', or Muscle Clean Position 4. The difference between **MS 4** and **MC 4** is that because of the wider grip, the bar sits higher up on the leg—right into crook of the hip.

"On my command 'Go!', stand and shrug simultaneously into **MS 5**, then accelerate the bar by pulling into **MS 6**, before punching up to catch the bar in **MS 7**. Ready? Go!

"Congratulations! You've just performed a high-hang muscle snatch. Did the bar feel lighter that time? It's because the powerful extension of your hip put momentum on the bar that effectively made it lighter, and thus easier to pull overhead. This aggressive extension from **MS 4** to **MS 5** (what used to be called 'triple extension', and what we prefer to call 'FINISH') is the heart of the snatch."

Positional Drills

"4! 5! 6! 7! Reset!" Drill positions one at a time, making corrections as necessary.

"4! Go!" At the command "Go!", trainees move from **MS 4** through **MS 5, MS 6,** and **MS 7** in one smooth and aggressive motion.

Muscle Snatch Teaching Script, cont.

"We're now going to work our way down to pulling from the floor. The bumpers we use have an approximate diameter of 18". This is standard. An 18" diameter means the bumpers have a radius of 9". So although we're using PVC pipe, we're going to hold the bar 9" off the ground.

"Understand that each new stage we'll look at it is only setting you up for that explosion at **MS 4**.

"Squat down behind the bar until it's 9" off the floor. Unlike the deadlift, allow the bar to travel out until it's over the point at which your big toe meets your foot—usually, about where your laces begin. The weight is slightly in front of the middle of the foot, the knees flared out. The gaze is forward, the spine is in 'absolute' extension. Arms are straight, and when viewed from the side, vertical, with the leading edge of the shoulder slightly in front of the bar. Elbows are turned out, wrists curled under. This is **Muscle Snatch Position 1 (MS 1)**, or 'floor'.

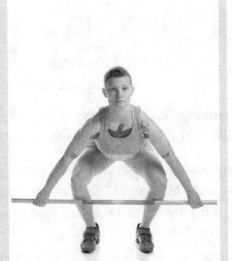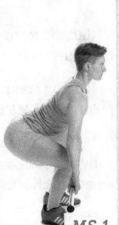

MS 1

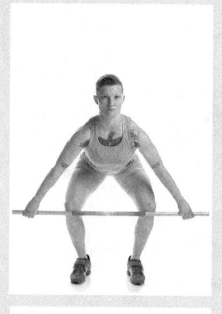

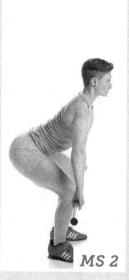

MS 2

"Driving with the legs, NOT with the hips, stand until the bar touches the bottom of your kneecap. The back angle should be maintained. Flaring the knees out wide as the bar rises helps. In this position, your gaze is forward, your back is flat, your shoulders are over the bar. This is 'hang below the knees'—**Muscle Snatch Position 2 (MS 2).**

"Be patient! Take your time with the pull from 'floor' to 'low hang'.

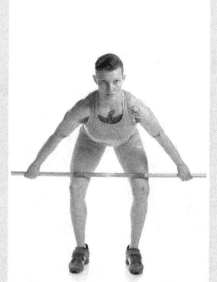

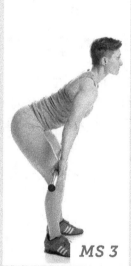

MS 3

"Next, push with the legs only while simultaneously sweeping the bar back toward the body. As your knees straighten, your hips will rise, and your shoulders will come out slightly in front of the bar. The tension in your hamstrings should increase markedly. The bar will rise about 1/4 the way up the thigh. This is 'hang' or 'extend'—**Muscle Snatch Position 3 (MS 3).**

"Lift the torso to vertical while simultaneously sitting down on your heels. The bar moves into the crook of your hip. We've returned to **Muscle Snatch Position 4.**

"On my command 'Go!', you're going to explode upward into **MS 5**, accelerate the bar by pulling into **MS 6**, and then punch the bar to **MS 7**.

"At this point it's worth emphasizing that the order of action is HIPS then ARMS. Don't pull early as you move from **MS 4** to **MS 5**. And make sure when you do pull into **MS 6** , you display what Coach Mike Bergener calls 'junkyard dog intensity'. Give it everything you have.

"Ready? Go!"

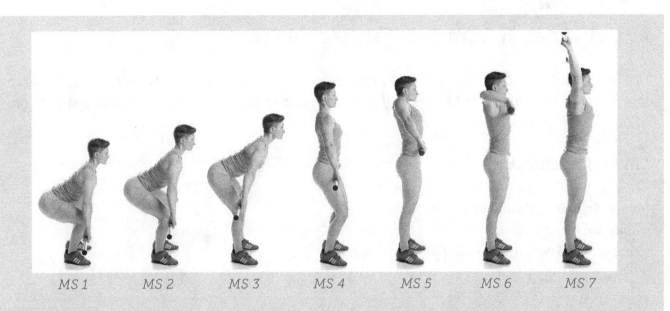

MS 1   MS 2   MS 3   MS 4   MS 5   MS 6   MS 7

"Once you get comfortable accelerating from MS 4, try starting from MS 3, then MS 2. Finally, starting from MS 1, smoothly execute the full movement to completion.

"Remember, the different phases of the lift (commonly referred to as the first, second, and third pulls) occur at different rates. The first pull, the transition from **MS 1** to **MS 2**, is relatively deliberate. From **MS 2** through **MS 3** heading for **MS 4**, there is an acceleration. **MS 4** to **MS 5**, the second pull, is an explosion. The third pull begins when the arms bend and lasts until the bar is received—in this case, the initiation of **MS 6** before resolving in **MS 7**."

Positional Drills

"1! 2! 3! 4! 5! 6! 7! Reset!" Drill positions of the muscle snatch one-at-a-time, making corrections as necessary.

"1! 2! 3! 4! Go!" Muscle snatch from the high hang. When using barbells, trainees should feel the bar is noticeably lighter from the force created by rapidly extending the hips.

"1! 2! 3! Go!" Muscle snatch from the mid-hang. Trainees should concentrate on getting all the way back on the heels and lifting the torso to vertical before exploding upward.

"1! 2! Go!" Muscle snatch from the low hang. Trainees should concentrate on shifting the knees back and getting over the bar in the transition from **MS 2** to **MS 3**.

"1! Go!" Muscle snatch. Make sure your athletes understand that like the clean, the snatch has three phases: a slow and deliberate pull from floor to below the knees, an acceleration from below the knee to above, and then an explosion as the torso shifts to vertical for the jump.

Muscle Snatch Common Faults and Fixes

All faults and fixes common to the muscle clean apply, including deadlift set-up, hips rise too soon, jumping from in front of knees, not sweeping bar in, reverse curling bar, pulling too soon, and not finishing, as well as...

1. Weak lockout.

Muscle Snatch Position 7 violation. Bar must be caught overhead with straight arms. Encourage the trainees to apply more force during the arm pull of MS 6

 "Punch up!"

 Demonstrate a correct MS 7.

 With athlete holding in MS 7, press in on elbows to straighten her arms.

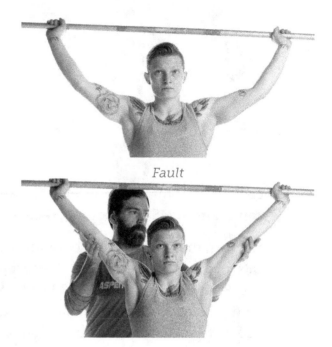

Fault

Tactile

Fault

Correct MS 6 to MS 7 transition

2. Knee rebend/half-ass power snatch.

Dumbbell Muscle Snatch Position 7 violation. Trainee performs a perfunctory knee bend as bar goes overhead. To get the greatest training benefit from this movement, arm pull must be strong enough that the bar is received overhead with legs straight. If this is impossible, either do a real power snatch or lighten the load. NOTE: this fault also applies to the muscle clean.

 "Stand up! No dip!"

 Demonstrate proper transition from MS 5 to 6 to 7.

The Dumbbell Muscle Snatch

The dumbbell snatch is a one-handed variation on the barbell snatch. A dumbbell is pulled from the floor to lock out overhead. It's less likely to bang up the forearms of an under-experienced but over-enthusiastic trainee than the kettlebell snatch, and it's easier to teach to a group. For the sake of consistency we'll use the same basic seven positions of the barbell muscle snatch.

"Stand with a light dumbbell between your feet. Hinge back at the hips and bend your knees to lower your right hand to the dumbbell. Grasp the handle with the pinky side of your hand next to the loading plate. Keeping your chest up and your back flat, rotate your torso so that your shoulder is in line with your hand. Your left arm should come up and out for balance, with fingers splayed or fist squeezed tight. This is **Dumbbell Muscle Snatch Position 1 (dMS 1).**

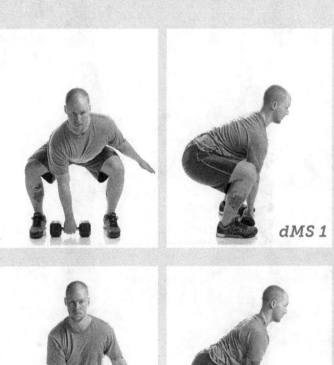

dMS 1

"Driving through the heel, squat the dumbbell to just below the knees. This is **Dumbbell Muscle Snatch Position 2 (dMS 2).**

dMS 2

"Continue pushing with the legs, driving the hips up. The dumbbell rises above your knees. **Dumbbell Muscle Snatch Position 3 (dMS 3).**

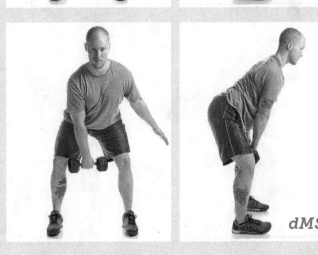

dMS 3

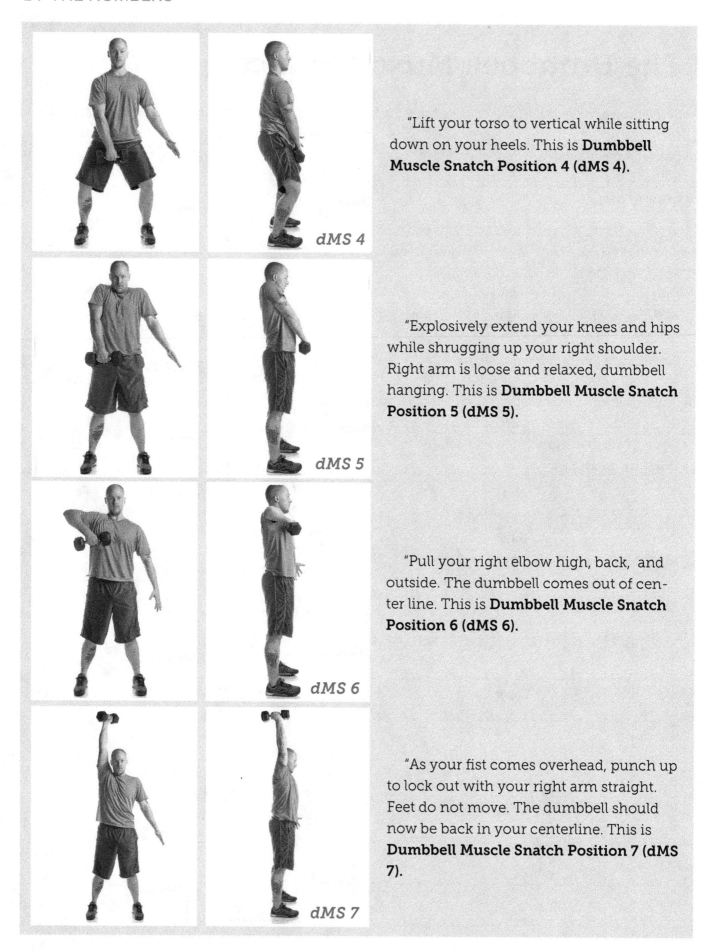

"Lift your torso to vertical while sitting down on your heels. This is **Dumbbell Muscle Snatch Position 4 (dMS 4).**

dMS 4

"Explosively extend your knees and hips while shrugging up your right shoulder. Right arm is loose and relaxed, dumbbell hanging. This is **Dumbbell Muscle Snatch Position 5 (dMS 5).**

dMS 5

"Pull your right elbow high, back, and outside. The dumbbell comes out of center line. This is **Dumbbell Muscle Snatch Position 6 (dMS 6).**

dMS 6

"As your fist comes overhead, punch up to lock out with your right arm straight. Feet do not move. The dumbbell should now be back in your centerline. This is **Dumbbell Muscle Snatch Position 7 (dMS 7).**

dMS 7

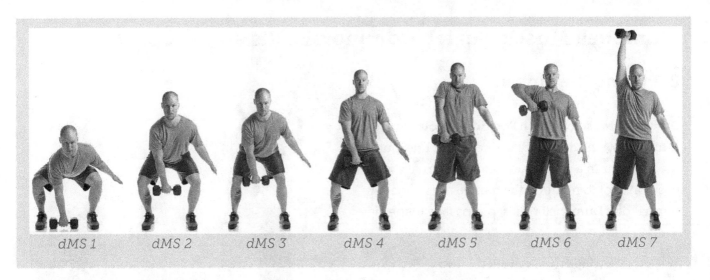

dMS 1   dMS 2   dMS 3   dMS 4   dMS 5   dMS 6   dMS 7

Positional Drills

"1! 2! 3! 4! 5! 6! 7! Reset!" Drill positions of the dumbbell muscle snatch one-at-a-time, making corrections as necessary.

"4! Go!" Dumbbell muscle snatch from the high hang. Trainees should feel the bar is noticeably lighter from the force created by the rapid extension of the hips.

"1! Go!" Dumbbell muscle snatch. Make sure your trainees understand that like the dumbbell clean, the dumbbell snatch has three phases: a slow and deliberate pull from floor to below the knees, an acceleration from below the knee to above, and then an explosion as the torso shifts vertical for the jump.

Dumbbell Muscle Snatch Common Faults and Fixes

1. Early arm pull.

Dumbbell Muscle Snatch Position 4 violation.
Arm must remain loose and relaxed until hip is fully extended.

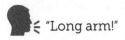 "Long arm!"

👁 Demonstrate a correct dMS 4

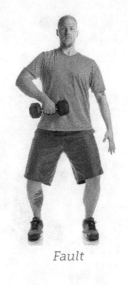

Fault

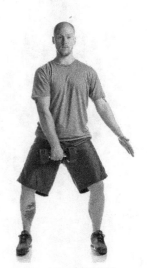

Correct dMS 4

Dumbbell Muscle Snatch Common Faults and Fixes, cont.

2. Pulling the zipper.

Dumbbell Muscle Snatch Position 6 violation.
Athlete pulls the dumbbell up the center line, putting the shoulder in a potentially painful internally rotated position. Not to mention the trainee risks knocking himself out! Dumbbell needs to pass face to the side.

 "Elbow high and outside!"

 Demonstrate a correct dMS 5.

 With athlete holding in MS 7 adjust position as desired.

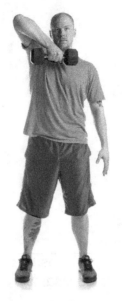

Fault

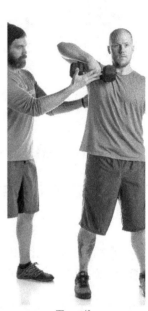

Tactile

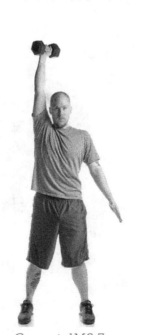

Fault

3. Bad overhead position.

Dumbbell Muscle Snatch Position 7 violation.
Dumbbell needs to be lined up close to the body's centerline—straight arm, biceps close to the ear.

 "Straight overhead!"

 Demonstrate proper dMS 7.

 With athlete holding in MS 7 adjust position as desired.

Correct dMS 7

Our fifth benchmark, "Sluggo", is a couplet: running and overhead squats. When first written, only one weight was specified. It's by tradition that we take about 70% of that weight to establish a prescribed load for female athletes—65lbs.

"Sluggo"

Five rounds for time of
Run 400m
14 Overhead squats 95/65lbs

Prescribing Correct Load and Level of Movement Complexity

USING PRACTICE MODE TO DETERMINE PROPER LOADING FOR PERFORMANCE MODE

In the past, MMGPP athletes and instructors alike simply made their best guess when it was time to scale (or not) the load for these benchmark WODs. But no more! Here are two methods to determine the load your athlete should use for a given workout.

The first is using a percentage of an athlete's rep max for the barbell movement upon which the WOD is based. So for today's WOD, after dynamic warm-ups and positional drills, I can give my athletes 15 minutes to work their way up to the heaviest overhead squat he or she can handle for three reps. Not a rep max, necessarily; not a PR. Just what they can do today. They'll then take that weight and run it through this formula to determine an estimated one rep max:

$$\text{weight x reps x .0333 + weight} = \text{E1RM}$$

Generally speaking, BtN recommends using 70% of E1RM for workouts of 30 reps or less, 50-60% E1RM for workouts of 40-50 reps, and 30-40% for WODs in which a given exercise exceeds 50 reps. Given "Sluggo"'s relatively high volume of overhead squats (70), 40% of that number is what they'll use for today's workout (assuming that 40% isn't higher than the prescribed 95/65lbs, in which case the athlete simply uses the Rx'd weight).

But...

Last week Harry's lack of shoulder flexion became more apparent than ever when I tried to teach him to overhead squat. He has a lot of mobility work to do before I'll let him overhead squat anything heavier than 12 oz of PVC pipe. So what should he do for "Sluggo"? Well, he *could* try to do 70 bad overhead squats with PVC...or he could default back through the hierarchy of complexity to find the movement he *can* do that preserves the desired training stimulus (in this case, squatting). So today he'll front squat. Remember our rule of thumb: *always prefer a simple exercise performed well to a more complex movement executed poorly.*

During the strength training portion of today's program, Harry does front squat triples. He squats 255lbs for a strong set of three. Applying the formula above, Harry establishes a front squat E1RM of 280lbs (255lbs x 3 reps x .0333 + 255lbs = 280.47lbs). Taking 40% of that and rounding down (always a good idea when loading for conditioning), his version of "Sluggo" will have front squats @ 110lbs.

Amy, while strong and flexible, only learned the overhead squat last week, so no rep maxes for her today. Instead she'll use an empty barbell (the 15kg [33lbs] women's bar) for "Sluggo". That's the second method: start with the empty bar. It's that simple. If that weight is so light she easily "beats" the workout (e.g., completes 2k of running and 75 overhead squats in less than 15:00), next time she can add 10lbs. Because each benchmark WOD comes up every twelve weeks or so, if she keeps going at that rate, nine months from now she'll be doing "Sluggo" as prescribed. She may get there even sooner if in three or four months she "tests out" by setting an overhead squat rep max.

Although Tim's squat mechanics are rapidly improving, both the overhead squat and the front squat are still out of reach for him, and I prefer not to have him do conditioning work with a barbell on his back. I assign him 15lbs dumbbell squats—no more than 10 per round. If he finishes before the three minutes of a given round is up, he can rest. His running has improved a lot, so I'll let him run the full 400m.

Establishing Correct Volume

For the non-firebreathing MMGPP athlete, I've determined the optimal time domain for "Sluggo" is 12:00, which is broken down into five 3 minute cycles.

"By the Numbers Testing 'Sluggo'"

Five cycles of three minutes of
Run 400m
AMRAP Overhead squats. If you get to 14 OHS before three minutes is up, immediately head back out on the next run. If you finish 14 OHS before time is up in the last 3 minute cycle, you're done.

The athletes have three minutes to complete their 400m run and their 14 squats. At each 3 minute mark, whether or not they've completed all squat reps, they head back out to run. By establishing a strict time limit for each cycle, the trainee is constrained to the volume she can achieve in one or two sets, minimizing the amount of time she'll spend, in later rounds, standing still and staring at a barbell she just doesn't want to pick up again. It also helps regulate the weight an athlete should use in subsequent efforts: if the athlete only gets 40 reps in today's effort, she should probably go a little lighter next time. Sixty reps, and when "Sluggo" returns in the programming, she should repeat at that weight. If she gets 70, she needs to go heavier next time, or, if she's using the prescribed weight, she can record a legitimate "Sluggo" score. Only then does time to completion mean anything.

LAST MINUTE POINT OF CONCERN

Before everyone sets up their barbells or other implements with their assigned weight, I make sure to review how they'll be getting the bar from the floor to the correct working position. Harry and Tim are fine—they'll simply use the muscle clean they learned last week.

Amy needs a little more explanation. Later in her development, she'll be able to snatch the weight into place. Today, however, I tell her to muscle clean the bar to her shoulders, push press it up and lower behind her neck, then move her hands out to the proper width for overhead squats before snatch push pressing the bar into support. I have her practice this with the empty barbell, and once I'm satisfied she's got it down, she's allowed to put weight on the bar.

"3...2...1...GO!"

Harry

Harry's customized "Sluggo" thrashed him, but good. Of course he rocketed through the first couple runs, but the front squats quickly took the starch out of him—catching your breath with 110lbs sitting on your chest is not easy! He completed 14 squats the first round, 13 the second, then 11, 10...when time was called, he collapsed to the deck. Where he goes next with "Sluggo" is really up to him. If he works very hard on his mobility, he might be ready to overhead squat when this workout returns in our programming, about 12 weeks from now. If Harry's OS hasn't improved, he'll just front squat again, at the same weight, to try to get all 70 reps before the clock runs out. Is it still a good workout, even if he's only front squatting? You can ask him...when he comes to.

Amy

Amy was doing a fine job with her overhead squats, but when she returned from her third run, she complained that her right shoulder was starting to ache. To be safe, I recommended that she switch to front squats for the remainder of the workout. The empty bar she had been using was probably a little light for front squatting, but there wasn't time to increase the weight, but in the end it didn't matter. Fatigue was catching up with her, and she finished the fifteen minutes with a total of 61 squats. She'll repeat at the same weight next time, hopefully with overhead squats all the way through.

Tim

This was the first time I saw Tim really pushed into the red. He managed to complete three full rounds before it seemed like it was definitely time for him to take a break. Rather than run 400m on his fourth trip out, I had him walk once around the building (which took about the same time), do ten squats on his return, and then walk one more lap to cool down. He was resistant at first—for a sedentary academic of a certain age, he's starting to get the Eye of Tiger—but I reminded him that he was paying me to keep him safe. He appreciated that, and afterwards, was effusive with his thanks.

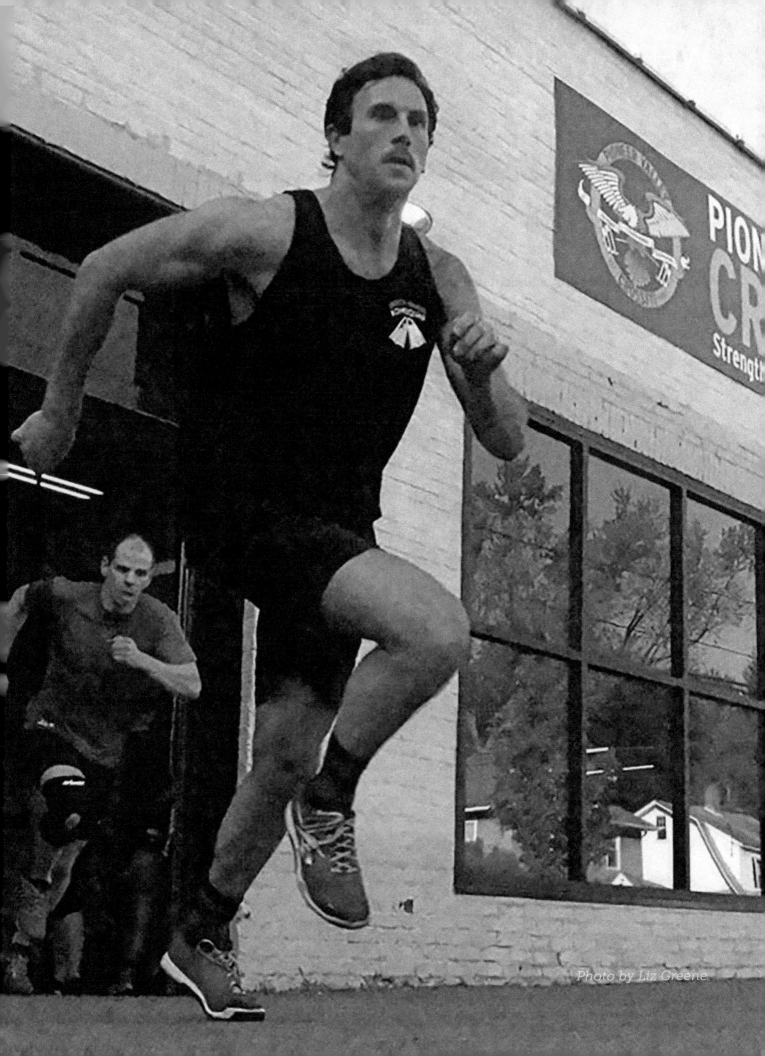

THE CLEAN

Category: Pull Object (ground to shoulder)

Movement screen: Front Squat Position 3 test

Ability screen: Power clean and land in perfect FS 2 (power clean + front squat), power clean + front squat x 5 (clean)

Building on the power clean, the clean (sometimes referred to as the "squat clean") allows an athlete to move the heaviest possible weight from ground to shoulder by jumping the barbell up to about navel height, receiving the bar at the bottom of a well-organized full front squat, and then standing the load up to completion.

If the day's programming includes squat cleans in the WOD, and a given athlete is still developing competence with the movement, break it into simpler components: muscle cleans and front squats, or power cleans and front squat. Nothing good comes from doing dozens of badly performed cleans.

Harry and Amy, of Team Space Monkey fame, both have solid front squats and power cleans, so they're ready for the full clean. Tim isn't ready for a ballistic drop into a squat, but adding a dumbbell squat to his dumbbell power clean will preseve much of the intended training stimulus.

A note about repetition in the teaching scripts: I deliberately repeat details regarding set-up and execution several times while I'm instructing complex movements like the clean and snatch. I believe it's necessary to help the information "stick" in trainees' minds. Later, when practicing and training, I want them to hear my voice in their heads!

Clean Teaching Script

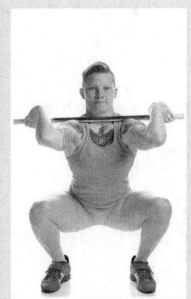
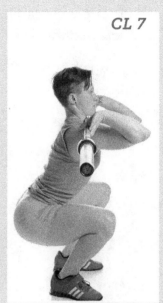

CL 7

"The clean is a power clean taken to its logical conclusion. As the weight you're cleaning gets heavier and heavier, your catch position gets lower and lower, until you are receiving the bar in a full front squat. **Clean Position 7 (CL 7)** is Front Squat Position 3, full depth. All other positions are the same as in the muscle and power cleans.

"Landing in this front squat is the result of a rapid reversal of direction from the upward impetus created by exploding from **Clean Position 4** into **Clean Position 5**. As the arms pull into **Clean Position 6**, the feet shift from under the hips to under the shoulders. In that transition, the lifter is in free fall for a split second, which allows her to work against the inertia of the bar to accelerate herself toward the floor. The load is received as her shoulders pass below the bar. Its descent is slowed and then arrested by the squat.

"Any flaw in your front squat technique will make completing your clean very difficult. You must have a vertical torso, a rigidly braced midline, a tight upper back, and high elbows if you want to stand up a heavy weight to completion in **Clean Position 8 (CL 8).**

"Let's practice that footwork. You remember the drop squat we practiced for the power clean? This time, we'll take it all the way down.

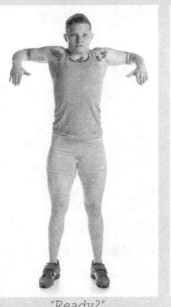
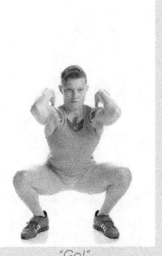

"Stand tall with your feet under your hips. Pull your elbows up and back to approximate the 'scarecrow' position of PC 6. On my command 'GO!', slide your feet out to shoulder width and drop into a full squat, whipping your elbows around to bring your thumbs to your sholders. Ready? GO!

"Reset, and repeat until you've got it."

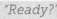 *"Ready?"*   *"Go!"*

"The best way to bridge the challenging increase in complexity between the power clean and the clean is to perform power cleans with an added front squat. Here's what I mean:

"Pick up your barbell. Hit 'reset' for me: clean-width grip with hooks in, feet under the hips, and screwed into the floor, midline braced, shoulders back, elbows out, wrists curled under.

"Set up in **Power Clean Position 4.** On my command 'Go!', explode up into **PC 5**, then shift your feet out into receiving stance. Simultaneously pull hard with your arms (**PC 6**), working off the inertia of the bar to accelerate your descent into **PC 7**. Freeze there. Ready? GO!"

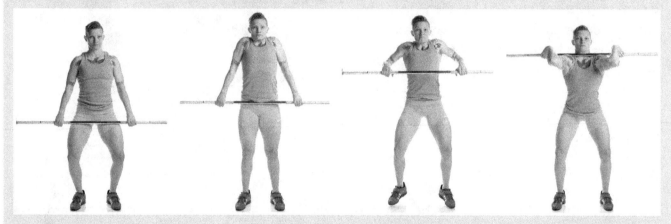

Power clean from the high hang

"Self-assess. Is your weight on the balls of your feet, are your knees too forward, or caving in? Are your elbows pointing anywhere but straight ahead? Whatever it is, adjust until you are in an ideal **PC 7**.

"Now, **PC 7** is identical to Front Squat Position 2. So once your **PC 7** is looking good, simply sit down into FS 3—which, you'll remember, is now **CL 7**, and then stand to completion in **CL 8**.

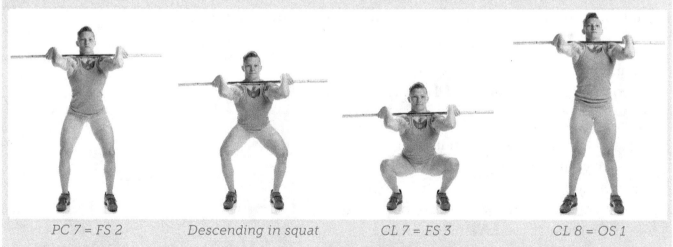

PC 7 = FS 2   *Descending in squat*   *CL 7 = FS 3*   *CL 8 = OS 1*

"The trick is to only squat once you are sure your position is correct. This is a great option if you're taking on a WOD like 'Elizabeth', which calls for full cleans. If you can't reliably catch a squat clean in good form and good balance, catch it in the power position, get organized, and then squat.

"Now you're ready to try for a clean from the high hang.

"Pick up your barbell. Hit 'reset' for me, then set up in **CL 4.**

"On my command 'Go!', explode up into **CL 5**, then shift your feet out into receiving stance. Simultaneously pull hard with your arms (**CL 6**), working off the inertia of the bar to accelerate your descent into **CL 7**. Freeze there. Ready? GO!

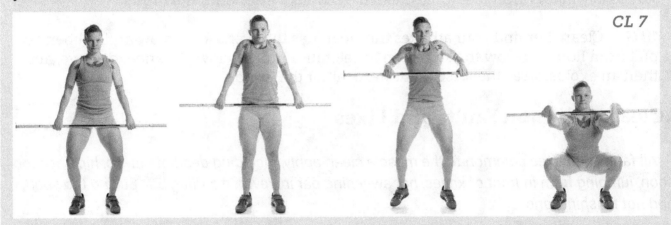

CL 7

"Self-assess. Do you look like you just took your time sitting down into a perfect front squat? If you don't, get into an ideal **CL 7** before standing up the bar through Front Squat Position 2 and finishing in **Clean Position 8 (CL 8).**

"Once you can reliably land in a well-organized front squat, you won't wait in CL 7. Instead, you'll use the stretch of your hamstrings in that deep front squat to help propel you to stand.

"Finally, here is the complete clean from the floor."

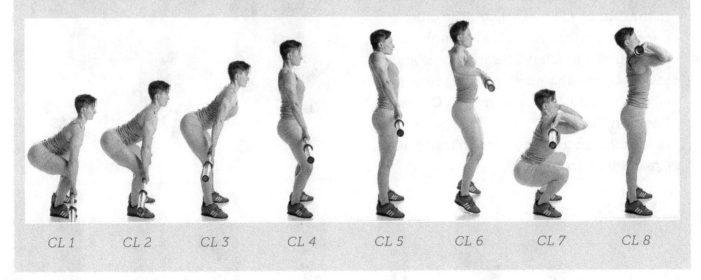

CL 1   CL 2   CL 3   CL 4   CL 5   CL 6   CL 7   CL 8

Positional Drills

"1! 2! 3! 4! 5! 6! 7! 8! Reset!" Drill positions of the clean one-at-a-time, making corrections as necessary.

"4! Go!" Clean from the high hang. When using barbells, trainees should feel the bar is noticeably lighter from the force created by rapidly extending the hips.

"1! Go!" Clean. Remind your athletes the clean has three phases: a slow and deliberate pull from floor to below the knees, an acceleration from below the knee to above, and then an explosion as the torso shifts vertical for the jump.

Clean Common Faults and Fixes

All faults and fixes common to the muscle clean apply, including deadlift set-up, hips rise too soon, jumping from in front of knees, not sweeping bar in, reverse curling bar, pulling too soon, and not finishing, and...

All faults and fixes common to the front squat apply, including all air squat flaws, as well as low elbows, collapsed rack position, and excessive forward lean.

Dumbbell Clean

"In the dumbbell clean the pull from the floor, the shift to jumping position, and the jump-and-pull are exactly the same as in the dumbbell power clean. The difference is that the dumbbells are caught in a full dumbbell squat. The dumbbells are racked on the shoulders, palms facing in, elbows in tight. This is **Dumbbell Clean Position 7 (dCL 7)**. The dumbbells are then stood up to completion in **Dumbbell Clean Position 8 (dCL 8)**."

dCL 7

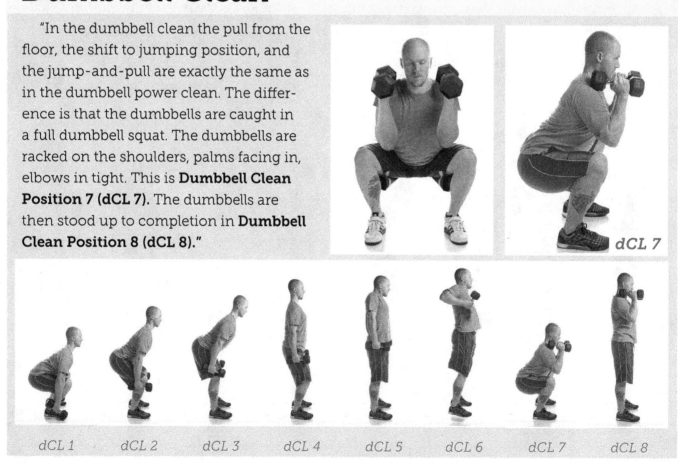

| dCL 1 | dCL 2 | dCL 3 | dCL 4 | dCL 5 | dCL 6 | dCL 7 | dCL 8 |

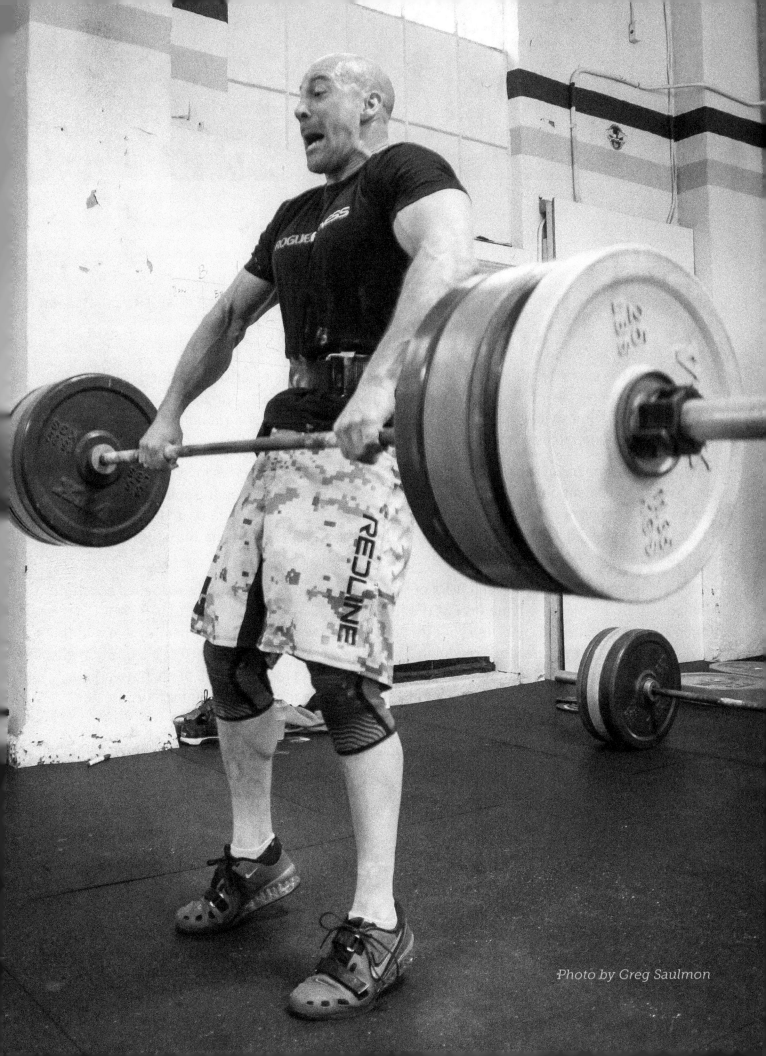

Photo by Greg Saulmon

Category: Hip and Trunk Flexion (seated)

Movement screen: N/a

Ability screen: Weighted sit-ups x 20 with 25/15lbs dumbbell (Roman chair sit-up), Roman

Similar to the classic Roman chair sit-up, the GHD sit-up has a very long range of motion. But instead of initiating the movement by contracting the abdominals to curl up the trunk, in the GHD sit-up the abdominals work to stabilize the midline, while a chain contraction of quadriceps and psoas pulls the torso to vertical.

Why change the basic action of the sit-up? I think the GHD sit-up was invented to create the hip-flexing equivalent of the hip extension (that is, an exercise in which the spine remains neutral while the pelvis moved with the spine), and found that firing the psoas with the kick could close the hip, freeing the abs to work at their most important job: keeping the spine in a neutral position.*

A word of caution: the extra-long ROM of the GHD sit-up means a greatly increased eccentric component of the movement means EXTREME SORENESS AND QUITE POSSIBLY RHABDO if too much volume is done too soon. Tell your trainees to start with 2-3 sets of 5 per day and gradually work up. When they are regularly doing 3 x 15, they'll be able to handle GHD sit-ups at higher volumes in WODs. Having said that, be wary of programming more than 75 or so in a workout. Even Chris Spealler, word has it, burns out at 100. And more than likely, your trainees are not Spealler.

Harry and Amy are both ready for GHD sit-ups. Tim, however, will stick with weighted sit-ups.

---

* As mentioned in Part I, although the GHD sit-up is in the Hip and Trunk Flexion (seated) hierarchy, there is no trunk flexion in the GHD sit-up.

GHD Sit-up Teaching Script

"Take a seat on the GHD bench. Insert your feet into the foot-anchor assembly. Ignore the plate and hook your feet around the pads. The assembly should be set close enough that you are sitting with your hips on the outside of the pad, with knees bent. Adjust as necessary.

"Lie back until your knees, hips, and shoulders are in a straight line. Then curl your trunk to sit up. This is called a **Roman chair sit-up.** It takes you through a longer range of motion than a traditional sit-up, and is initiated by the abs flexing your spine.

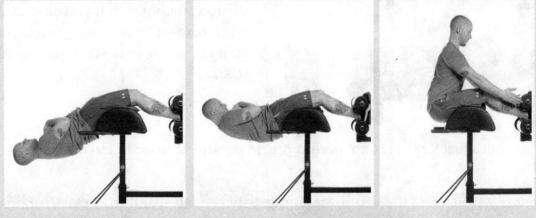

"In a GHD sit-up, however, the abdominals play a different role. Instead of curling the trunk, they work to keep the spine neutral. Imagine a string running from your navel to your solar plexus. Keep the string taut by sitting up tall, with your shoulders packed.

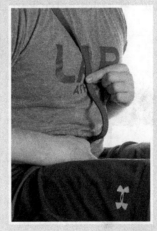
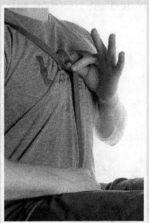

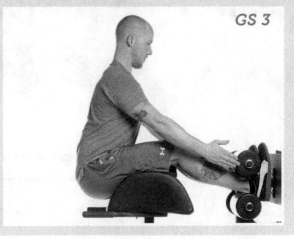

GS 3

"Keeping your shoulders back and down, hinge forward from the hips to tap the pads. Your knees should be bent, your feet hooked around the pads. This is **GHD Sit-up Position 3 (GS 3).**

"The GHD sit-up is initiated by kicking the shins into the pad. If you've ever used a Nautilus leg extension machine, the action is quite similar. The kick up into the pad results from a powerful contraction of the quads, which tug on the hip flexors. These in turn pull on the spine, drawing your torso upright. The key to executing the GHD sit-up, instead of just a flailing Roman chair sit-up, lies in feeling this subtle muscular interaction.

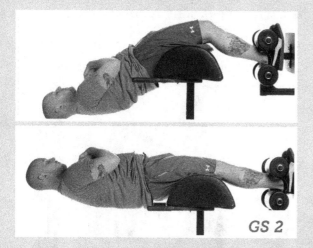

"Lie back until you are parallel to the floor. WITHOUT TRYING TO SIT UP, slowly but firmly kick your shins up into the foot anchor pad. If you do it correctly, your torso will rise. When your legs are straight, you're in **GHD Sit-up Position 2 (GS 2).**

GS 2

"Once you get a feel for it, kick up more aggressively and sit up to touch the foot anchor pads.

"Remember, at the top of the sit-up, the 'string' between navel and solar plexus should be pulled taut—so sit tall, with shoulders back and down. No slouching!

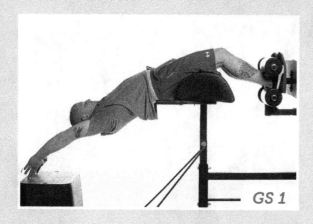

"Gradually work your way to lying back until you are starting with knees, hips, shoulders and head in a line. Your knees are still bent. This is **GHD Sit-up Position 1 (GS 1).** If you wish to set a standard of touching the ground on each rep, that's fine, but if, due to the height of the GHD bench, you cannot touch the floor without hyperextending your spine, place a box at the proper height."

GS 1

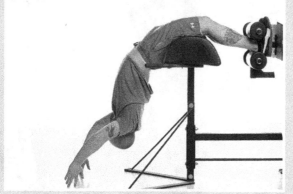

DO NOT ALLOW ATHLETES TO HYPEREXTEND THEIR SPINES. It puts unnecessary compression on the lower spine and may result in injury.

This is bad. Don't do it.

"You can fold your arms across your chest, or keep your hands at your temples. If you want to reach overhead in **GS 1**, touch your shoulders in **GS 2**, then tap the pads in **GS 3**."

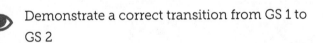

GS 2

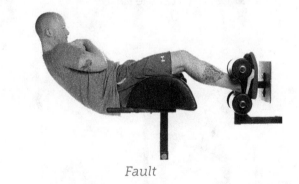

GS 3

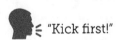

GS 1

Positional Drills

"1! 2! 3!" Drill positions of the GHD sit-up one-at-a-time, making corrections as necessary.

GHD Sit-up Common Faults and Fixes

1. Sitting up first.

GHD Sit-up Position 2 violation. Sometimes a trainee will not understand how to initiate the GHD sit-up, and reverts to an overly enthusiastic Roman Chair sit-up.

🗣 "Kick first!"

👁 Demonstrate a correct transition from GS 1 to GS 2

✋ Take the athlete back to the parallel kick-up drill so he can learn to feel how the extension of the knee helps lift the torso.

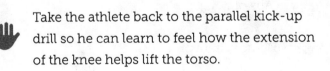

Fault

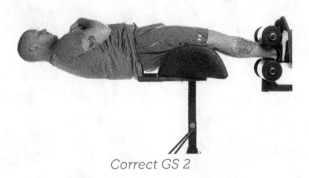

Correct GS 2

413

GHD Sit-up Common Faults and Fixes, cont.

2. Driving legs down instead of kicking up into pad.

GHD Sit-up Position 2 violation. Some trainees, seeing the powerful extension of the knee, mistakenly think the initiating movement of the GHD sit-up is driving the heel into the plate. Not so! Driving the shin up into the pad creates a closed kinetic chain, which makes for a more efficient transfer of power. Have the trainee practice the kick up into the pad until he gets the hang of it. For this, he'll be relying on your feedback, as he learns to distinguish a successful effort from missed attempts.

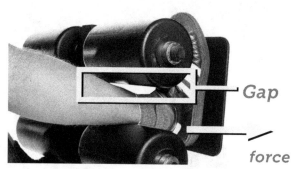

Bad: pushing the heel forward creates an open kinetic chain

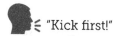 "Kick first!"

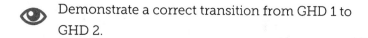 Demonstrate a correct transition from GHD 1 to GHD 2.

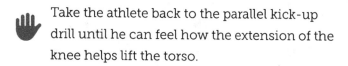 Take the athlete back to the parallel kick-up drill until he can feel how the extension of the knee helps lift the torso.

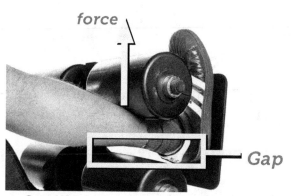

Good: kicking up into the pad creates a closed kinetic chain

3. Lower back crunches.

GHD Position 1 violation. Athlete overextends his spine in order to reach the ground. The athlete should strive to maintain a straight line from knee to shoulder.

 "Abs on!"

 Demonstrate proper GS 1.

 Hold your hand underneath the trainee's back to provide a barrier beyond which they cannot go.

Fault

Tactile

Category: Hybrid (squat, push away from object [horizontal], jump and land)

Movement screen: N/a

Ability screen: Air squat x 5, Box push-up x 10 (box burpee), push-up x 10 (step-up burpee), step-up burpee x 10 (burpee), burpee x 10 (kipping burpee)

This is a big day for Amy and Tim—they're getting introduced to the burpee. Harry is all too familiar with this brutal exercise from his days in the Marine Corps!

The burpee is a stylized way to move from standing to prone and back. At its simplest, the burpee is pure function, a movement pattern necessary for survival. Its most challenging variation is the "king of bodyweight conditioning exercises," developing tremendous stamina and endurance, as well as upper body pushing and hip explosiveness.

I am a sworn enemy of the sloppy, sprawl-out-and-lurch-back-up-to-your-feet-as-fast-as-you-can burpee that is all too common in MMGPP training. Please don't let your trainees be unduly influenced by the way burpees are performed in competition. Explain that the strict movement is safer and has a better training ROI. Done poorly, the burpee is an embarrassing flail-a-thon that can aggravate lower back issues. Executed correctly, the burpee blends the squat, push-up, and jump into a seamless whole. I'm convinced the only burpee worth training is the one that preserves these elements in recognizable form.

Box Burpee Teaching Script

"From a standing position **(Box Burpee Position 1 [bBU 1]),** hinge back at the hip and plant your hands at the edge of the box **(bBU 2).**

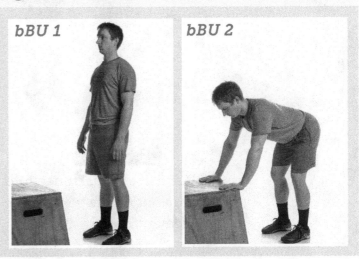

bBU 1 bBU 2

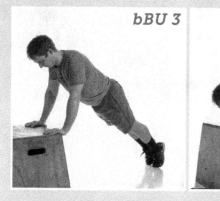

bBU 3

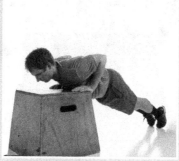

bBU 4

"Step back into well-organized plank (**bBU 3**): feet together, straight line from ankle to shoulder, shoulders packed.

"Execute a box push-up (down to **bBU 4**, back up to **bBU 3**).

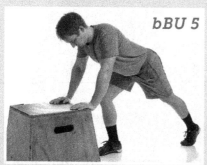

bBU 5

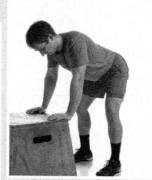

"Step up right (**bBU 5**), step up left to return to **bBU 2**.

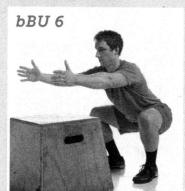

bBU 6

"Execute a full squat (**bBU 6**).

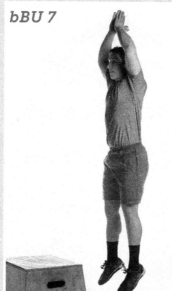

bBU 7

"Jump and clap your hands overhead (**bBU 7**).

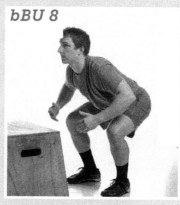

bBU 8

"Land in a partial squat (**bBU 8**). Plant your hands on the box to cycle the movement, starting at **bBU 2**."

Burpee Teaching Script

If the box burpee is easy and the trainee has the requisite 10 strict push-ups, introduce him to the standard burpee.

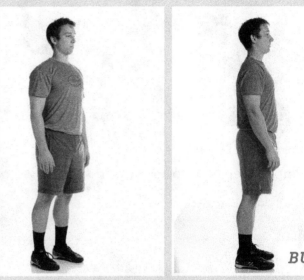

"The burpee begins in a full stand, with feet screwed into the floor, midline braced, and shoulders packed. This is **Burpee Position 1 (BU 1).**

BU 1

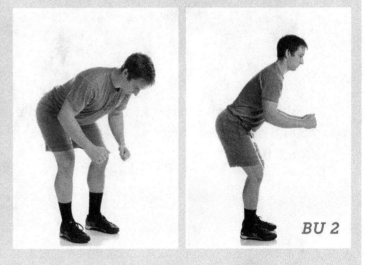

"Hinge back at the hip, keeping your shins vertical. This is **Burpee Position (BU 2).**

BU 2

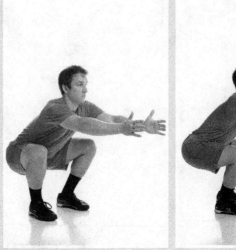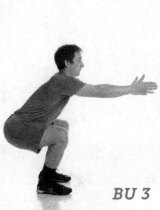

"Sit down until the crease of your hip is below the top of your knee. This is **Burpee Position 3 (BU 3).**

BU 3

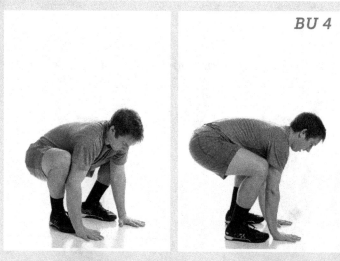

BU 4

"Plant your hands on the ground in front of your feet. This is **Burpee Position 4 (BU 4).**

"Jump or step back to a rigid, arms-extended plank position. This is **Burpee Position 5 (BU 5).**

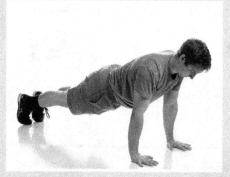
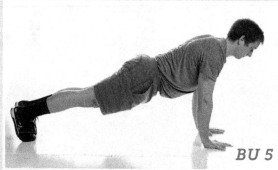

BU 5

"Keeping a straight line from ankle to shoulder, and keeping the shoulder blades partially retracted and depressed, lower yourself until your chest and chin brush the floor. This is **Burpee Position 6 (BU 6).**

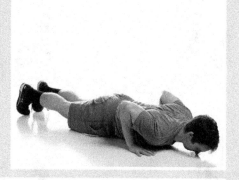
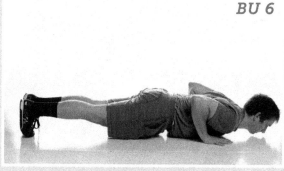

BU 6

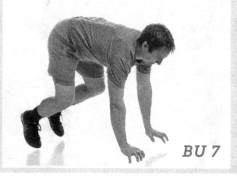

BU 7

"From the bottom of this push-up, you must explode up through **BU 5** into **Burpee Position 7 (BU 7)**, a mid-air passing position that sees you lifting your chest as you hop forward. Land in **BU 3**: feet flat and set shoulder width, knees pushed out, hip crease below the knee, chest up, etc.

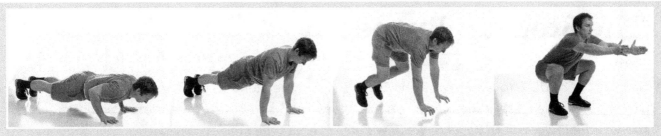

Landing in a good squat depends on exploding out of the push-up.

"Now jump straight up, passing through **BU 2** and **BU 1** to get airborne with arms extended over head. This is **Burpee Position 8 (BU 8).** YAY BURPEES!

"Finally, land in a well-organized partial squat. You've returned to **BU 2**, and you're ready to cycle into the next repetition."

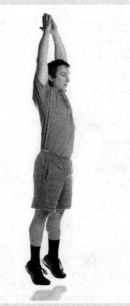
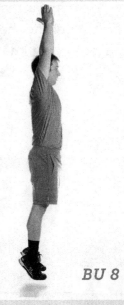

BU 8

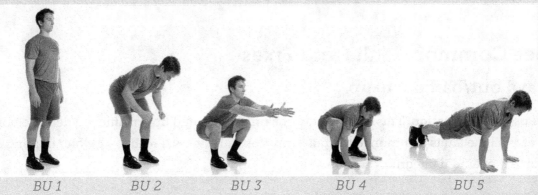

| *BU 1* | *BU 2* | *BU 3* | *BU 4* | *BU 5* |

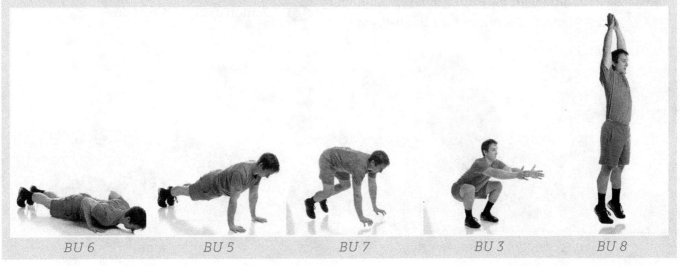

| *BU 6* | *BU 5* | *BU 7* | *BU 3* | *BU 8* |

The Step-up Burpee

Athletes lacking sufficient strength, or even strong athletes as they tire, will have difficulty blasting out of BU 6 to land in a sound BU 3. Instead they tend to land on the balls of their feet, which puts unnecessary shear force on the knees, or in a hugely lumbar flexed position, which stresses the lower back. We have these athletes execute the step-up burpee.

"From the arms extended plank position of **BU 5**, step your right foot forward and out to line up just behind the right hand. Then step up your left foot to match. By lifting your chest and pushing your knees out, you are now in a pretty good squat, and can complete the sequence.

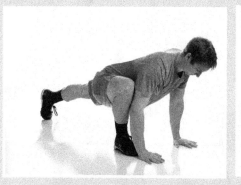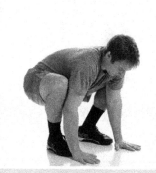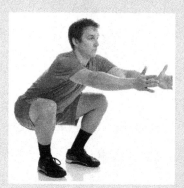

"In the course of an extended effort, stepping up out of the burpee allows you to accomplish the same amount of work as jumping into bad positions does, but at much less risk."

Burpee Common Faults and Fixes

1. Sprawl out/bad push-up.

Burpee Position 4 violation. This can include "snaking" down and up, insufficient depth, elbows flaring out, etc—all the faults common to the push-up. Your athletes will realize a greater training effect if you enforce movement integrity.

 As appropriate for the error... "Abs on!", "Straight body!", "Lower!", "Screw in your hands!", etc.

 Demonstrate a correct push-up.

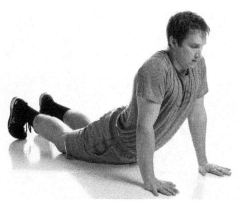

Fault (concentric or eccentric)

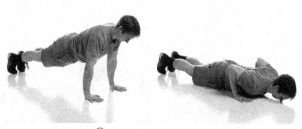

Correct sequence

Burpee Common Faults and Fixes, cont.

2. Hyperflexed lumbar.

Burpee Position 3 violation (transitioning out of BU 5). If the athlete fails to apply enough explosive power to his push-up as he jumps forward, he'll land a squat marred by a pronounced forward lean and lost lumbar curve. If the athlete simply lacks the necessary upper body strength, he should step up out of the push-up.

 "Explode up!" and "Chest up!"

 Demonstrate a proper transition from BU 5 back to BU 3.

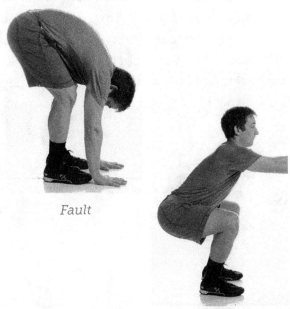

Fault

Correct BU 3

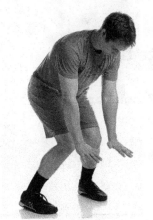

Fault (front view)

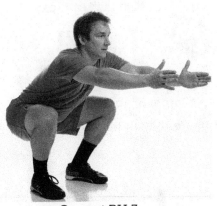

Correct BU 3

3. Landing in a bad squat.

Burpee Position 3 violation. Athlete jumps forward out of the push-up to land with knees knocking, or feet tight together, or up on the balls of his feet, or some unholy combination thereof. The athlete must try to land in a well-organized Air Squat Position 3— heels shoulder width, knees pushed out, hip crease below the knee, etc.

 Verbal cues as appropriate to the air squat flaw on display.

 Demonstrate a proper transition from BU 5 back to BU 3.

Burpee Common Faults and Fixes, cont.

4. Landing in a partial split.

Burpee Position 3 violation. Athlete jumps forward into a splay-legged stance. This is a pernicious variation developed by competitive CrossFit athletes. All well and good for them, but it's a corner-cutting measure that is not a best practice for everyday people trying to get fit.

 "Land in a good squat!"

 Demonstrate a proper transition from BU 5 back to BU 3.

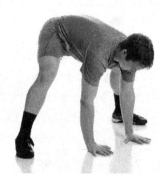

Fault

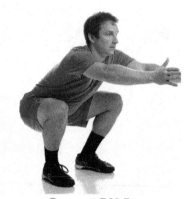

Correct BU 3

5. Incomplete finish.

Burpee Position 7 violation. Athlete fails to leave the ground, completely extend his hip, or fully reach overhead to hit Burpee Position 7. Remind him he may occasionaly be required to jump to a target 6" above his reach, as in Reebok CrossFit Games Open WOD 12.1. He may as well train to be ready for it.

 "Full jump!" or "Get tall!" or "Reach high!"

 Demonstrate a correct transition from BU 3 to BU 7.

 Set up a target 6" above the athlete's reach and require them to jump up to touch it on every rep.

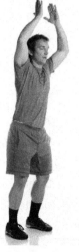

Fault

Correct BU 7

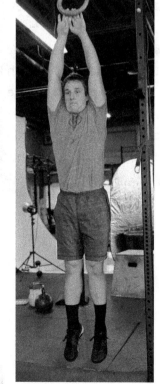

Orthosis

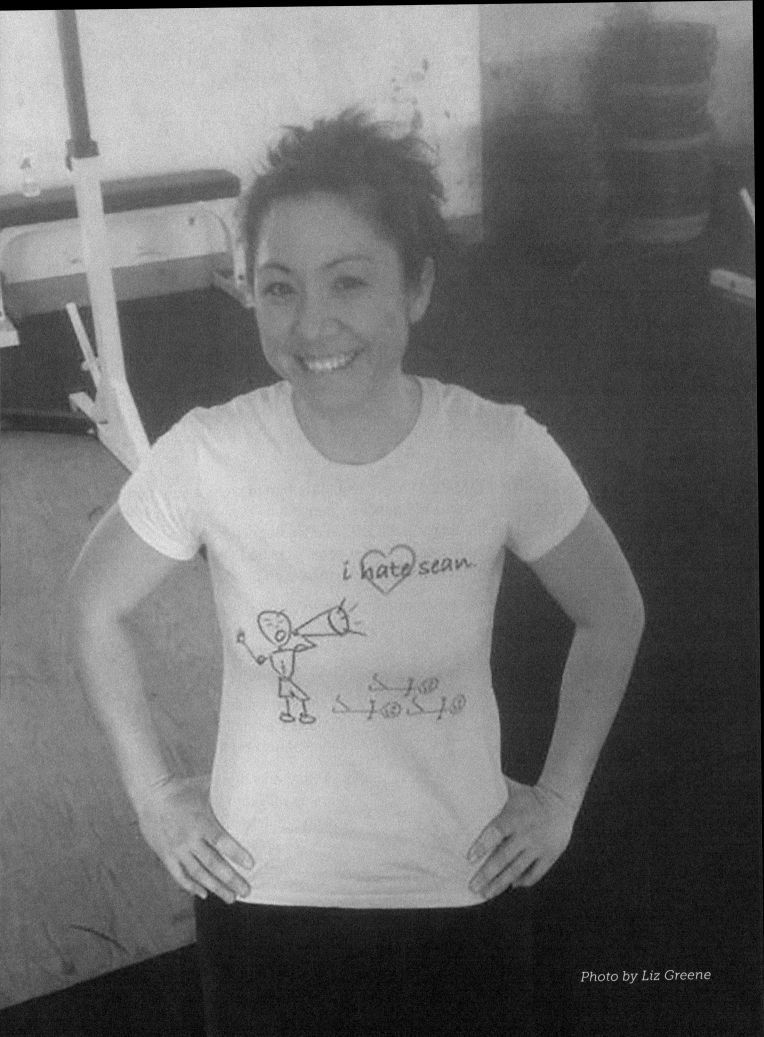

Photo by Liz Greene

Category: Push Object (vertical)

Movement screen: Clean-grip overhead squat Position 2 test

Ability screen: Push press x 5

The push jerk builds on the action and positions of the push press. But now, instead of pressing the load overhead, once the athlete has launched the bar into the air with the force generated by his knees and hips, he pushes himself down to receive the bar in a clean grip, partial overhead squat. In this locked-out position, his arms and shoulders are able to support more weight than they can actually produce force to move. The athlete then stands the weight up to complete the lift.

Should your athlete push jerk? Here's a simple test: have him to press a light barbell overhead. Then ask him to hinge back into Overhead Squat Position 2. If he cannot easily hit this clean-grip, partial overhead squat, he should not push jerk. Injuries happen at end range-of-motion, and ballistic movements in particular need a "buffer zone" of extra ROM. If your athlete doesn't have the requisite flexibility, don't force (or allow) him to take an unnecessary risk.

When push jerks come in up your programming, have this hypothetical, inflexible athlete press or push press instead. Meanwhile, he can do extra mobilization homework until he can push jerk comfortably and safely.

You can teach the push jerk with PVC if you like, but light barbells give a better sense of moving the body around the load.

Today, only one member of Team Space Monkey will learn the push jerk: Amy. Harry will continue to push press, and Tim can dumbbell press.

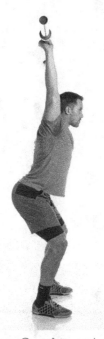
Good to go!

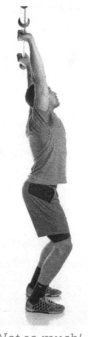
Not so much!

Push Jerk Teaching Script

"When a weight becomes too heavy to push press because the triceps aren't strong enough to lock out the elbows in the last phase of the movement, it's time to use the push jerk. In the push jerk, after the hip has completely extended in the dip/drive, you rapidly reverse direction to drop under the bar and catch it in a partial, clean-grip, narrow-stance, overhead squat. You then stand up the bar to complete the lift.

"Pick up your light barbell and press it overhead. With your feet hip-width, hinge back into a clean grip, partial overhead squat with the pipe lined up in the frontal plane. This is **Push Jerk Position 4 (PJ 4)**.

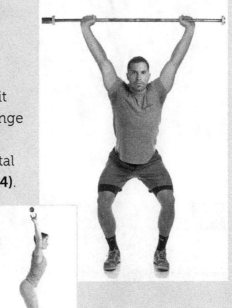
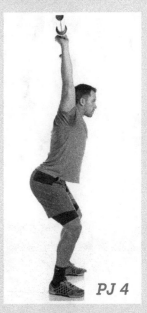

PJ 4

"Notice the similarity between **PJ 4** and Overhead Squat Position 2. From the side, they are identical.

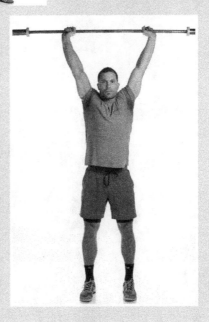

"Keeping your barbell in the frontal plane, stand up tall, completely extending the knees and hips. Push up through the shoulder blades, but don't shrug your shoulders up into your ears. Brace your midline and try to 'snap' the pipe in half by rotating your thumbs back. This is the finish, **Push Jerk Position 5 (PJ 5)**—also the finish of the press and push press.

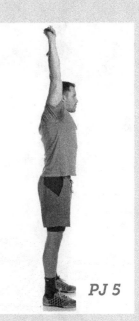

PJ 5

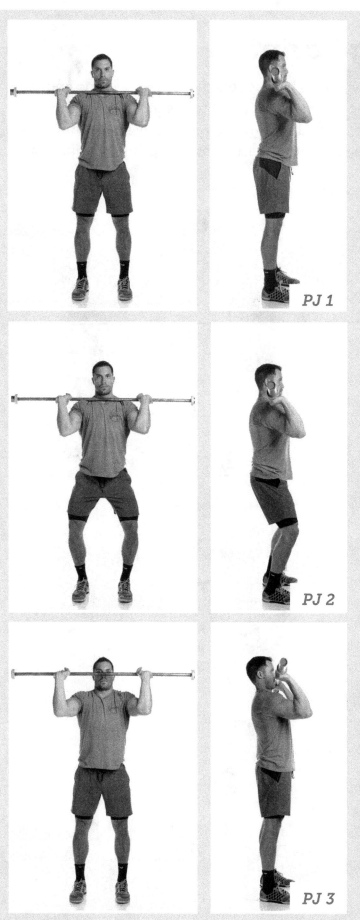

PJ 1

PJ 2

PJ 3

"Okay, now set up in Push Press Position 1: bar seated firmly on upraised shoulders, as in the push press, full-fist grip outside the shoulders, elbows elevated so the forearms are at about 45 degrees relative to the ground, mid-line braced, feet under the hips. This is now **Push Jerk Position 1 (PJ 1).**

"With weight on your heels, and keeping your torso vertical, flare your knees out so that you sit straight down 2-4". This dip is **Push Jerk Position 2 (PJ 2).**

"Return to **PJ 1.**

"Now pull your head back (sexy double chin!) and press the bar up in front of your nose. This is **Push Jerk Position 3 (PJ 3).**

"On my command 'Go!' shove the bar into overhead support position as you simultaneously push yourself down into a quarter squat. I want you to freeze in your landing position. Ready? Go!

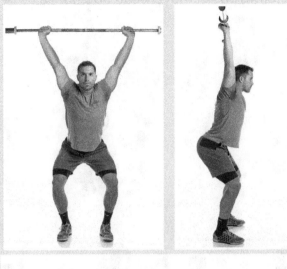

"You've returned to **PJ 4**. Self-assess: are your arms locked out straight? Are your hips hinged back, knees pushed out, shins close to vertical, weight back toward your heels? If so, stand to **Push Jerk Position 5**. If not, correct your position, and then stand."

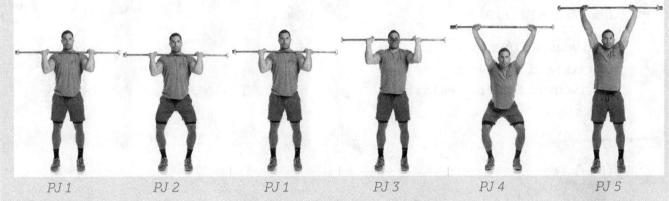

PJ 1   PJ 2   PJ 1   PJ 3   PJ 4   PJ 5

Positional Drills

"3! 4! 5!" At this point, the set-up, dip, drive, and overhead support positions should be familiar from the push press. The trainee needs to drill pushing under the barbell in the transition from **PJ 3** to **PJ 4**. Emphasize the violent push under the bar, the necessity of pausing to assess and correct one's receiving position (**PJ 4**), and standing to complete the rep before lowering the bar.

"1! 2! Go!" Bring trainee from set-up to dip position. On the command "Go!", the athlete initiates an aggressive drive upward before retreating under the bar to receive in **PJ 4**. Emphasize the importance of fully extending the hips in the drive from **PJ 2** through **PJ 1** toward **PJ 3**.

"1! Go!" The full movement. Remind the trainee that in the descent from **PJ 1** to **PJ 2**, the knees should push out, rather than the hips hinge back, in order to maintain a vertical torso. Rebounding from **PJ 2** is an explosion that drives the shoulders into the bar. The athlete must then actively push down under the bar, rather than just dropping, to catch it in a well-organized, partial-depth, clean-grip, narrow-stance overhead squat.

Push Jerk Common Faults and Fixes

All faults and fixes common to the push press apply, including leaning forward in dip, knees caving in during dip, muted hip function, early press, interally rotated overhead position, and

1. Incomplete hip extension.

Push Jerk Position 1 violation. If the athlete fails to hit PJ 1 on his way up from PJ 2 to PJ 3, he robs himself of potential power production. Remind your athlete he has to shoot upward like a rocket, completely extending his hips as he drives his head toward the ceiling.

 "Squeeze your butt!" or "Big jump!"

 Demonstrate a proper transition from PJ 2 to PJ 1 to PJ 3.

 Hold your hand just above your trainees head, and tell him to hit your hand with the top of his head as he drives up.

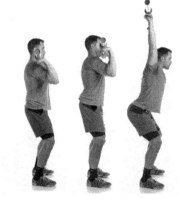

Fault

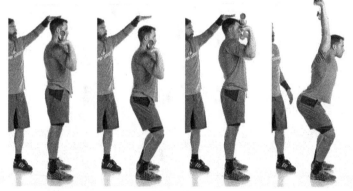

Tactile

2. Soft elbows.

Push Jerk Position 4 violation. If the athlete lands in PJ 4 with soft elbows, he'll have to press to lock out, which is a disqualifying fault in the weightlifting world. Even worse, his soft elbows might not be able to support the weight going overhead, and he'll dump the bar.

 "Punch under!"

 Demonstrate a correct PJ 4.

 With athlete holding in PJ 4, press on his elbows to straighten them.

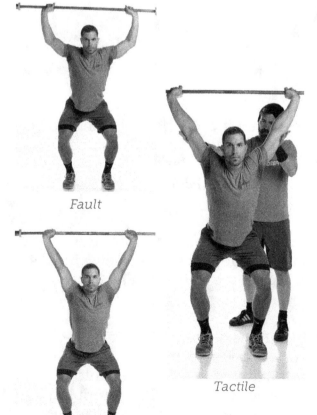

Fault

Tactile

Correct PJ 4

Push Jerk Faults and Fixes, cont.

3. Feet come out too wide.

Push Jerk Position 4 violation. An athlete reluctant to sit down under a large load will sometimes try to get lower by jumping to a wide stance. This is aesthetically displeasing as well as bad for the knees.

Note that there is another variation of jerk called the "power jerk" in which the feet move from under the hips to shoulder-width. If your athlete prefers to move his feet, that's fine; just make sure they don't go any wider than hip width. Also, the athlete should be aware that correctly performed, the power jerk is probably inferior to the push jerk in terms of cycle time in a metcon workout. The footwork of the power jerk will necessarily slow down repetition speed.

 "Sit down!" or "Feet don't move!"

 Demonstrate a proper PJ 4.

Place two boxes or two stacks of plates just outside width of athlete's stance. If he tries to jump wide, they will block him, quickly teaching him what is allowable width. Make sure the blocks are high enough the athlete can't inadvertently jump *on* them and twist an ankle.

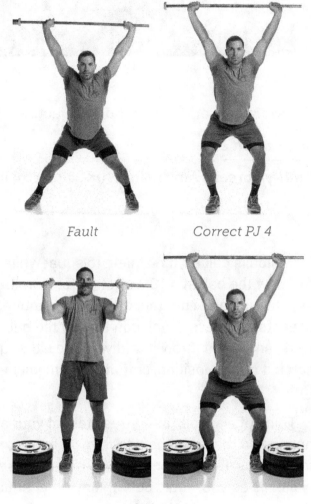

Fault   *Correct PJ 4*

Orthosis

WALLBALLS

Category: Hybrid (squat, push object [vertical])

Movement screen: N/a

Ability screen: Air squat x 5 (medicine ball front squat), medball front squat x 5 (wallball)

Wallballs call for the athlete to squat while holding a medicine ball, then stand hard and fast to throw the ball at a 10' target (9' for women). While wallballs are primarily a tool for developing stamina and endurance, they also require accuracy—one of the most neglected of the ten aspects of fitness. If you don't throw the ball so that it hits the target, you don't get credit for the work, and if you throw it wildly, you're either going to have to interrupt your smooth cycling to catch it out of position, or that 20lbs medicine ball just might end up punching you in the face. Oof!

Think of wallballs as a stress test of your athletes' squat. Putting a medicine ball in their hands and requiring them to throw it at a target should change NOTHING about their squat mechanics. Exhaustion is not an excuse. Be as relentless about correcting squat faults during wallballs as you would be with any other squatting movement.

Harry, Amy, and Tim will all throw some wallballs today. Tim has an air squat now, and his lack of overhead flexibility isn't nearly the issue with wallballs it is when he tries to press a barbell. At no point will he have to lock out the medicine ball in the frontal plane, so he's in.

Wallball Teaching Script

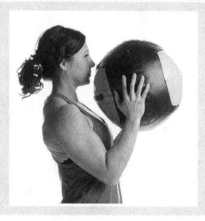

"Stand arms-length from the post or wall that supports the target. Hold the medicine ball just under your chin and close to your chest. Screw your hands into the ball—right hand counterclockwise, left, clockwise. Keep your elbows in and your shoulders back and down.

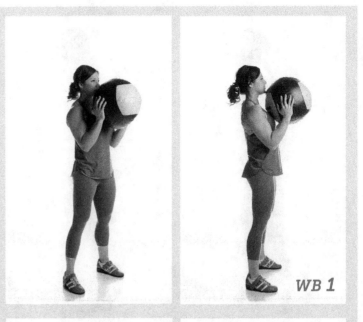

WB 1

"Set your feet shoulder-width and screw your feet into the floor. This is **Wallball Position 1 (WB 1).**

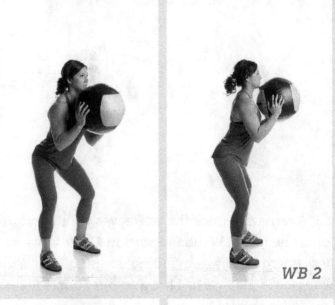

WB 2

"Unlock your knees and sit back. Knees bend but do not come forward. This is **Wallball Position 2 (WB 2).**

"Sit into a full squat. Keep your head position neutral, your torso vertical, and the medicine ball racked under your chin against your chest. This is **Wallball Position 3 (WB 3)."**

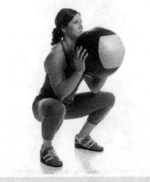

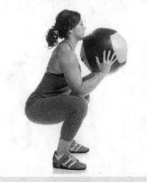

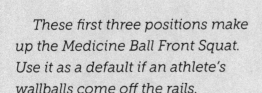

These first three positions make up the Medicine Ball Front Squat. Use it as a default if an athlete's wallballs come off the rails.

"As you come up out of the squat, accelerate to drive your chest into the ball. Just as your hit **WB 1**, throw the ball at the target. Understand that this is not a two-part movement; the squat is blended into the press, like in the thruster.

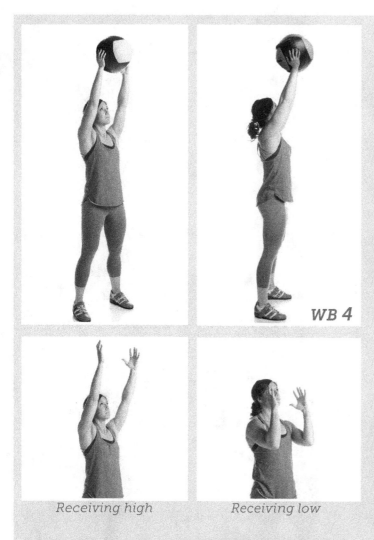

WB 4

Receiving high   Receiving low

"The moment just before the medicine ball leaves your hands is **Wallball Position 4 (WB 4).**

"Try to throw the bar into the target so that it bounces back to you. Accuracy is an important component of the wallball exercise.

"It's okay to tilt your head back a little as you look up at the target during the throw. But during the squat, keep your gaze forward and your head position neutral.

"Once you've thrown the ball at the target, you have two options as to how you receive it on the return.

"You can leave your arms overhead, with hands framing the target, to catch the ball high in **Wallball Position 4**. You then pull it into your chest you descend into the next rep, passing through **Wallball Position 1.**

"Alternately, once the ball leaves your hands, drop your arms, and then catch the ball at chest height in **Wallball Position 1**. The advantage of this is that it makes the movement a little less energetically demanding; keeping your hands above your head is exhausting. The disadvantage is that the ball has another couple feet to accelerate as it hurtles down toward you. Be ready for impact."

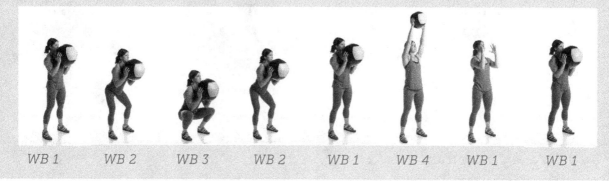

WB 1   WB 2   WB 3   WB 2   WB 1   WB 4   WB 1   WB 1

Positional Drills

"1! 2! 3! 4! 1!" Most athletes pick up the wallball without additional positional practice, but if a trainee is having trouble with sequencing, try having her practice the four positions of the wallball with an imaginary medicine ball.

Wallball Common Faults and Fixes

All faults and fixes common to the air squat apply, as well as...

1. Failure to hit target.

For rep to count the ball must impact the designated target, traditionally set at 10' for men and 9' for women.

 "Throw harder!"

 Demonstrate what a target hit looks like.

 If necessary, give the athlete a lighter medicine ball.

2. No rebound.

If your athlete does not throw the ball horizontally as well as vertically, it will drop straight down, defeating any attempt to smoothly cycle the movement. The athlete must throw the ball into the wall to get it to bounce back.

 "Throw into the wall!"

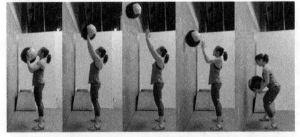

Fault: ball drops straight down from target

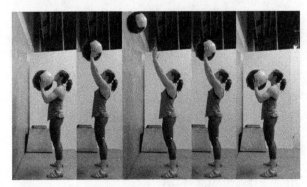

Correct: ball bounces off wall back to hands

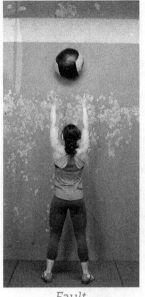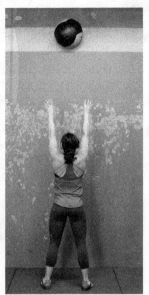

Fault   *Correct*

3. Compromised rack position.

Wallball Position 3 violation. An athlete with an immature squat, or an exhausted athlete of any level, may start folding forward and lowering the medball to her hips as she sits into WB 3. Cue her through WB 1, WB 2, WB 3; if reminding her of the proper positions doesn't help, do away with the throw and have her medball front squat.

 "Chest up!" or "Ball on chest!"

 Demonstrate a correct wallball front squat.

 If necessary, give the athlete a lighter medicine ball.

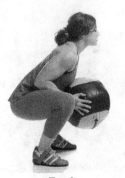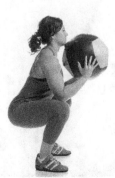

Fault   *Correct WB 3*

THE STRICT TOES-TO-BAR

Category: *H*ip and Trunk Flexion (hanging, straight leg)

Movement screen: N/a

Ability screen: supine knee draw x 5 (supine leg raise), supine leg raise x 5 (incline or

The strict toes-to-bar is a core-strengthening exercise borrowed from the world of gymnastics. It requires strong abs, a strong back, and good body awareness. It's as necessary to doing the more commonly seen kipping toes-to-bar as strict pull-ups are to kipping pull-ups...which is to say, not absolutely, but still a good idea, for reasons of safety and efficiency.

To perform a strict toes-to-bar, the athlete hangs from the bar with arms straight, raises his extended legs until his toes touch the bar, then lowers them. Many trainees will not have the strength or flexibility, at least initially, to perform this feat, so it's important to progress them through a series of exercises that maintain the stimulus—hip flexion with the difficulty increased by the lever arm length of straight legs—while at the same time remaining accessible enough for the trainee to perform competently.

One might ask, if knees-to-elbows are a prerequisite for toes-to-bar, why aren't they part of its movement hierarchy? I put them in two different categories because they progress to different gymnastics movements: the KTE to skin-the-cats and then front and back levers, and the toes-to-bar to the glide kip.

Of Team Space Monkey, only Harry currently has sufficient upper body strength for this exercise. Amy and Tim will both figure out which version of the toes-to-bar is appropriate for them as we work our way through the progression.

Toes-to-Bar Teaching Script

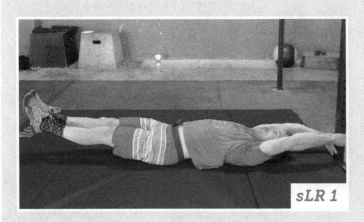

sLR 1

"Take a seat on the floor about 2' in front of a pull-up bar post. Lie down and assume a hollow body hold, extending your legs in front of you and your arms overhead to grab the post for an anchor. Make sure your arms are straight, your glutes and abs engaged, your feet together and your toes pointed. This is **Supine Leg Raise Position 1 (sLR 1).**

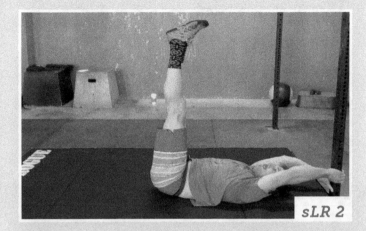

"Keeping your legs straight, lift your feet until your hips are flexed to 90 degrees. This is **Supine Leg Raise Position 2 (sLR 2).**

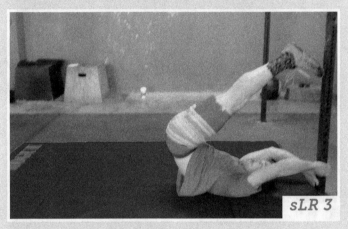

"Holding tight to the post for leverage, contract your abs to curl your trunk until your toes touch the post behind you. Keep your weight on your back—don't roll up onto your neck. This is **Supine Leg Raise Position 3 (sLR 3).**

The jump in difficulty between the supine leg raise and the toes-to-bar is quite drastic. The incline straight leg raise is a great way to bridge the gap. It increases the challenge of the supine leg raise by gradually moving the torso towards vertical. Use stall bars and an incline board, or you can build an incline by propping one end of a utility bench on bumpers in front of a post.

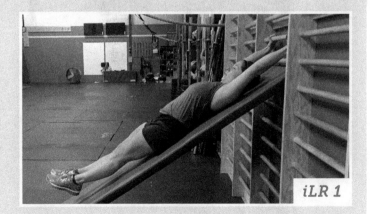

"Set an incline board up on your stall bars at the desired angle. Lie down and assume a hollow body hold, extending your legs in front of you and your arms overhead to grab the post for an anchor. Make sure your arms are straight, your glutes and abs engaged, your feet together and your toes pointed. This is **Incline Leg Raise Position 1 (iLR 1).**

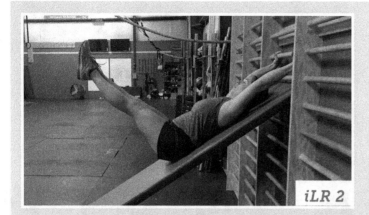

iLR 2

"Keeping your legs straight, lift your feet until your hips are flexed to 90 degrees. This is **Incline Leg Raise Position 2 (iLR 2).**

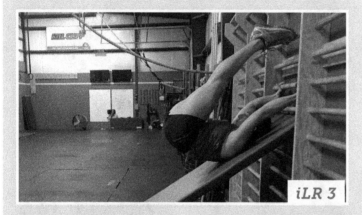

iLR 3

"Holding tight to the post for leverage, contract your abs to curl your trunk until your toes touch the post behind you. Keep your weight on your back—don't roll up onto your neck. This is **Incline Leg Raise Position 3 (iLR 3).**

"When this gets too easy, raise the board to increase your angle relative to the floor."

If your gym doesn't have stall bars and improvising an incline board with materials at hand seems impractical, you can use the hanging leg raise as a progression between supine leg raise and toes-to-bar. While the incline leg raise has the benefits mentioned earlier, the hanging leg raise teaches the first two positions of the toes-to-bar, and builds grip strength, besides.

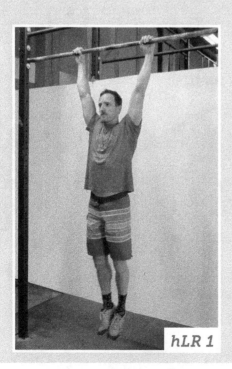

hLR 1

"Begin in an active hang from the pull-up bar: hands shoulder-width, a full-fist (thumbs around) grip with pinky knuckles pointing to the ceiling. Shoulders should be active, midline hollow, legs straight, feet together, toes pointed. This is **Hanging Leg Raise Position 1 (hLR 1).**

"Keeping the legs straight, lift your feet until your hips are flexed to at least 90 degrees. This is **Hanging Leg Raise Position 2 (hLR 2).** Note that this is the same position as the L-hang you practiced last week.

"The ability to get your toes all the way to the bar depends in large part on the your lat strength. You must be able to extend your shoulders strongly enough to lift your chest and hips.

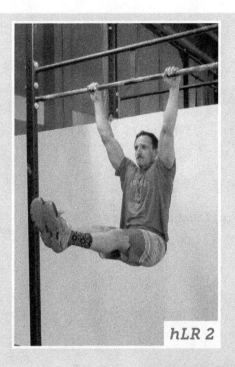

hLR 2

"**Toes-to-bar Position 1 (TB 1)** and **Toes-to-bar Position 2 (TB 2)** are the same as Positions 1 and 2 of the Hanging Straight Leg Raise.

"Then, as the feet rise higher than your hips, push down on the bar while keeping your arms straight, extending your shoulders and lifting the chest toward the ceiling. This additional elevation allows you to touch your toes to the pull-up bar. This is **Toes-to-Bar Position 3 (TB 3).**

"Lower to **TB 2**.

"Return to **TB 1**."

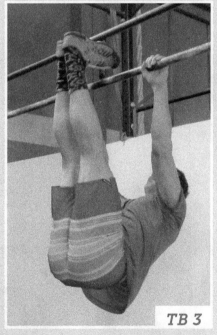

TB 3

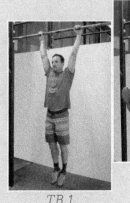

TB 1

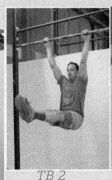

TB 2

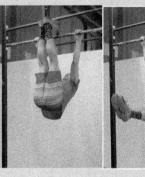

TB 3

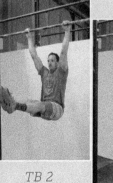

TB 2

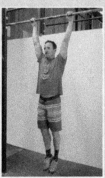

TB 1

Positional Drills

"1! 2! 3! 2! 1!" Practice positions of the toes-to-bar one at a time, making corrections as necessary.

Toes-to-bar Common Faults and Fixes

1. Swinging up.

Toes-to-bar Position 1 violation. The exercise must be initiated with flexion of the hips, not a swing of the legs.

 "No swinging!" or "Stay strict!"

 Demonstrate correct line of action for the strict toes-to-bar.

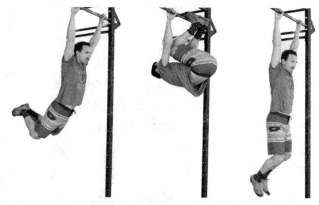

Faulty sequence

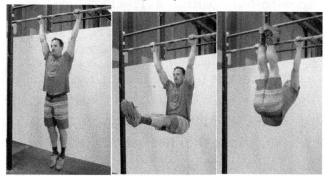

Correct sequence

2. Bent knees.

Toes-to-bar Position 3 violation. Trainee bends his knees as he raises his feet to the bar, shortening the lever arm. Part of the challenge of the strict toes-to-bar is that the legs must be kept straight throughout the movement, which both increases demand on flexibility and adds to the load, as the lever being lifted from the fulcrum of the hip is longer.

 "Straight legs!"

 Demonstrate a correct TB 3.

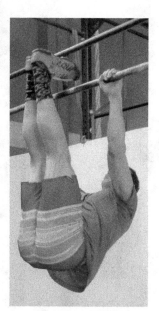

Fault

Correct TB 3

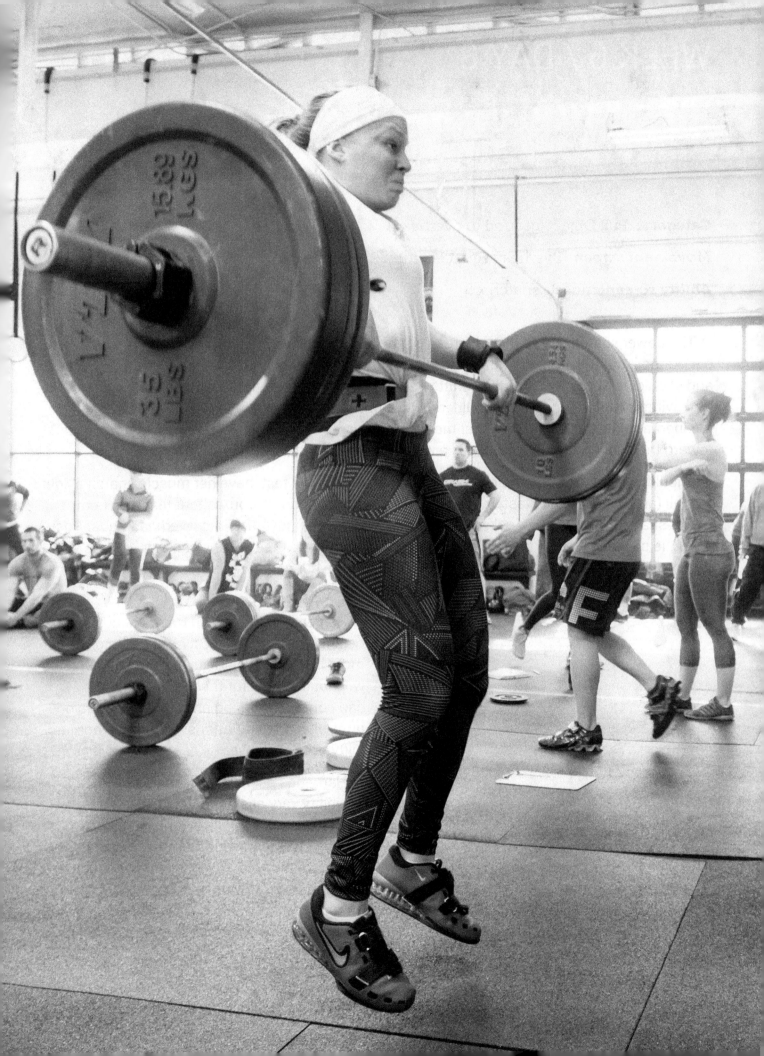

THE POWER SNATCH

Category: Pull Object (ground to overhead)

Movement screen: Overhead squat Position 2 test

Ability screen: muscle snatch x 5

The power snatch allows the athlete to put heavier loads overhead by adding a drop under the bar. At the instant the athlete "finishes" (hitting Snatch Position 5, with knees and hips extended and shoulders shrugged), she then shifts her feet from "jumping" position (under the hips) to "receiving" position (under the shoulders) while pulling powerfully on the bar. Working against the inertia of the bar during this brief moment of free fall allows the athlete to accelerate herself toward the floor and receive the bar in a well-organized partial overhead squat.

Should you teach your athlete to power snatch? Here's the test: have her muscle snatch a light barbell (and if she hasn't mastered the muscle snatch, then don't worry about teaching her the power snatch). With the bar locked out overhead, have her hinge back into Overhead Squat Position 2. Is she able to keep the bar lined up over the front of her heel? If she can't, or if she is visibly straining to stretch her shoulders into position, have her continue to muscle snatch, while mobilizing with the goal of increasing her shoulder flexibility.

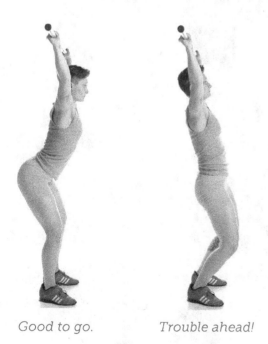

Good to go.   *Trouble ahead!*

Remember: *there is no rush*. As movements become more complex, it becomes more and more likely that your less experienced athletes will not be ready for them. That's fine! They can continue working on the simpler versions until whatever limitations—incompetence, mobility, etc.—improve.

Harry has been working on his overhead flexibility very assiduously, so even though he still can't pass a clean-grip OS 2 test, with a wider, overhead squat grip, he does much better. So today he'll learn the power snatch along with Amy. Even with a single dumbbell, though, Tim is unable to hit a partial overhead squat, and he'll be better served to work on his db muscle snatch.

Power Snatch Teaching Script

"The first five positions of the power snatch: **Power Snatch Position 1**, **Power Snatch Position 2**, **Power Snatch Position 3**, **Power Snatch Position 4**, and **Power Snatch Position 5** are the same as in the muscle snatch. **Power Snatch Position 6** is a little different: now the third pull will be initiated whil you are in mid-air, as your feet move from under your hips to under your shoulders.

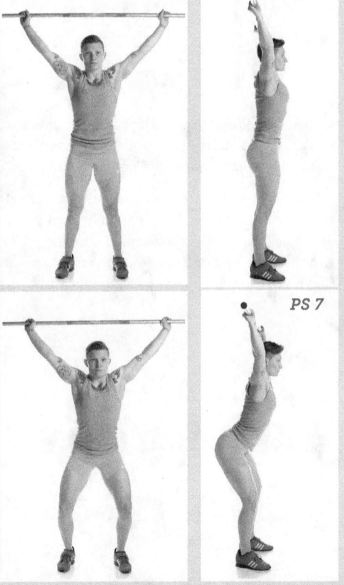

PS 7

"**Power Snatch Positions 7** and **8** are different, too.

"Set up for an overhead squat: wide grip, bar in frontal plane, falling slightly back in your wrists as you try to 'snap' it in half. Brace your midline and set your feet shoulder-width. **This is Power Snatch Position 8 (PS 8),** which is the completion of the lift.

"Now hinge back at the hips. With the weight toward your heels and kneels pushed out, you should be in Overhead Squat Position 2, or as we'll now refer to it, **Power Snatch Position 7 (PS 7).**

"Bars down. Let's review the footwork of the drop squat. Stand tall with your feet under your hips.

"When I say, 'Go!', slide your feet out until they are under your shoulders. Arrest your fall with your hips hinged back, weight on the center of your feet, knees pushed out.

"Move your feet back under your hips. On my command 'Go!', drop into that partial squat, and freeze. Ready? Go!

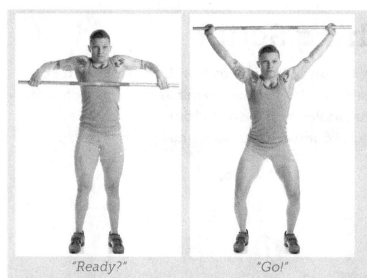

"Ready?"   *"Go!"*

"Reset.

"Hit **Muscle Snatch Position 6**, which will now be **Power Snatch Position 6 (PS 6).**

"On my command 'Go!', drop into a partial overhead squat as you spin the bar overhead—that is, hit **PS 7.** Ready? Go!

"Self-assess. Are you in a good partial overhead squat? Weight back toward the heel, fairly neutral toe position, knees out, hips hinged back, chest up, arms locked straight? Armpits forward? If not, get organized. Then stand up into **Power Snatch Position 8.**

"From here we'll use positional drills to build the movement until you are executing a power snatch from the floor. Move carefully from **PS 1** to **PS 2**, build tension with **PS 3**, get back on your heels for **PS 4**. As you explode up into **PS 5**, your knees and hips fully extending, keep your head neutral and your gaze fixed on a point before you. Remember that **PS 6**, like **Power Clean Position 6**, is now a passing position—you are pulling on the bar as your feet slide from

(cont. on next page)

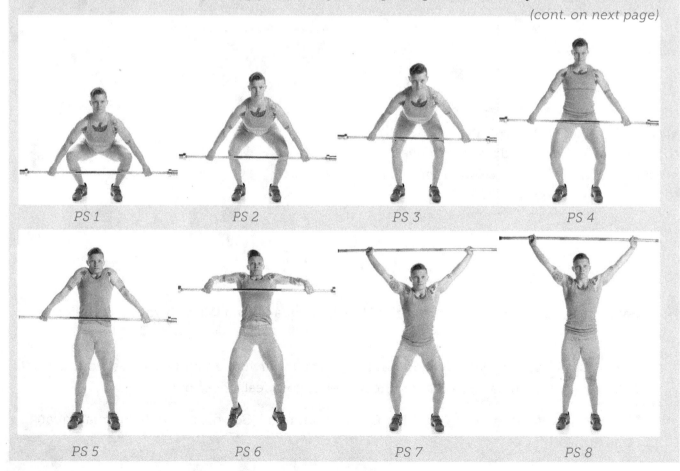

PS 1   PS 2   PS 3   PS 4

PS 5   PS 6   PS 7   PS 8

under your hips (or 'pulling' position) to under your shoulders ('receiving'). In **PS 6**, you are in free fall, not standing on the ground. Remember Newton's Third Law of Motion? For every action, there is an equal and opposite reaction. So use the aggressive upward arm pull you learned from the Muscle Snatch to accelerate yourself downward. Catch the bar in **PS 7** with elbows locked straight. Then stand to complete the rep in **PS 8**."

Positional Drills

"5! 6! 7! 8!" Practice the positions of the power snatch turnover one at a time, making corrections as necessary.

"4! Go!" Practice the high hang power snatch. Pause in **PS 7** to self-assess and correct before standing up the bar.

"3! Go!" Practice the hang power snatch. Pause in **PS 7** to self-assess and correct before standing up the bar.

"2! Go!" Practice the low hang power snatch. Pause in **PS 7** to self-assess and correct before standing up the bar.

"1! Go!" Practice the power snatch. Pause in **PS 7** to self-assess and correct before standing up the bar.

Power Snatch Common Faults and Fixes

All faults and fixes common to the muscle snatch apply, including deadlift set-up, hips rise too soon, jumping from in front of knees, not sweeping bar in, reverse curling bar, pulling too soon, and not finishing, and...

All faults and fixes common to the overhead squat apply, as well as...

1. Throws head back.

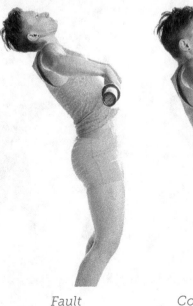

Power Snatch Position 6 violation. Seeking to maximize her extension in the finish, the athlete hyperextends her spine and throws her head back to the point she's looking at the ceiling. Head should remain in a neutral position with gaze directed at a point directly in front.

 "Chin down!" or "Eyes forward!"

 Demonstrate correct transition from PS 5 to PS 6.

Fault   *Correct PS 6*

Dumbbell Power Snatch

Screen your athlete for the db power snatch as you would the barbell power snatch: test his capacity to do a partial one-arm dumbbell overhead squat. If he can't do it, have him stick with the dMS.

"In the dumbbell power snatch the first six positions are the same as the muscle variation. The difference is that the dumbbell is caught in a partial overhead squat. This is **Dumbbell Power Snatch Position 7 (dPS 7)**. The dumbbells are then stood up to completion in **Dumbbell Power Snatch Position 8 (dPS 8)**."

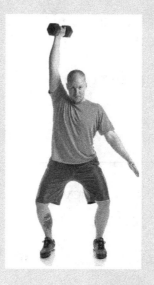
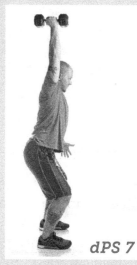

dPS 7

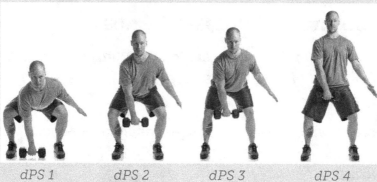

dPS 1   dPS 2   dPS 3   dPS 4

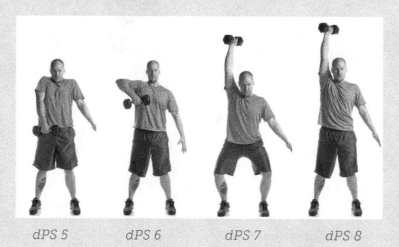

dPS 5   dPS 6   dPS 7   dPS 8

"Kukla, Fran, and Ollie" was one of the first children's shows broadcast on television. It had been one of my dad's favorites when he was a kid, so naturally, when I was young he was excited to introduce me to it, too. Unfortunately, after he popped the tape into the VCR and hit "play", I was so horrified by puppet figures like "Beulah Witch" and "Madame Oglepuss" that I to this day I can't hear certain names without going cold with terror. I guess that's why I named this week's benchmark workout

"Kukla"

20-15-10 reps for time of
Thrusters 95/65lbs
Pull-ups

Prescribing Correct Load and Level of Movement Complexity

"Kukla" tests your ability to crank out 45 barbell thrusters and 45 pull ups in a certain amount of time (ideally, four minutes or less). For the developing athlete, the appropriate load and movement choice is whatever allows them a fair shot at accomplishing that goal.

With that in mind, the load for the thruster should be light, especially at first exposure. So today's session starts with a technique review (five positions of the thruster, which our crew studied last week), segues into five minutes of deliberate practice of the thruster (moving from position to position slowly and methodically, self-assessing and correcting each pose), all in preparation for fifteen minutes of weight training. Harry works up to a 1 rep max thruster. I have Amy work up to a challenging set of three. Tim practices dumbbell thrusters.

Harry manages to thruster 175lbs. I tell him to take 50% of that weight (85lbs, rounding down) and use that for "Kukla". He objects—he's done a similar workout with 95lbs before. What was his time? I ask. "About five minutes," he says. Just try it my way, I tell him. If, afterwards, he thinks it was too easy, he can have the satisfaction of saying "I told you so," and I won't argue with him again. He grudgingly agrees.

Working out of the rack, Amy gets up to 63lbs for a triple. This gives her an E1RM of about 69lbs. 50% of that is 34lbs, which, by astounding coincidence, is almost exactly the weight of one of our 15kg women's bars—the load I was going to recommend for today's "Kukla". Funny how things work out sometimes!

Over by the dumbbell rack, Tim has worked his way up to a set of five dumbbell thrusters with 25lbs in each hand. For today's workout, he'll use 15lbs dbs, and I'll keep the 10s handy, just in case.

Establishing Correct Volume

After experimenting with a four-minute "Kukla"*, I've found that for a general population, a six-minute version is a lot more doable. Most of your athletes will be scaling their pull-ups, and those doing band-assisted pull-ups need a little more time for their transitions. We want to give everyone a fair chance to complete their 20-15-10 reps and advance. The goal remains to "blast through without stopping", so that when the workout is over they'll be in a state of total oxygen debt, that miserable, aching, post-workout gasping that proves so addictive.

"By the Numbers Testing 'Kukla'"

AMRAP :75 thrusters. If you get to 20 before time is up, move on to...
AMRAP :75 pull-ups. If you get to 20 before time is up, move on to...
AMRAP :60 thrusters. If you get to 15 before time is up, move on to...
AMRAP :60 pull-ups. If you get to 15 before time is up, move on to...
AMRAP :45 thrusters. If you get to 10 before time is up, move on to...
AMRAP :45 pull-ups. If you get to 10 before time is up, you're done.

One of the things I really like about the hectic pace these intervals imply is it teaches how to work with intensity. There's simply no time to stand around staring at the bar, and there's no time to dawdle during the transitions from thrusters to pull-ups and back. The athletes quickly learn that finishing this workout in the allotted time is really mostly about making up their mind to do it.

If a new athlete beats "Testing Kukla" by getting, say, all 20-15-10 thrusters and ring rows, then the next time "Kukla" comes up, he can put ten pounds more on the bar and use a more challenging pull-up sub. Eventually he'll work his way up to using prescribed movements and loads—at that point, he'll actually be ready to handle them. If he didn't get all 45 reps of each, then he'll repeat at the same level of challenge each time "Kukla" comes up, until he successfully completes it in six minutes.

If you want to train the four minute version, use intervals of :50, :40, :30, and Godspeed!

"3...2...1...GO!"

Harry

Once again, Harry's enthusiasm for going hard initially trumped the requirement that he do it right. His very first thruster rep saw the bar way out in front at completion, rather than locked out over the front of his heel.

"Harry, PULL BACK ON THE BAR!" I yelled—a verbal cue.

His next two reps landed in the same place.

"LIKE THIS!" I said, miming pulling the bar back until my arms blocked my ear. Visual cue.

Two more reps out front.

"Goddammit," I grumbled. Because now I had to make a choice. Harry was in Performance Mode; I was Coaching for Performance. He was making an error of execution (not finishing in a correct Thruster Position 5) and I had given him two cues that had failed to fix it. So, under BtN guidelines, I COULD make him stop, taking him out of Performance Mode and back, temporarily, into Practice Mode, so I could make sure he understood his error. I knew he would be mad, but ultimately, that's not my problem! If he persisted with his sub-par execution, his time for this workout would be meaningless, anyway.

But in a flash of inspiration, I decided to try one more cue: a tactile one. Moving behind him as he worked, I said, "Hit my hand with the bar!" As he pressed it overhead, he pulled the bar back to slap against my palm. Success! Now he understood. He performed his last three reps of that set to standard and then jumped for the pull-up bar.

Harry stayed ahead of the clock and called time at 3:33. As he lay there gasping, I stood over him and asked, "So? Too easy?" Without opening his eyes, he raised his shaking right hand and lifted one finger (not his index) in response. Another satisfied customer! And I'm satisfied as well. He worked ferociously hard, and his movements (after a few corrections) were impeccable. Next time he can add ten pounds, and if he beats the clock again, the time after that he can go as RX'd.

Amy

Amy finished her last band-assisted pull-up just before time ran out. She also managed to complete all 20-15-10 reps, "...although the middle fifteen," she said between gasps for breath, "that was pretty close." Next time she'll go at least ten pounds heavier, and hopefully won't be using any assistance for pull-ups at all.

Tim

Tim also finished the assigned work. 20-15-10 reps of dumbbell thrusters was a challenge for him, but the ring rows were surprisingly easy. Each round he finished his rows with time to spare, which let him get a jump on his next set of thrusters. Good to know! I tell him he's promoted off of ring rows; now he can split his time between piked ring rows and band-assisted pull-ups. I think that I'll probably try to direct him toward assisted pull-ups in practice and piked ring rows for performance; despite his remarkable progress, Tim is still a bit stiff and uncoordinated, and I worry about him rushing to get his foot in and out of the assistance band while standing on a box.

Category: Pull Object (ground to overhead)

Movement screen: Overhead squat Position 3 test

Ability screen: Power snatch and land in perfect OS 2 (power snatch + overhead squat),

Building on the power snatch, in the snatch (sometimes referred to as the "squat snatch"), the athlete receives the bar overhead in a well-organized full overhead squat.

If the WOD includes snatches, and a given athlete is still developing competence with the movement, break it into simpler components that can be performed well, but preserve the stimulus: muscle snatch and overhead squat, or power snatch and overhead squat. If the athlete doesn't have the flexibility to overhead squat, have her clean instead. Not everybody needs to snatch.

Of our Team Space Monkey crew, only Amy, relative newbie that she is, will start learning the full snatch today. Harry and Tim will work on power snatches and dumbbell muscle snatches, respectively.

Snatch Teaching Script

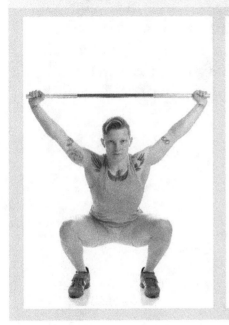

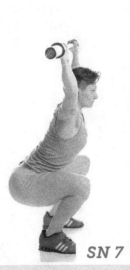

SN 7

"The snatch is a power snatch taken to its logical conclusion. As the weight you're snatching gets heavier and heavier, your catch position will get lower and lower, until you are receiving the bar in a full overhead squat. **Snatch Position 7 (SN 7)** is the same as Overhead Squat Position 3. Otherwise all positions are the same as in the muscle and power snatch.

"Any flaw in your overhead squat technique will make completing your snatch very difficult. You must have a vertical torso, a rigidly braced midline, a tight upper back, and straight elbows, with the bar balanced in the line of gravity, if you're going to complete the lift by standing up into **Snatch Position 8**.

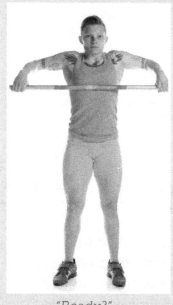

"Ready?"

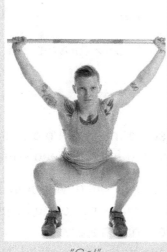

"Go!"

"Let's practice that footwork. Get into **Snatch Position 6** for me: feet under the hips and screwed in to the ground, midline braced, bar held at chest height, close to the body, elbows up and back.

"On my command 'Go!', slide your feet out to shoulder width. Simultaneously, whip the bar overhead as your drop into **SN 7**. Freeze in your catch position. Ready? Go!

"Self-assess. If your position is good, stand.

"The best way to bridge the challenging increase in complexity between the power snatch and the snatch is to perform power snatches with an added overhead squat. Here's what I mean:

"Pick up your barbell. Hit 'reset' for me: overhead squat-width grip with hook grip, feet under the hips and screwed into the floor, midline braced, shoulders back, elbows out, wrists curled under.

"Set up in **Snatch Position 4**. On my command 'Go!', explode up into **SN 5**, then shift your feet out into receiving stance. As your arms pull into **Snatch Position 6**, the feet shift from under the hips to under the shoulders. In that transition, you are in free fall for a split second, which allows you to work against the inertia of the bar to accelerate yourself toward the floor. The load is received with the arms locked straight in **PS 7**. Freeze there. Ready? Go!"

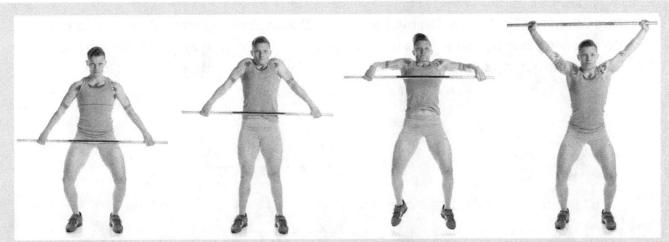

Power snatch from the high hang

"Self-assess. Is your weight on the balls of your feet? Are your knees too forward? Caving in, maybe? Is the bar anywhere but in the frontal plane? Are your elbows pointing back? Whatever the issue is, adjust until you are in an ideal **PS 7.**

"Now, **PS 7** is identical to **Overhead Squat Position 2**. So once your **PS 7** is looking good, simply sit down into **OS 3**—which, you'll remember, is now **SN 7**, and then stand to completion in **SN 8.**

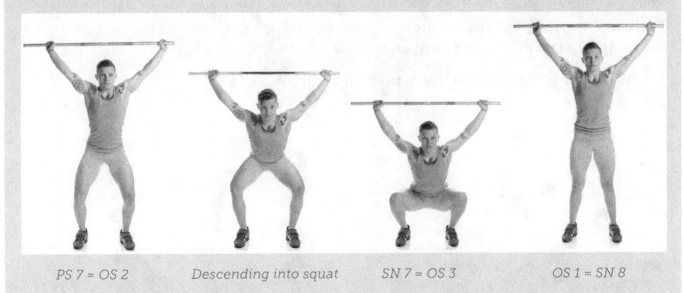

PS 7 = OS 2   *Descending into squat*   *SN 7 = OS 3*   *OS 1 = SN 8*

"The trick is to only squat once you are *sure* your position is good. This is a great option if you're taking on a WOD like 'Amanda', which calls for full snatches. If you can't reliably catch a snatch in good form and good balance, catch it in the power position, get organized, and then squat.

"Now you're ready to try for a full snatch from the high hang.

"Pick up your barbell. Hit 'reset' for me.

"Set up in **Snatch Position 4.** On my command 'Go!', explode up into **SN 5**. Shift your feet out into receiving stance, and at the same time, pull hard with your arms (**SN 6**), working off the inertia of the bar to accelerate your descent into **SN 7**. Freeze there. Ready? Go!"

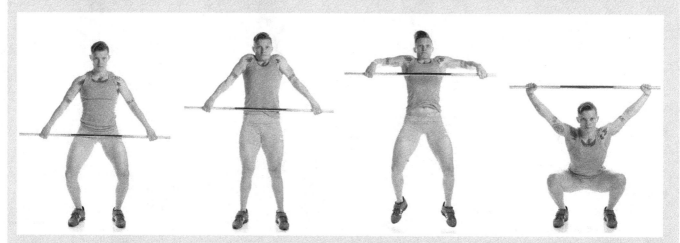

"Self-assess. Is your receiving position ideal? If so, stand up. If not, get into a perfect Snatch Position 7 before squatting up the bar through **Overhead Squat Position 2** to finish in **Snatch Position 8** (same as **Overhead Squat Position 1**)."

"Once you can reliably land in a well-organized overhead squat, you won't wait in **Snatch Position 7**. Instead, you'll use the stretch of your hamstrings as you hit the bottom position to help propel you up into **Snatch Position 8.**

"Finally, here is the complete snatch from the floor."

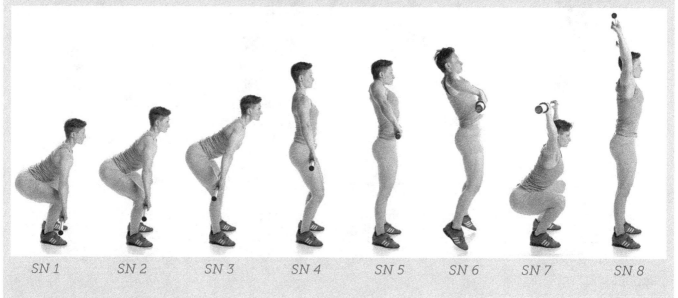

| SN 1 | SN 2 | SN 3 | SN 4 | SN 5 | SN 6 | SN 7 | SN 8 |

Positional Drills

"1! 2! 3! 4! 5! 6! 7! 8! Reset!" Drill positions of the snatch one at a time, making corrections as necessary.

"4! Go!" Snatch from the high hang. When using barbells, trainees should feel the bar is noticeably lighter from the force created by rapidly extending the hips and knees.

"1! Go!" Snatch. Make sure your trainees understand that like the clean, the snatch has three phases: a slow and deliberate from floor to below the knees, an acceleration from below the knee to above, and then an explosion as the torso shifts vertical for the jump.

Snatch Common Faults and Fixes

All faults and fixes common to the muscle and power snatch apply, including deadlift set-up, hips rise too soon, jumping from in front of knees, not sweeping bar in, reverse curling bar, pulling too soon, and not finishing, and...

All faults and fixes common to the overhead squat apply, including all air squat flaws, as well as soft elbows and ship's figurehead fault.

Dumbbell Snatch

! *Screen your athlete for the db snatch as you would the barbell snatch: test his capacity to do a full one-arm dumbbell overhead squat. If he can't do it, have him stick with the dPS.*

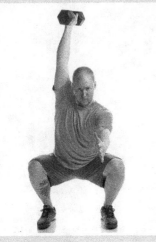
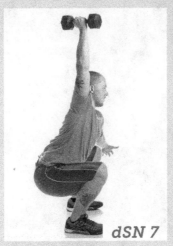

dSN 7

"In the dumbbell snatch the pull from the floor, the shift to jumping position, and the jump-and-pull are exactly the same as in the dumbbell power snatch. The difference is that the dumbbell is caught in a full overhead squat. This is **Dumbbell Snatch Position 7 (dSN 7).** The dumbbell is then stood up to completion in **Dumbbell Snatch Position 8 (dSN 8).**"

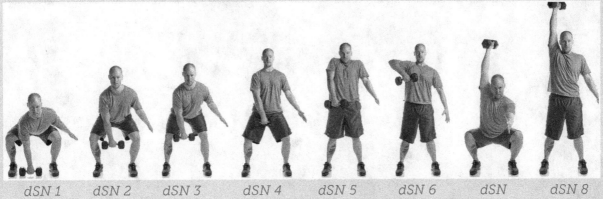

dSN 1   dSN 2   dSN 3   dSN 4   dSN 5   dSN 6   dSN   dSN 8

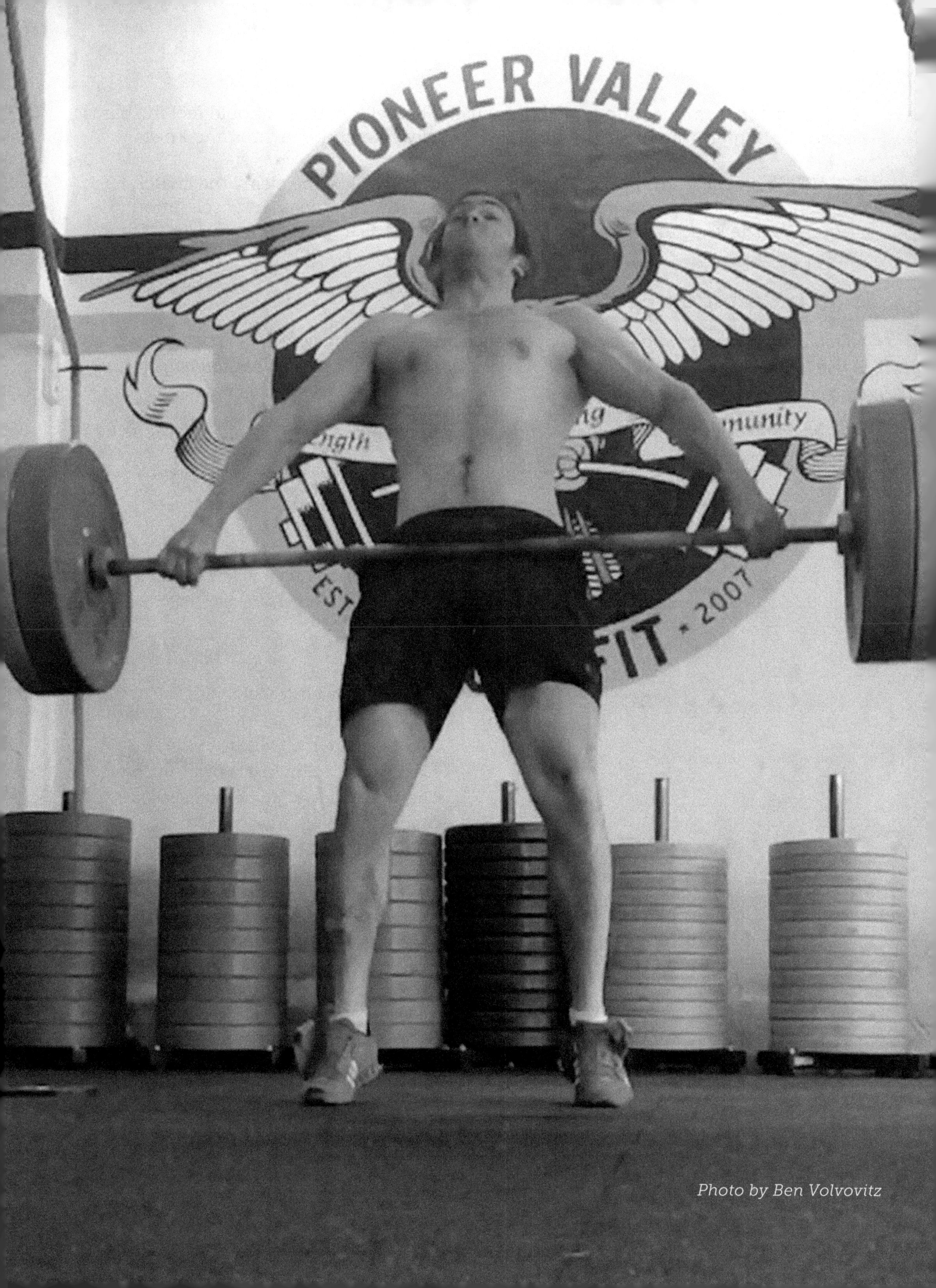

Photo by Ben Volvovitz

WEEK 7 / DAY 1
THE PISTOL

Category: Single-leg squat

Movement screen: Ankle flexibility test

Ability screen: N/a (box step-up), forward lunge x 5 (reverse lunge), reverse lunge x 10 (hanging leg pistol from box), hanging leg pistol from box to below parallel x 4 (elevated leg pistol from box), elevated leg pistol from bumper plate x 4 (pistol)

The pistol is a single-leg squat that can help identify strength imbalances between the two legs, and generally speaking improves proprioception as the athlete learns to activate the smaller, stabilizing muscles of the leg and hip.

It should go without saying that an athlete should have a very solid air squat before attempting pistols. But even an athlete with a decent two-legged squat may find pistols prohibitively difficult due to tight ankles, hips, and hamstrings.

Here's a simple test: Have your trainees stand tall with feet close together. Then have them squat down on their heels, pushing their knees out. It will quickly be obvious who has the requisite ankle flexibility for pistols, and who doesn't.

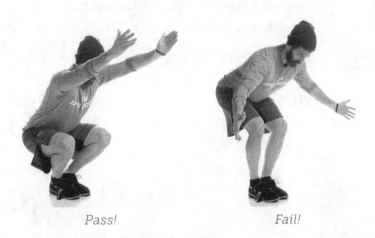

Pass!   *Fail!*

Those athletes lacking the necessary ankle flexibility to execute a pistol can simply increase the load on their forward and reverse lunges to train single-leg strength. When they can pass the Ankle Flexibility Test, they may begin working toward pistols.

Instead of teaching the positions of the pistol through a reduced range-of-motion, and then gradually having the athlete work toward full ROM, By the Numbers first builds the strength necessary to squat on one leg through full ROM, and then gradually develops the flexibility and balance necessary to perform the pistol.

I think Harry and Amy will do quite well with the pistol. Most likely, Tim will end up sticking with the first exercise in our pistol progression, the reverse lunge.

Pistol Teaching Script

The best place for trainees to begin their progression toward the pistol is with the reverse lunge. It puts a higher strength demand on the individual leg than does the air squat, while helping developing balance and proprioception in a safe environment (i.e., on the ground.)

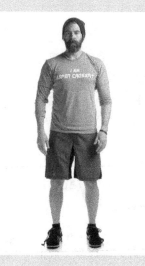
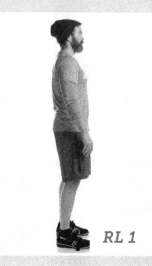

RL 1

"Stand tall with your feet under your hips. Screw your feet into the ground, squeeze your butt, lock your ribs down, pack your shoulders. **This is Reverse Lunge Position 1 (RL 1).**

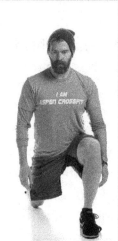
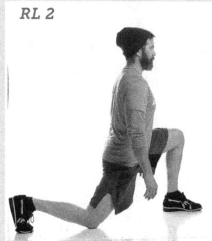

RL 2

"Take a long step back and slightly out. Slightly internally rotate this leg, kicking the heel out. Sink the knee to the floor. The knee of the forward leg should be lined up over the ankle. The torso should remain vertical. Weight should be centered between the legs. This is **Reverse Lunge Position 2 (RL2).**

"Push off the ball of the rear foot and down through the front heel to return to **RL 1**."

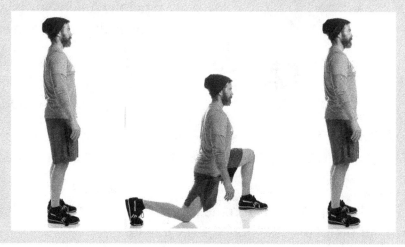

If your trainee can handle the reverse lunge, s/he may begin working toward the pistol.

"Stand on one foot atop a 12" box. Allow your other leg to hang straight toward the floor. This is **Hanging Leg Pistol from Box Position 1 (hPI 1).**

"Being careful to keep your foot screwed into the box with your weight back toward the heel of your standing foot, sit back. This is **Hanging Leg Pistol from Box Position 2 (hPI 2).** If your foot has already made contact with the floor, stand back up.

"Otherwise continue until the foot of your hanging leg makes light contact with the floor. Don't come to rest--keep all of your weight on your standing leg. This is **Hanging Leg Pistol from Box Position 3 (hPI 3).**

"If that's relatively easy, try again, this time on a taller box.

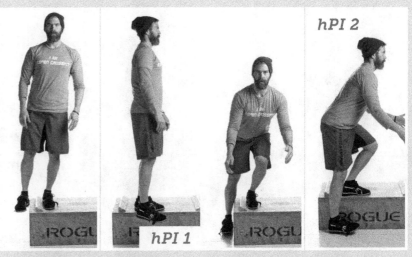

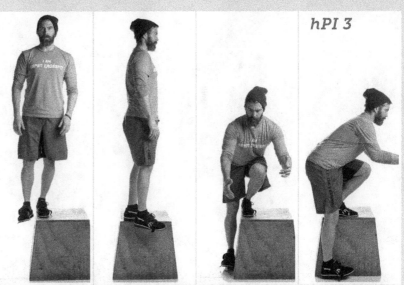

"Use taller and taller boxes until you are squatting below parallel. Then begin elevating the extended leg and working your way back down, using shorter boxes. At that point you are doing **Elevated Leg Pistol from Box (ePI).**"

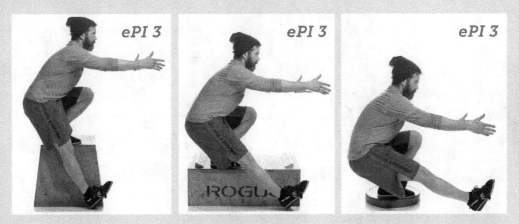

"When you can hit **ePI 3** from a bumper plate, you're ready to try a real pistol."

"Shooting the duck" is a trick familiar to those who ice- or rollerskate. It's also a great way to build strength and stability in the bottom position of the pistol.

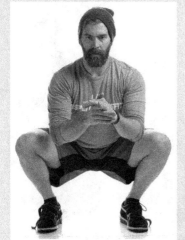 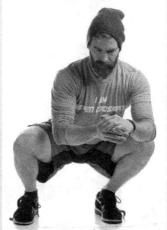

"To begin, get down into **Air Squat Position 3.**

"Shift your weight onto one foot.

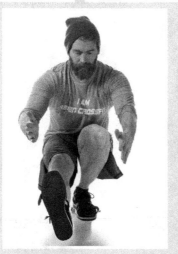

"Stand slightly, to give your hips a bit of room to move, and then extend the other leg, keeping your foot off the ground. Sink back into a full squat on one leg. Remain in this position for a count of five, concentrating on trying to hit a perfect pose: leg straight and pointing straight ahead, toes pointed, chest up, lumbar curve maintained, external rotation on the supporting leg (e.g., knee is pushed out, not caving in). Then switch sides.

Like the air squat, the pistol has three positions: stand, hinge, and squat.

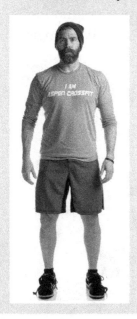 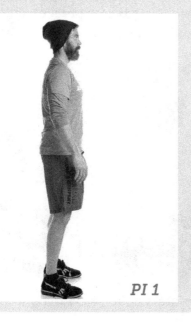

PI 1

"Stand tall in reset position: feet under your hips, toes gripping the floor, weight back toward the heel, screwing your feet into the floor, midline braced, shoulders packed, gaze forward. This is **Pistol Position 1 (PI 1).**

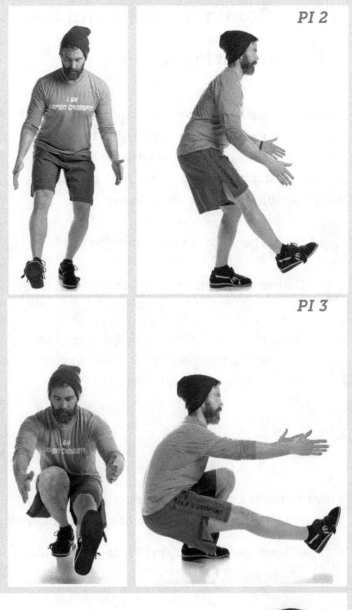

PI 2

PI 3

"Hinge back at the hip, elevating one leg. Keep the knee straight and the toe pointed. Lift your hands as counterbalance. This is **Pistol Position 2 (PI 2).**

"Sit all the way down until the crease of your hip is below the top of your knee. The knee of the supporting leg should be tracking over the foot; the opposite leg should be fully extended, and the back as straight as possible while keeping your weight over your foot. This is **Pistol Position 3 (PI 3).**

"Drive through the heel to return to **PI 2.**

"Fully extend the knee and hip of your standing leg before setting your elevated foot down in **PI 1.**

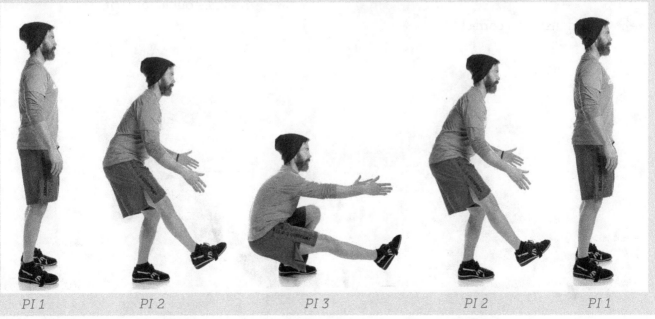

| PI 1 | PI 2 | PI 3 | PI 2 | PI 1 |

Pistol Common Faults and Fixes

1. Initiating at knee.

Pistol Position 2 violation. The pistol is a species of squat, and must be initiated by hinging back at the hip. If the athlete breaks at the knee too soon, he'll end up standing on the ball of the foot, putting potentially harmful shear force on the knee.

 "Hinge back!" or "Sit back!" or "Hips first!"

 Demonstrate correct transition from PI 1 to PI 2.

 As he begins his pistol, block the knee of the trainee's standing leg with the back of your hand as he transitions from PI 1 to PI 2.

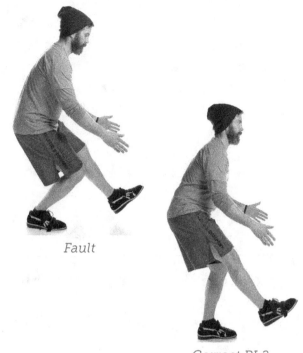

Fault

Correct PI 2

2. Knee collapses in.

Pistol Position 3 violation. In the bottom position of the pistol, the athlete allows the knee of his standing leg to trail in toward his centerline, committing a valgus fault.

 "Screw your feet in!" (in PI 1) or "Push your knee out!" (PI 2).

 Demonstrate a correct PI 3.

 Place the back of your hand in the desired position and tell the athlete to push his knee out to touch it.

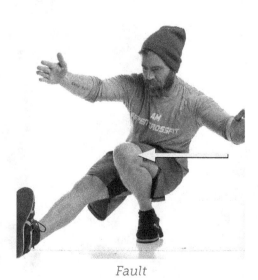

Fault

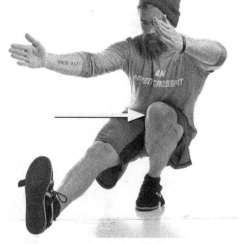

Correct PI 3

Pistol Common Faults and Fixes, cont.

3. "Competition pistol" (Abduction and internal rotation of extended leg).

Pistol Position 3 violation. Athlete sends his leg out to the side, with toe pointing in toward his centerline. Could be caused by hip impingement, failure to fire the glutes, or some combination thereof.

 "Toe out!" or "Squeeze your butt!"

 Demonstrate a proper PI 3.

 Return athlete to box pistols, find the elevation at which the athlete can execute a pistol and keep his extended leg in correct position.

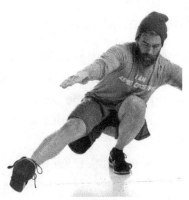

Fault

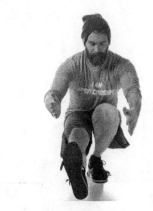

Correct PI 3

4. Holding foot.

Pistol Position 3 violation. An athlete who lacks the flexibility and balance to keep his extended leg straight and off the floor will grab his foot to hold it up. It's a pragmatic solution but not one that leads toward long-term improvement.

 "No holding!"

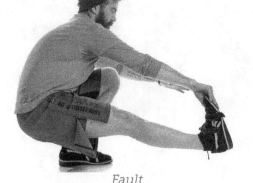

Fault

Demonstrate a correct PI 3.

Have the athlete loop a band around the extended foot and practice pistols, gradually introducing slack into the band to wean himself from holding up his foot.

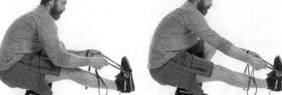

Gradually increase slack to wean

Pistol Common Faults and Fixes, cont.

5. Falling backward.

Pistol Position 3 violation. After initiating squat, athlete falls backward. Assuming he has passed the ankle flexibilty test, this occurs because he failed to keep his weight evenly distributed over his area of base. At all times during the pistol the athlete must keep his weight over the center of his foot; failing to stretch forward the arms or lifting the torso to vertical too soon will send him sprawling backward.

 "Reach forward!" or "Keep reaching!"

 Demonstrate how to lean forward and extend arms to keep weight over foot.

 Give the athlete a light kettlebell or dumbbell to hold at arm's length. The weight will act as a counterbalance, and can be reduced over time until he can perform a pistol without aid.

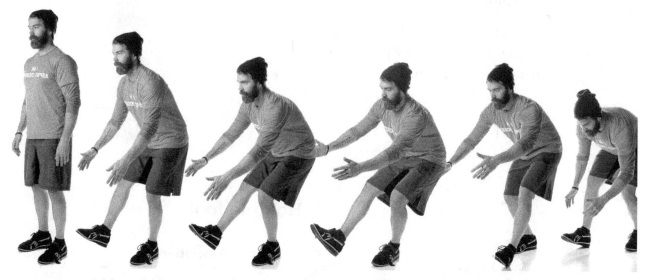

Athlete initiates pistol, but after PI 2 loses balance and falls backwards.

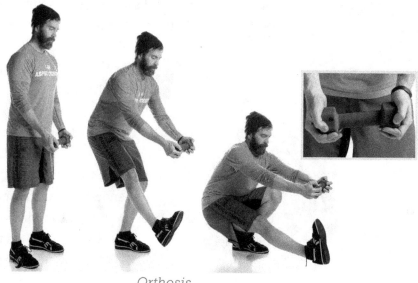

Orthosis

THE ROPE CLIMB

Category: Hybrid (squat, pull to object)

Movement screen: N/a

Ability screen: Ring row x 10 (rope climb from seated), rope climb from seated x 3 (plank

In MMGPP programs, we climb ropes because a) it's a nice break from constant pull-ups (and for those who don't have strict pull-ups yet, the seated climb and the plank climb from the floor help build strength in the bottom position, where bands offers the most assistance), b) it builds self-confidence—we love to see the joy in people's faces the first time they make it to the top of the rope, and c) rope climbing is a potentially life-saving skill that every adult should have. Not to mention it's fun!

What follows is BtN's standard teaching progression for the rope climb. It begins with a climb from seated on the floor (to build grip strength), then a climb from the floor in plank position (increased grip and upper body load), and then finally teaches the trap-and-stand technique. Using one of these three variants, virtually all of your trainees will be able to do some version of the rope climb.

Finally, please note that there are many ways to climb the rope. I like this one because it's easy to learn and minimizes rope burns. (Don't forget to warn your athletes ahead of time to wear long pants or tall socks while climbing.) But feel free to teach any technique you find effective, as long as you can break it down positionally.

Today, all three of our Team Space Monkey athletes will be climbing ropes. It's a nice break for me as their instructor—I don't have to try to coach three different movements at once!

Rope Climb Teaching Script

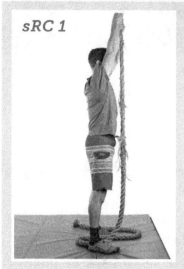

sRC 1

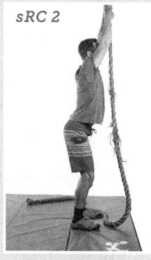

sRC 2

"Standing about a foot back from where the rope hangs to the floor, grasp the rope in both hands as high up as you can reach. Squeeze your butt, lock your ribs toward your hips, set the shoulders back and down. This is **Seated Rope Climb Position 1 (sRC 1).**

"Holding tight to the rope, hinge at the hip, pulling the rope toward you. This is **Seated Rope Climb Position 2 (sRC 2).**

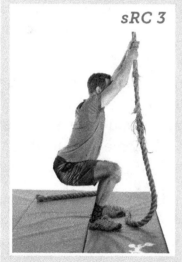

sRC 3

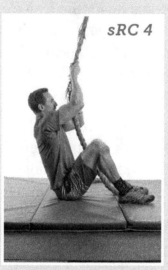

sRC 4

"Walking your hands down the rope, sit down in a squat. This is **Seated Rope Climb Position 3 (sRC 3).**

"Tilt back and lower yourself hand under hand on the rope until you are seated on the floor. This is **Seated Rope Climb Position 4 (sRC 4).**

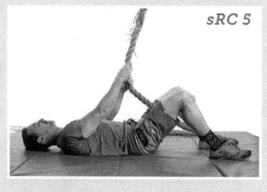

sRC 5

"Continue your descent until you are flat on your back. This is **Seated Rope Climb Position 5 (sRC 5).**

"To return, pull yourself up hand-over-hand to return to **sRC 3**, and then use your legs as necessary to return to **sRC 2** and then **sRC 1**."

If the seated rope climb is easy for your trainees, introduce them to the plank climb.

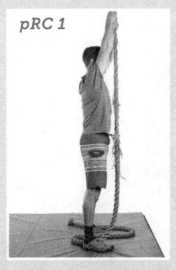

pRC 1

"Standing about a foot back from where the rope hangs to the floor, grasp the rope in both hands as high up as you can reach. Set your feet shoulder-width. Squeeze your butt, lock your ribs toward your hips, set the shoulders back and down. This is **Plank Rope Position 1 (pRC 1).**

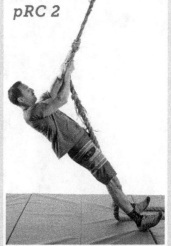

pRC 2

"Maintaining a straight line from ankle to shoulder, rock back on your heels until your arms are completely extended. This is **Plank Rope Climb Position 2 (pRC 2).**

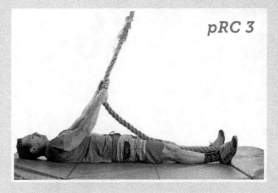

pRC 3

"Lower yourself hand-under-hand until you are supine on the floor. This is **Plank Rope Climb Position 3 (pRC 3).**

"Still maintaining a straight line from ankle to shoulder—you'll really have to concentrate on keeping your glutes and abs locked to prevent sagging hips—climb up from the floor hand-over-hand through **pRC 2** to return to **pRC 1**."

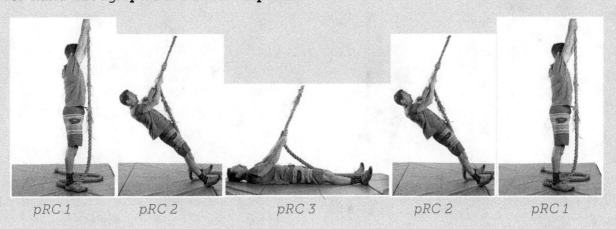

pRC 1   pRC 2   pRC 3   pRC 2   pRC 1

The standard rope climb is more about technique than raw upper body strength. As such it is accessible and safe even for those trainees who may not yet have strict pull-ups.

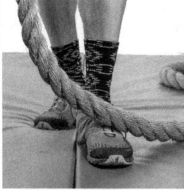

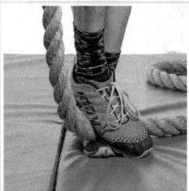

"The standard rope climb is built on the technique of trapping the rope between your feet and using it as a base of support. Start in a stand directly under the rope, with the rope trailing to the left over your left foot.

"Step on the rope with your right foot, toes to the left, heel to the right. The rope should be between the sole of your right foot and the instep of the left—basically, you're standing like a little kid who really has to go to the bathroom. This is your trap. Being able to reset this position while hanging from the rope is the key to efficient climbing.

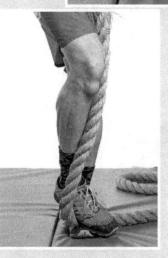

"Now draw the rope inside your right knee. This is to keep the rope in place so that it will thread smoothly between your feet.

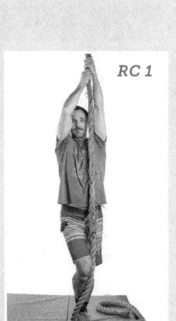

RC 1

"Reach up with both hands and hold on tight to the rope. With the rope secured between your feet, and threaded around your knee, you are now in **Rope Climb Position 1 (RC 1).**

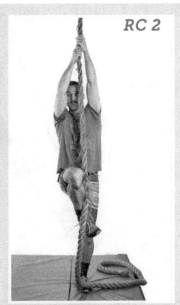

"Keeping your left foot on the floor, pull your right knee high. This is **Rope Climb Position 2 (RC 2).**

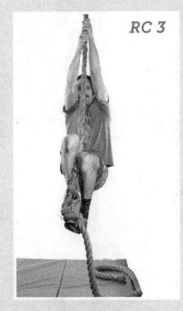

"Now, holding on for dear life, lift your left foot and slide it up along the rope until its instep traps the rope against the sole of your right foot. This is **Rope Climb Position 3 (RC 3).**

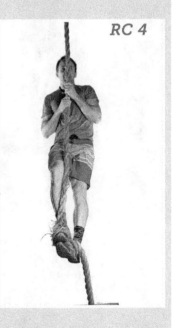

"With the rope trapped between left instep and right sole, stand up tall. Your hands will be at about chest height. This is **Rope Climb Position 4 (RC 4).**

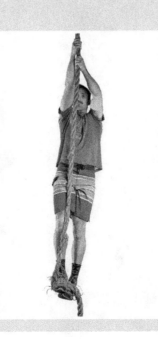

"Now walk your hands up the rope one at a time until your arms are fully extended. You've returned to **RC 1.** Repeat the process until you've climbed to the desired height (15' is standard).

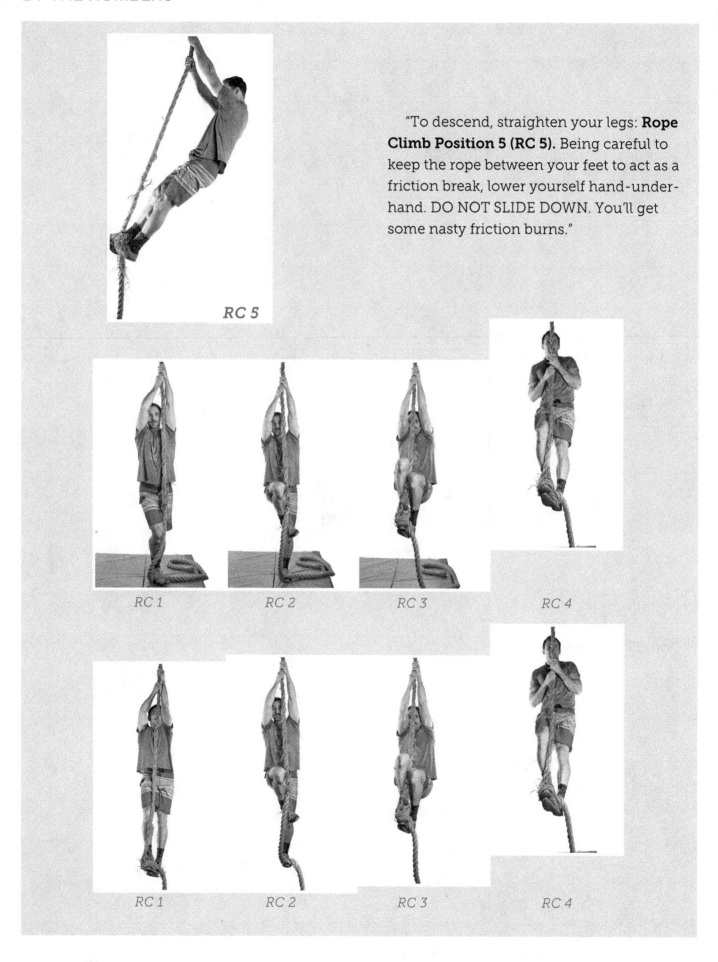

"To descend, straighten your legs: **Rope Climb Position 5 (RC 5).** Being careful to keep the rope between your feet to act as a friction break, lower yourself hand-under-hand. DO NOT SLIDE DOWN. You'll get some nasty friction burns."

RC 5

RC 1   *RC 2*   *RC 3*   *RC 4*

RC 1   *RC 2*   *RC 3*   *RC 4*

Advanced athletes can work on legless rope climbs—truly legit, old-school training.

"Standing directly under the rope, grasp the rope with one hand below your chin, and the other arm at full extension. This is **Legless Rope Climb Position 1 (lRC 1)**. Pull strongly with the extended arm and shoot your low hand up to grab the rope above your head. This is **Legless Rope Climb Position 2 (lRC 2)**.

"Continue alternating **lRC 1** and **lRC 2** until you've climbed 15' or until fatigue requires you to return to to the ground. During your descent, use hands only, or use **RC 5**, depending on strength, experience, and level of fatigue."

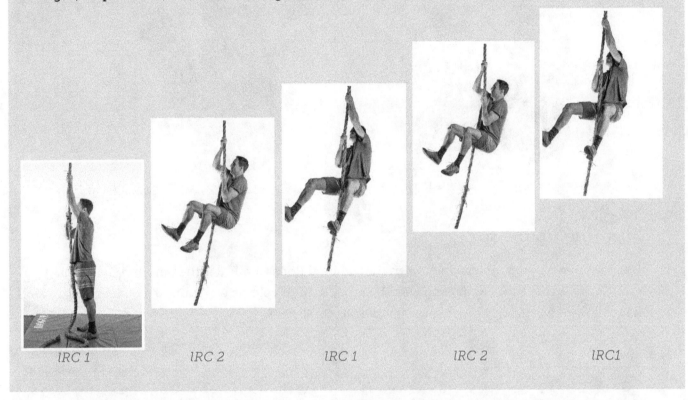

lRC 1   lRC 2   lRC 1   lRC 2   lRC1

"**IMPORTANT SAFETY WARNING: It is possible that you could fall off the rope and be badly injured or even die. That's why it is absolutely essential you do not attempt to climb the rope in WODs if there is the slightest doubt that you are fresh and strong enough to make it up and down safely. If you become exhausted in a workout, please, please let discretion be the better part of valor, and default back to a simpler movement in the hierarchy of Rope Climbs.**"

Rope Climb Common Faults and Fixes

1. Bad trap.

Rope Climb Position 1 violation. Feet are side-by-side with rope held weakly between them. Trappng the rope securely between the feet is key for efficient climbing. The rope should fit snugly between the sole of one foot and the instep of the other.

"Foot on top!"   Demonstrate a correct RC 1 foot trap.

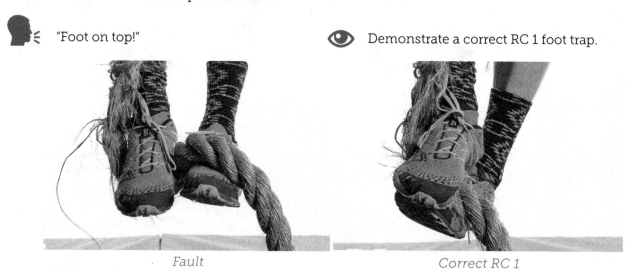

Fault   *Correct RC 1*

2. Chinning up the rope.

It's important that trainees understand that in the standard Rope Climb, it is the trap-and-stand that moves the body up the rope, not pulling with the arms. In high volume workouts, the athlete relying too much on his arms will quickly become too fatigued to climb safely.

"Trap and stand!" or "More legs!"   Demonstrate the proper way to trap and stand up on the rope. If you want, take one hand off to show it is the trap that supports the body's weight.

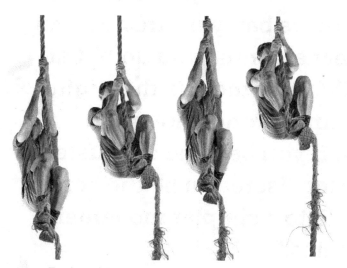 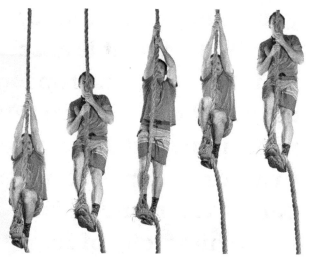

Fault: athlete uses arms only to ascend   *Correct: athlete traps rope and stands up*

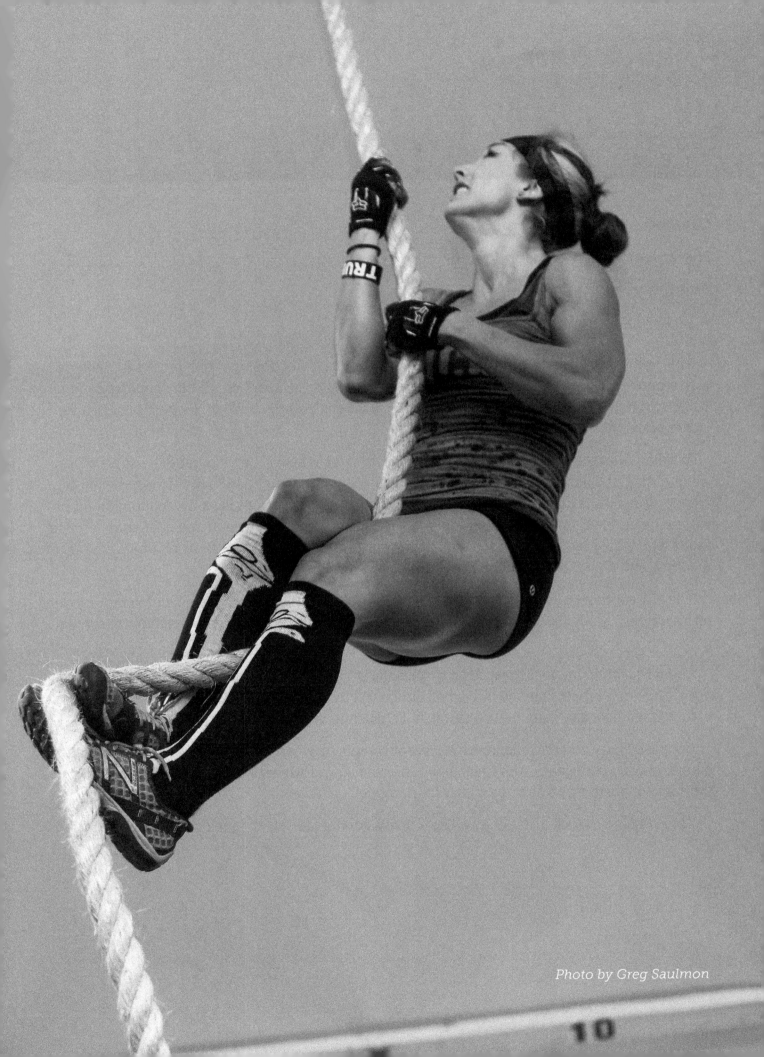

Photo by Greg Saulmon

THE SPLIT JERK

Category: Push Object (vertical)

Movement screen: Samson stretch

Ability screen: Forward lunge x 10, push jerk x 5

The split jerk allows the athlete to receive the bar in a lower position than most can manage with a push jerk. This means that even larger weights can be launched off the shoulder and then stood to a finish. The split position also creates a longer, broader base of support, which makes it easier to balance a load overhead.

Training the split jerk is useful even for those athletes who will never pursue the sport of weightlifting. It's a tremendous developer of speed, balance, and coordination; these benefits are increased if the athlete trains the split position on both sides. It's also the foundation for fun variations on the way the lifts are traditionally performed, e.g., split clean and split snatch (*pace* those who would remind me that it's really the split variations that are the traditional versions of the lifts), and dumbbell variations thereof.

There are many ways to teach the split jerk: this is mine. It's a good example of what I call "entertrainment": goofy fun as the spoonful of sugar that helps the medicine of legitimate technique go down.

Today will be tough for Tim and Harry, for different reasons. Tim doesn't have very good balance, and I don't think jumping into a half-lunge will be good for him. I'll have him practice stepping into a lunge, and dumbbell pressing. It'll challenge his balance and flexibility in a safe way.

Because Harry couldn't pass the movement screen, he wasn't allowed to push jerk. And because he can't push jerk, I won't teach him the split jerk. However, I will teach him the foot work for the split position; he can use it later for dumbbell split cleans.

Amy is going to rock the split jerk. She's quick, and has terrific balance and coordination.

Split Jerk Teaching Script

"We'll begin by establishing your dominant foot. Close your eyes, and then let yourself tip forward until you start to fall. Whatever foot involuntarily shoots out to keep you from hitting the ground is your dominant foot. Learn the split position with that foot in front.

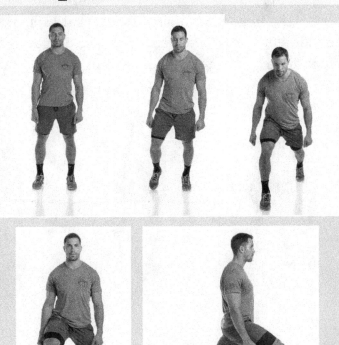

"Start with your feet shoulder-width. Step your dominant foot straight foot forward and your subordinate foot straight back. The knee of your leading foot should be lined up over the ankle. The knee of your trailing leg should be 'soft'—a quarter bent—with the ball of the foot on the floor, the heel raised and kicked out.

"This internal rotation of the rear leg is very important to maintaining hip stability. To understand this, rotate the heel back toward the body's centerline and observe how the hip twists. Then move the heel back out to 'square' the hip."

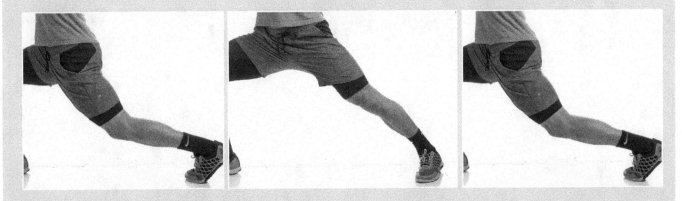

"This is your basic split position. One note about split position: once you understand it, begin practicing it on both sides, simply to avoid imbalances and to improve your coordination.

"Okay. Now stand with your feet under your hips, midline braced, shoulders back, etc. Put your hands on your hips. On my command 'Go!', dip down (as in **PP 2**), jump (as in **PJ 3**), and then land in your dominant-foot forward split position...an action that rather resembles a dance step choreographed by Michael Flatley, of 'Riverdance' fame. Important note! The rear foot hits a split second before the front. Think 'Step through!' Ready? DANCE!

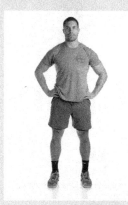 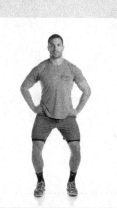 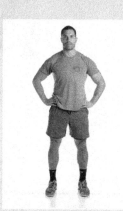 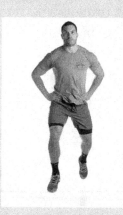 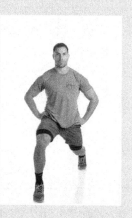

RIVERDANCE! drill

"Once you can confidently jump into split position, now try jumping to split position while punching your hands overhead, a la Mary Katherine Gallagher in the movie 'Superstah!' Ready? SUPAHSTAH!

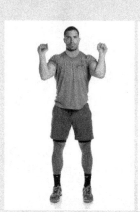 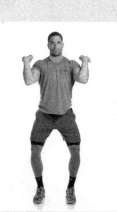 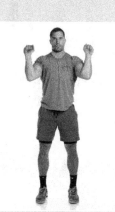 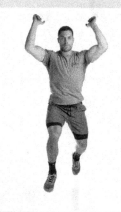 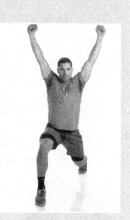

SUPAHSTAH! drill

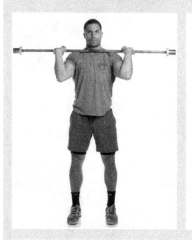 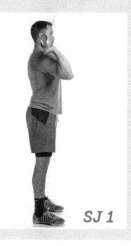

SJ 1

"Once 'Superstah!' has been mastered, pick up a light barbell and set up as you would for a push jerk: feet under the hips, midline braced, bar on the upraised shoulders, elbows elevated. This is **Split Jerk Position 1 (SJ 1)**."

"With your weight in your heels, flare your knees out to sit 2-4". Keep the torso vertical and the elbows high. **This is Split Jerk Position 2 (SJ 2).**

"**Return to SJ 1.** In execution, the transition from SJ 2 back to SJ 1 is extremely aggressive. Pushing from the heels, drive your shoulders into the bar to launch it into the air.

"**Split Jerk Position 3 (SJ 3)** is similar to Push Jerk Position 3: head pulled back, bar rising up past the face. But the feet are moving rapidly from under the hips to their positions in the split. For a split second, you and the bar are in free fall at the same time. Working off the inertia of the bar, shove yourself straight down toward the floor.

"Rear foot hits first as you step into your dominant-foot forward split position and press yourself down under the barbell to lock it out overhead. Feet should be shoulder width, front foot flat, toes forward, knee lined up over the ankle. Rear leg should be up on the ball of the foot, heel kicked out, knee soft. Weight should be distributed roughly 60/40 front-to-back. This is **Split Jerk Position 4 (SJ 4).**

"Let me be specific: even though you are 'stepping through', you are *not* stepping forward! Your COG should not translate forward at all. Go straight down under the bar.

"To recover, step your front foot back to the middle. This is **Split Jerk Position 5 (SJ 5).**

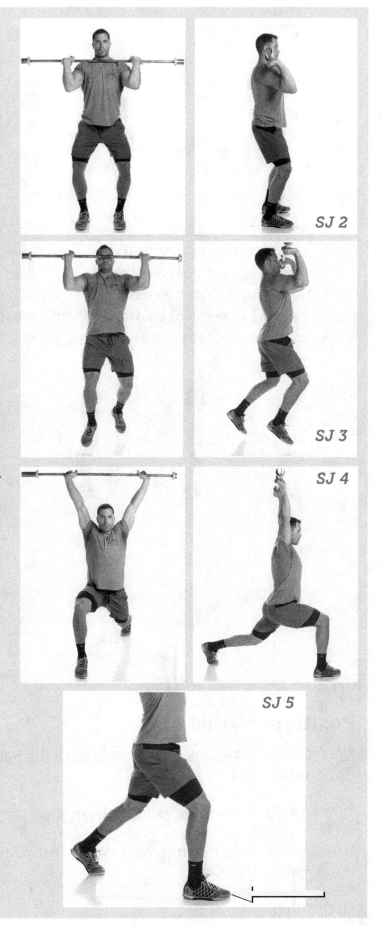

SJ 2

SJ 3

SJ 4

SJ 5

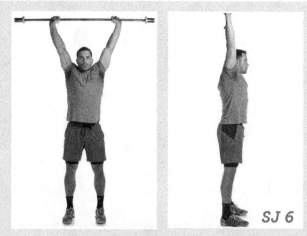

SJ 6

"Step your rear foot forward to line up with the front. This is **Split Jerk Position 6 (SJ 6),** the conclusion of the lift. Make sure you hit **SJ 5,** *then* **SJ 6**. When recovering with a load overhead, stepping with the rear foot first will tend to put a forward impetus on the bar that could cause a missed lift.

"To execute the split jerk, simply perform the 'SUPAHSTAH!' drill with the barbell in your hands. Make sure your elbows are nice and high at the start. Keep your torso vertical and your weight in your heels as you dip. Pushing from the heels, fully extend your hip as you drive your shoulders into the bar. As the bar rises, shove yourself beneath it. Send your feet forward and back. Rear foor lands first. Catch the bar with arms locked straight. Pause to self-assess your position, then recover by stepping your front foot back and your rear foot forward."

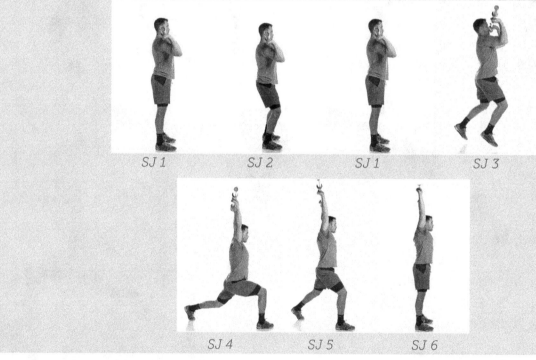

SJ 1   SJ 2   SJ 1   SJ 3

SJ 4   SJ 5   SJ 6

Positional Drills

"1! 2! 1! 3! 4! 5! 6!" Practice the positions of the Split Jerk one at a time, making corrections as necessary.

"1! 2! 1! 3! Go!" Take trainees to **PJ 3**. On "Go!" they explode downwards under the bar.

"1! 2! Go!" Practice moving from set-up to dip. If dip position (**SJ 2**) looks good, have them split jerk under the bar.

"1! Go!" Split jerk.

Split Jerk Common Faults and Fixes

1. Not getting low enough.

Split Jerk Position 4 violation. The split jerk is for getting under the bar, not pushing it up. The heavier the load, the lower you have to go. It takes commitment to shove oneself down under the bar—rear and front foot must travel further in demonstration of that commitment.

 "Get lower!" or "Step longer!" or "Commit!"

 Demonstrate a correct SJ 4.

 While athlete holds in SJ 4 adjust his position—push his rear foot back and front foot forward, then push down on his shoulder until his front knee lines up over his front ankle.

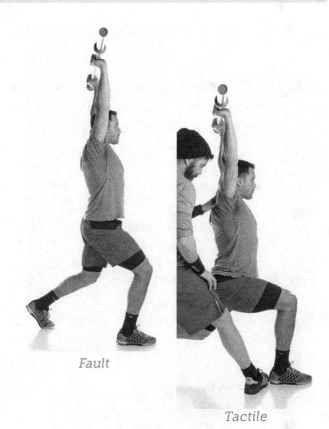

Fault

Tactile

2. Soft elbows/ press to lockout

Split Jerk Position 4 violation. Athlete receives the bar with bent elbows and must press to lock out. Remind him he must receive bar with arms locked out straight. Remind the athlete he must work off the inertia of the bar to push himself toward the floor.

 "Punch under!" or "Arms straight!"

 Demonstrate a correct PJ 4.

 While athlete holds in PJ 4 adjust his position.

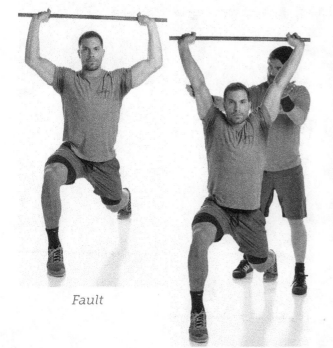

Fault

Tactile

Split Jerk Common Faults and Fixes, cont.

3. Knee jammed forward over foot.

Split Jerk Position 4 violation. Front knee should line up over the ankle. Can be caused by athlete taking a short step. Can also be caused by the athlete driving forward rather than pushing himself straight down toward floor.

 "Step through!" or "Longer step!" or "Straight down!" as appropriate.

 Demonstrate a correct SJ 4.

 While athlete holds in SJ 4 adjust his position.

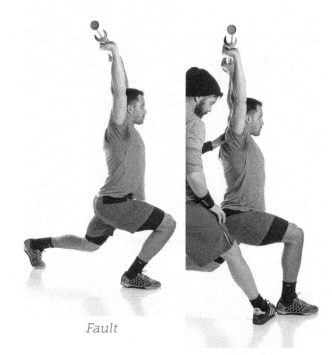

Fault

Tactile

4. Rear heel turned in.

Split Jerk Position 4 violation. Rear foot must be up on ball of the foot with heel kicked out.

 "Rear heel kick out!"

 Demonstrate a correct SJ 4.

 While athlete holds in SJ 4 adjust his position.

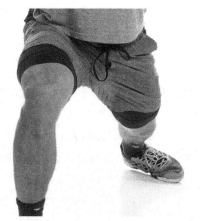

Fault

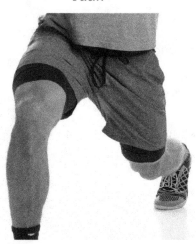

Correct SJ 4

Split Jerk Common Faults and Fixes, cont.

5. Tight tope walking.

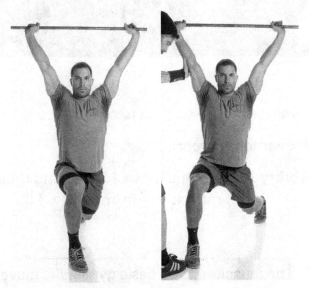

Fault   *Tactile*

Split Jerk Position 4 violation. Front foot moves toward centerline in split position. For maximum lateral stability, the feet in split position should be approximately shoulder-width.

 "Step out!"

 Demonstrate a correct SJ 4.

While athlete holds in SJ 4 adjust his position.

Using chalk on the rubber mat, draw desired finish position for feet. (Don't draw on wooden platforms with chalk—it's a possible safety hazard, as the chalk will make the polished wood slippery.)

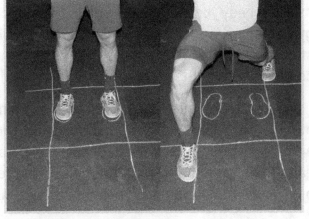

Orthosis

6. Rear knee hits floor.

Split Jerk Position 4 violation. There's such a thing as *too* low. Athlete slams rear knee into floor. Bar must be caught in in a tense half-lunge.

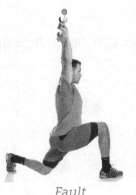

Fault

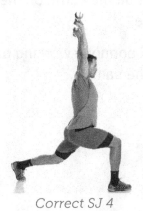

Correct SJ 4

 "Step through and hold!"

 Demonstrate a correct SJ 4.

While athlete holds in SJ 4 adjust his position.

THE MUSCLE-UP

Category: Hybrid (pull to object [strict, vertical], push away from object [vertical])

Movement screen: N/a

Ability screen: Pull-ups x 10 and ring dips x 10 and false-grip ring row x 10 (muscle-up from floor), muscle-up from floor x 3 (band-assisted muscle-up), skinniest band-assisted

The muscle-up is a basic gymnastic movement that takes an athlete from hanging beneath a pair of suspended rings to holding herself in full support atop them.

When I say "basic", I mean basic: the muscle-up is considered a move so elementary in the gymnastics world it's not even given a difficulty rating. It's just what you do to get into position to start your ring routine...which makes it somewhat ironic that so many in the MMGPP community consider getting their first muscle-up a rite of passage that can't come soon enough.

In their impatience, people will try every gimmicky progression that promises to make their muscle-up dreams come true. But in truth, there's only one way to get a muscle-up: be strong enough to muscle-up. It makes me wince to see people swinging their bodies wildly to build up enough momentum to carry them through the transition, only to then kick and squirm up to lock-out. That's not a progression, that's corner-cutting, a workaround—not the stuff of virtuosity.

The following muscle-up instruction assumes the trainee can meet minimum strength standards: 10 strict pull-ups and 10 strict ring dips. There is no point in training the muscle-up with athletes who do not (yet) meet those standards. Don't use valuable class time trying to teach this progression to those have no realistic hope of implementing it, just because "...they're doing MMGPP training, they should be working on their muscle-up". For those developing athletes, pull-ups and dips will continue to provide all the stimulus they need. And that's fine. You don't need a muscle-up to be a MMGPP athlete.

Today is Harry's day to shine. Amy will continue working on her strict pull-ups (she's up to five!) and her bar dips. Tim will work on the same.

Muscle-up Basics

"To muscle-up, one must be able to maintain a strong false grip.

"This is how to set the false grip. Grasp the rings as you normally would, with the proximal phalanges of your fingers parallel to the ceiling. Now rotate your hand into the rings until the back of your hand faces the ceiling. The ring should sit diagonally across the palm, passing over the outside heel on the hand.

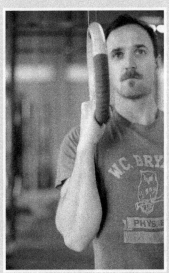

Neutral grip

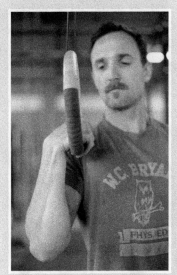

False grip

"Once you've got a feel for the false grip, try some false grip ring rows. You may find that by concentrating on squeezing your pinkies you're better able to maintain the grip.

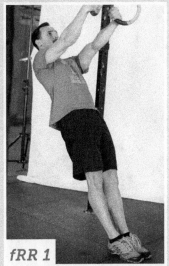

fRR 1

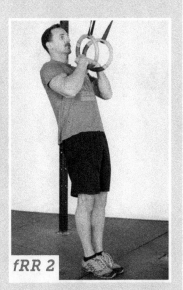

fRR 2

"Now we'll mime the muscle-up to learn its three phases: pull, transition, and dip.

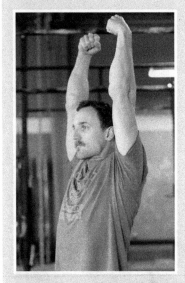

"Stand tall with your feet together, midline braced. Press your hands over your head, and then flex your wrists into false grip. Rotate your thumbs back slightly.

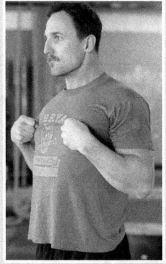

"Phase one: Drive your elbows down to draw your fists to your chest.

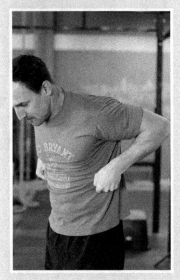

"Phase two: Elbows go around and back, head comes through. The knuckles of the thumbs should trace lines from clavicles to armpits. Think of Hulk Hogan tearing off his t-shirt. Or headbutting a soccer ball.

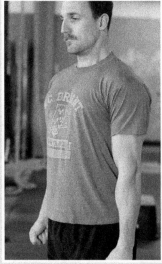

"Phase three. Press up to lock out.

"Next we're going to practice muscling up from the floor, using our legs for assistance.

"Kneel down. Press your fists, curled in as with the false grip, above your head until your bent elbows are at the height of your nose. Set your rings level with your fists.

"Return to kneeling. Get your false grip on the rings. This is **Muscle-up from the Floor Position 1 (fMU 1).**

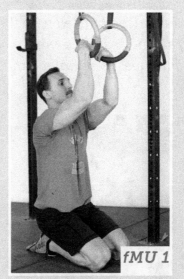

fMU 1

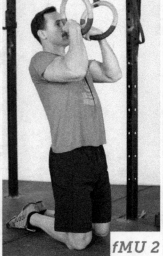

fMU 2

"Keeping the rings close together, pull toward your chest. This is **Muscle-up from the Floor Position 2 (fMU 2).**

"As the rings make contact with your chest, aggressively sit-up and drive your head forward as you pull the rings around your body. Push from your toes if you need assistance. Keep the rings close. You should wind up in a deep dip position. **Muscle-up from the Floor Position 3 (fMU 3).**

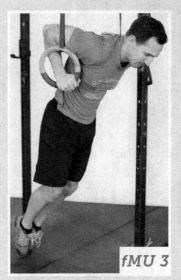

fMU 3

"Press to support. This is **Muscle-up from the Floor Position 4 (fMU 4)."**

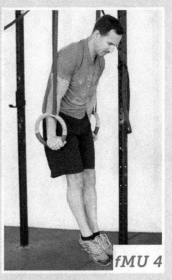

fMU 4

Once an athlete has familiarized himself with the basic mechanics of the muscle-up while safely on the floor, using a band assist is a great way for him to groove good movement patterns. Gradually weaning trainees to skinnier bands helps them build the strength necessary to muscle-up.

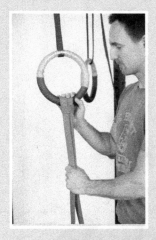 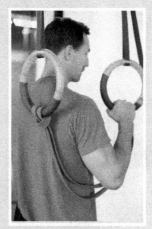

"Loop the band around one ring and hold the other, free end in place with your hand. If you need anything wider than a 1" band, you're not ready for this.

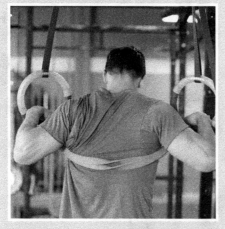

"String the band behind you.

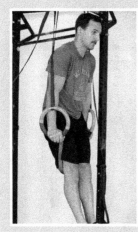 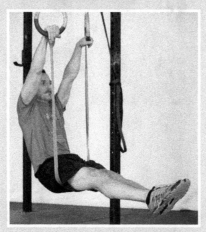

"Hop up to sit in the band like a sling.

"Legs should be held out straight. Feet should be off the floor. Don't surrender your false grip!

"Practice the three phases of the muscle-up: pull, transition, and dip. At first you'll want to pull hard and fast to generate some momentum to help you through the transition. As you get stronger, slow down the pull-and-transition phase to three full seconds ('One Mississippi, two Mississippi', etc.) and work on muscling through the transition."

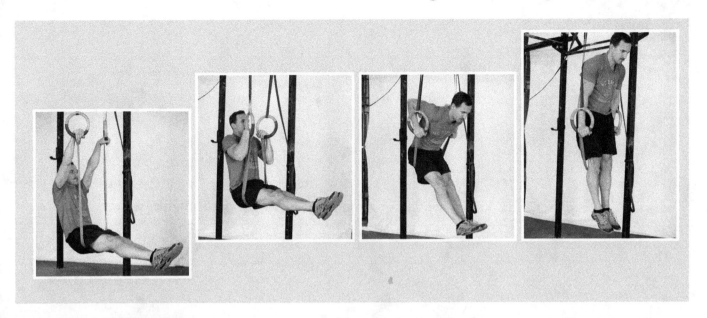

Positional Drills

"1! 2! 1! 3! 4!" Practice the positions of the band-assisted muscle-up one at a time, making corrections as necessary. Without momentum, the transition from **MU 2** to **MU 3** will be difficult, but the struggle will be more than worth it when moving to the full movement.

L-hang Muscle-up Teaching Script

"Once you've worked your way up to a slow transition on the 1/4" band, you may find that a strict L-hang muscle-up comes easily. When in an L-hang, the extended legs act as a counterweight, and will actually help tip you through the transition from pull to dip.

"Set your false grip on the rings, and then hit an L-hang: hips piked, legs held out straight in front of you, feet together, toes pointed. This **L-hang Muscle-up Position 1 (lMU 1).**

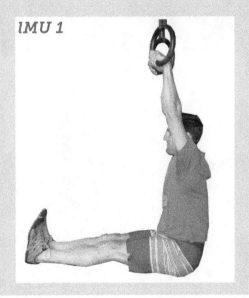

lMU 1

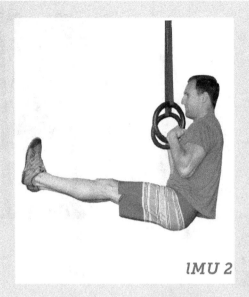

lMU 2

"Maintaining a strong L position, pull the rings to your chest. This is **L-hang Muscle-up Position 2 (lMU 2).**

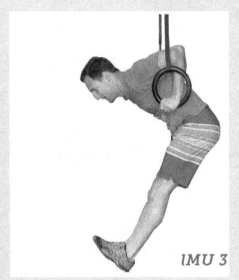

lMU 3

"As you press down on the rings and swing your elbows back, allow the weight of your legs to tip you forward through the transition. You should end up in the bottom of a ring dip. This is **L-hang Muscle-up Position 3 (lMU 3).**

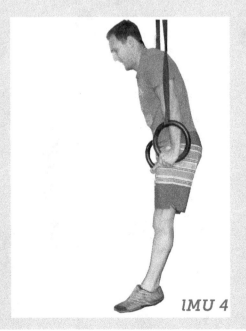

lMU 4

"Dip up to locked-out support. If you can hold a legitimate ring L-sit in this position, great! If not, allow your legs to drop so you end up in a well-organized Ring Dip Position 1. Either way, now you're in **L-hang Muscle-up Position 4 (lMU 5).**

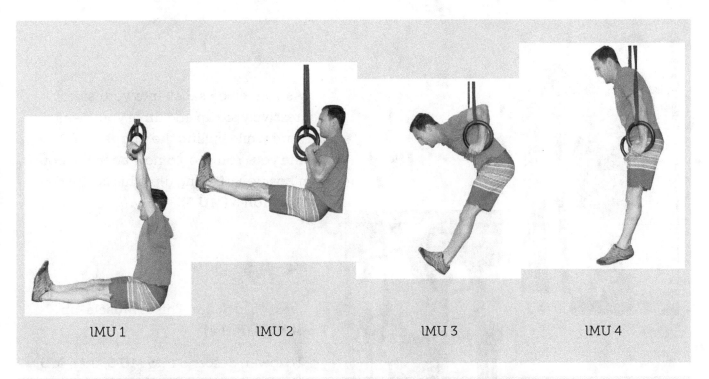

lMU 1   lMU 2   lMU 3   lMU 4

Muscle-up Teaching Script, cont.

"When you can do an L-hang muscle-up, you're ready for the real thing.

"Hang straight-armed from the rings with active shoulders. Body hollow, feet together, toes pointed. Take your false grip. This is **Muscle-up Position 1 (MU 1)**.

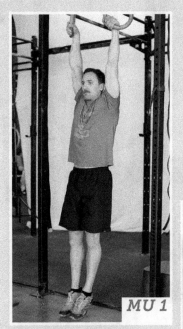

MU 1

"Keeping the rings close, pull them to your ribs. This is **Muscle-up Position 2 (MU 2)**.

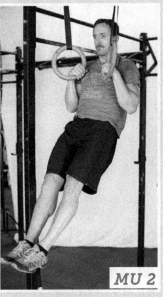

MU 2

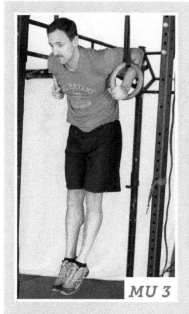

MU 3

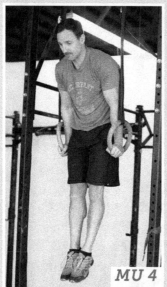

MU 4

"As your elbows tuck into your sides, aggressively sit-up and drive your head forward while pulling the rings around beside you. You should now be in the bottom position of a ring dip. This is **Muscle-up Position 3 (MU 3).**

"Press to lock out. This is **Muscle-up Position 4 (MU 4).**

"To lower, descend into **MU 3**, then **MU 2**, and reset in **MU 1.**"

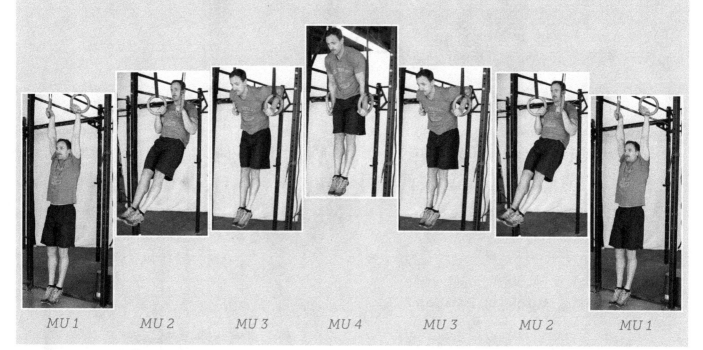

MU 1   MU 2   MU 3   MU 4   MU 3   MU 2   MU 1

Positional Drills

"1! 2! 3! 4! 3! 2! 1!" Practice the positions of the muscle-up one at a time, making corrections as necessary.

Muscle-up Common Faults and Fixes

Faults and fixes common to the pull-up apply, including midline breaks and failure to come to full extension in bottom position, as well as...

All faults and fixes common to the dip and ring dip, as well as...

1. No false grip.

Muscle-up Position 1 violation. Athlete hangs with a neutral grip. An athlete attempting a strict muscle-up without a false grip will not be able to get on top of the rings. The false grip is critical to the execuion of the muscle-up.

 "Roll your wrists through!"

 Demonstrate a correct false grip.

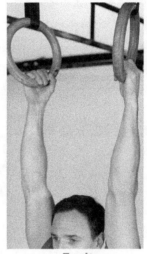

Fault

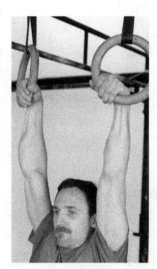

Correct MU 1

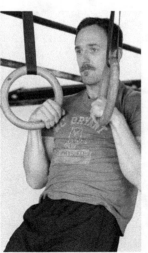

Fault

2. Pull isn't low enough.

Muscle-up Position 2 violation. If the trainee doesn't pull himself extra high, he won't have the clearance necessary for the transition phase. Athlete must pull rings to his chest.

 "Pull to your ribs!"

 Demonstrate a correct MU 2.

Correct MU 2

Muscle-up Common Faults and Fixes, cont.

3. Rings come away from body during transition.

Muscle-up Position 3 violation. Athlete cannot complete transition because he is attempting a half-assed iron cross. Rings must be kept close to the body, with knuckles of the thumbs tracing lines from the clavicles to armpits as the elbows move behind and above the torso.

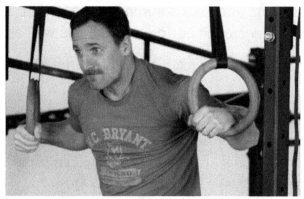

Fault

 "Keep the rings close!" or "Tear off your t-shirt!" or "Around and back!"

Demonstrate a correct transition from MU 2 to MU 3.

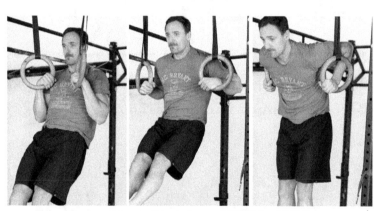

Correct transition from MU 2 to MU 3

4. No head through.

Muscle-up Position 3 violation. Athlete fails to complete the transition because he does not aggressively push his head "through the window" to get his shoulders in front of the rings.

 "Head butt!" or "Sit up!"

 Demonstrate a correct transition from MU 2 to MU 3.

Fault

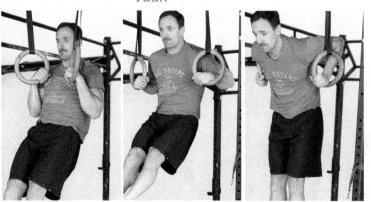

Correct transition from MU 2 to MU 3

Category: Hip and Trunk Extension

Movement screen: N/a

Ability screen: Back extension x 5

The hip-and-back extension is a back extension with the hips moving independently of the pad.

Hip/Back Extension Teaching Script

"Climb up onto the GHD bench.

"Facing the floor, fit your lower legs legs between the foot anchor pads and press your feet against the back plate.

"The foot anchor assembly of the GHD bench should be set at a length that puts your thighs atop the pad and your hips out in front as you set up with your body prone and parallel to the floor. Your mid-line should be strongly braced. Hands can be held at temples, crossed at the chest, or held behond your head. This is **Hip/Back Extension Position 4 (HB 4).**

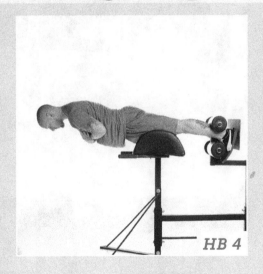

HB 4

"Now pike your hips so the top of your head is pointing at the floor. This is **Hip/Back Extension Position 1 (HB 1).**

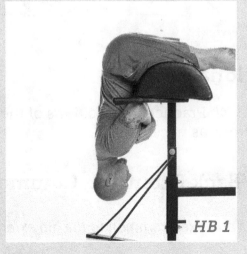

HB 1

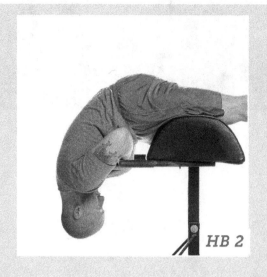

HB 2

"Begin by squeezing your glutes hard until your pelvis is parallel to the floor. parallel to the floor. We'll call this **Hip/Back Extension Position 2 (HB 2).**

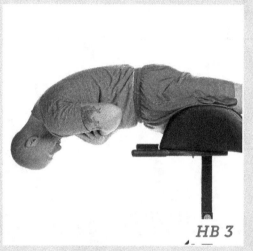

HB 3

"Vertebra by vertebra, lift your spine. Halfway up, your lower spine will have returned to neutral, but your upper spine is still in flexion. This **Hip/Back Extension Position 3 (HB 3).**

"Finally, lift your chest to extend the thoracic spine. This brings you back to **HB 4.**"

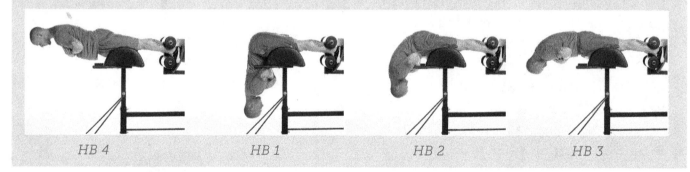

HB 4   HB 1   HB 2   HB 3

Positional Drills

"1! 2! 1! 3! 4!" Practice the positions of the hip/back extension one at a time, making corrections as necessary.

Hip/Back Extension Common Faults and Fixes

Faults and fixes common to the hip extension and back extension apply.

Our week seven WOD is a perennial favorite among our athletes. In my gym, we've always preferred to call it

"Charles Bronson"

For time:
49 Box jumps 24/20"
49 Jumping pull-ups
49 Kettlebell swings 35/25lbs
49 Walking lunges
49 Knees-to-elbows
49 Push press 45/33lbs
49 Hip extensions
49 Wallballs 20/14lbs
49 Burpees
49 Double-unders

Unlike most of our earlier benchmarks, in which movements were repeated in rounds, "Charles Bronson" is a chipper. That means all reps of a given exercise have to be completed before you can move on to the next exercise. As your stamina starts to flag, you've no choice but to continue to "chip away" until the assigned work is done.

Prescribing the Correct Level of Movement Complexity

The movements of "Charles Bronson" are not very technical, but I do make one modification from the original: the back extensions are now hip extensions. Back extensions should be slow and controlled, which defeats the purpose of this WOD. Also, because at my gym we have a limited number of GHD benches, I reserve the hip extension for the most experienced athletes. More junior athletes perform good mornings with an empty barbell.

Harry and Amy will be going "as Rx'd." Tim will use a 12" box, a 25lbs kettlebell swung Russian-style, supine knee draws, dumbbells for the strict presses, PVC pipe for the good mornings, and a 10lbs medicine ball.

Establishing Correct Volume

Chippers can be a lot of fun, but it's easy to over do it. "Charles Bronson" is 490 reps! (Ten exercises, 49 reps of each.) For many of your athletes, that is not a desirable training stimulus. It's a workout that can easily take 40 minutes, or longer, and by the end an athlete can be so depleted that he has little hope of using good exercise form. On the other hand, athletes of all levels do seem to take a certain satisfaction in persevering through such an epic beatdown. So how do we balance our desire to "entertrain" our athletes, while keeping them safe, *and* administering a dose of exercise stimulus that will increase their fitness?

Accomplished MMGPP athletes can complete "Charles Bronson" in less than 20 minutes, an achievement roughly the equivalent of a sub-three minute "Kukla". Using the time limitation technique we've used on other WODs, we could structure "Charles Bronson" as a 20 minute workout for our average athletes, or 25.* Time and experimentation have led me to make this workout thirty minutes long. This seems to preserve the "beat down" factor MMGPP athletes masochistically enjoy, while ensuring everyone does a volume of exercise appropriate for them.

"By The Numbers Testing Charles Bronson"

AMRAP 3 Box jumps 24/20". If you get to 49 before time is up, move on to...
AMRAP 3 Jumping pull-ups. If you get to 49 before time is up, move on to...
AMRAP 3 Kettlebell swings 35/25lbs. If you get to 49 before time is up, move on to...
AMRAP 3 Walking lunges. If you get to 49 before time is up, move on to...
AMRAP 3 Knees-to-elbows. If you get to 49 before time is up, move on to...
AMRAP 3 Push press 45/33lbs. If you get to 49 before time is up, move on to...
AMRAP 3 Hip extensions. If you get to 49 before time is up, move on to...
AMRAP 3 Wallballs 20/14lbs. If you get to 49 before time is up, move on to...
AMRAP 3 Burpees. If you get to 49 before time is up, move on to...
AMRAP 3 Double-unders. If you get to 49 before time is up, you're done!

Most people make it through the box jumps, jumping pull-ups, kettlebell swings, and walking lunges without a problem. Things slow down quite a bit with the knees-to-elbows, then pick up again with the push press and good mornings. At this point they are getting pretty tired, so the wallballs and burpees are like a brick wall. If they get through them, great. If not, no big deal, and honestly, do you want your athletes gutting out 49 sloppy burpees in an exhausted state? Not if you value their joint health, you don't. The final 49 double-unders are an opportunity to go out on a high note, if your athlete has double-unders, and if not, well, at least it's only 3 more minutes of misery.

---

* Use 2 minute intervals for a 20 minute version, and 2:30 for 25 minutes.

This is all well and good for Harry and Amy. Tim, though, seems a bit intimidated by having to perform 10 different exercises in one workout. I tell him to ignore the clock entirely and performs 3 sets of ten reps of each exercise from the box jumps to the wallballs. But Tim says he can handle it—he wants to do 30 reps of each exercise, all the way through. Hmm, dilemma! I agree, with the proviso he does box burpees. He can handle the push-ups; it's the stepping into the full squat part that worries me. Further, I tell him that if the wheels start to come off at any point, I'm going to pull him out. He nods, and we're both satisfied.

Setting Up for "Charles Bronson"

When setting up for your gym to run "Charles Bronson", it's unlikely you'll have enough equipment (or space) for each athlete in your group to have his or her own exclusive set of exercise stations. The best strategy is to set up a series of "courses": one (or more, depending on how many athletes you have to provide for) for male athletes going "as rx'd", one or more for females rx'd, one or more for male scaled (same as female rx'd), and etc. Our athletes write down all ten exercises in order on a 3 x 5 card which they are required to carry with them through the workout. All too often people dazed by the intensity of their effort will wander to the wrong station, messing things up for everyone else.

How you set up, and the route your athletes take from start to finish, depends entirely on how your gym floor is organized.

Have your athletes line up in ranks behind the boxes for the initial box jumps, with the fittest, most experienced athletes up front. At "3, 2, 1, Go!" these firebreathers will get to work on box jumps. As soon as they finish their 49 reps, the move on to jumping pull-ups. If they haven't finished 49 at 3:00, they move on anyway. The second rank steps up, but does not start until the 3:00 mark, at which point they get to work. If you had a third heat, they'd start at 6:00, etc.

Hopefully nobody in the first group flags. If they do, and the athlete behind them on their track is staying ahead of the clock and catches up, be ready with an extra barbell or medicine ball so there's not a traffic jam. One way or another, everyone in the first group is done by 30:00, everyone in the second group is done by 33:00, every one in the third by 36:00, and etc. Those who have managed to stay in front of the clock the whole time have an "as rx'd" score. Those athletes not completing all the required reps at a given station in the allowed time should write down how many reps they got before moving on. For instance, if they got all the reps on the first four exercises, but only got 39 knees-to-elbows, then got 50 push press and good mornings, but only 43 wallballs, 27 burpees, and 5 double-unders, the next time they're faced with "Charles Bronson", they'll have a clear goal: beat those numbers. By recording these scores with each exposure they'll be able to track their progress.

"3...2...1...GO!"

Harry

Harry has stamina to burn, so I knew that for him a good "Charles Bronson" was going to be largely dependent on his ability to keep the standards of performance for each movement in mind.

He had no problem with the 50 box jumps, but he did tend to forget to fully extend his knees and hips when he landed atop the box. I told him, "STAND UP!" Similarly, with the jumping pull-ups, he didn't always squat down far enough that his elbows completely straightened. My cue was, "STRAIGHT ARMS!" The kettlebell swings went well—he's doing a lot better with that American Swing Position 4—as did the walking lunges. All continued to go swimmingly until he got to the burpees. At roughly 21 minutes in, he had plenty of time. But in his zeal to finish in under 25:00, he reverted back to old ways best forgotten: throwing himself to the floor, peeling up, hopping forward to bend in half with his butt in the air, barely lifting his torso above parallel the ground to clap his hands behind his head before throwing himself down again.

"STRICT PUSH-UPS!" I said. "JUMP FORWARD INTO THE BOTTOM OF A SQUAT." When that failed, I told him, "STEP UP." But he's wasn't listening. I pull him out of Performance Mode and back into Practice Mode.

"Stop," I told him. He mad-dogged me, but did as I said. "Like this." And I demonstrated a burpee with a strict push-up and a step/step spiderman stand-up. "Do it like that, stay organized, and KEEP MOVING." Then I let him get back to work.

Did it slow him down a little? Yes. At the end of the workout, was he any less fit? Come on, do you really think so? "Power" is only one of the ten generally recognized aspects of fitness, along with stamina, endurance, strength, speed, balance, coordination, flexibility, agility, and accuracy. We're in this for the long haul, and I have to encourage my athletes to think that way too, even when they're young firebreathers like Harry. Working from well-organized position to well-organized position is ALWAYS going to be safer, and therefore more conducive to progress, in the long run.

Amy

Amy is more conscientious than Harry; she's very concerned with doing things right. So her box jumps, jumping pull-ups, kettlebell swings, and walking lunges all looked great.

The knees-to-elbows were a problem for her, though. "TO ELBOWS," I reminded her, because she was mostly doing knees-to-armpits. She struggled, but her performance didn't seem to improve. I took her into Practice Mode. Standing on her box, she paused to listen as I told her, "Press down on the bar. Try to lift your chest—your hips will rise and you knees will find the right place." Because that didn't work, either, I had her default back through the movement hierarchy to the Hanging Knee Raise. Those she was able to do without a problem.

Remember, during Performance, the goal, besides demonstrating movement skill, is to *keep moving*. Constant motion, even at a lighter load or reduced level of complexity, will increase power output more than single reps and long moments of static recovery.

The push presses went reasonably well for her, as did the hip extensions. But by the time she was halfway through the 3 minutes allotted to wallballs she was visibly exhausted, propping herself up against the wall with the medicine ball. When it was time for burpees, I had her do burpees with her push-ups on a 20" box. She only managed 28 in 3 minutes. But then she hammered 49 double-unders in a row! Talk about a comeback! When she threw down her rope, there were still almost 90 seconds left on the clock. She was so excited about her double-under streak that the beatings she took on the wallballs and burpees were already forgotten. She wanted to know, "When are we doing this again?!"

Tim

Honestly, Tim shocked me with his performance. He only jumped to a 12" box, but he got all 30 reps, and only 2 minutes into the workout he was already on to jumping pull-ups. Again, he got 30 reps with time to spare, and then moved on. He slowed down a bit with the walking lunges. For the knees-to-elbows, he did supine knee draws. For push press, he did dumbbell presses with 15lbs dumbbells. Good mornings were performed with PVC pipe. When he got to wallballs he finally got into trouble. Tim's air squats are his weakest movement, and trying to throw the ball at the target undid all the progress he's made the last six weeks. Without even trying to cue corrections, I had him default back to medicine ball front squats, which he did as five sets of five, resting for 15 seconds or so in between sets.

When he'd completed that work, he looked done in. Caught up in the spirit of the thing, he wanted to keep going, but honestly, between the box jumps, the walking lunges, and the medball front squats, he had done enough lower body work for one day. So I compromised one more time and gave him 30 push-ups to finish up with. Push-ups are in Tim's wheelhouse, and he got to work with relish. He called time at just under 27 minutes, a happy camper.

Category: Pull Object (ground to shoulder)

Movement screen: N/a

Ability screen: Clean x 5, dumbbell clean x 5

Weightlifters work to improve their technique by breaking down the clean and the snatch into their constituent components for concentrated practice. MMGPP programs use these partial movements, sometimes for the traditional purpose of honing strength, speed, and precision in various phases of the lifts, and sometimes as part of metabolic conditioning workouts. Learning these variants is easy in the By the Numbers system. Having mastered the eight positions of both the clean and the snatch, one need merely change their order to create a slew of new exercises.

Although there is some variation among weightlifting coaches as to nomenclature, here's the naming convention we use in BtN:

1. Any lift received with the knees and hips straight is a "muscle" version of the lift. For instance, "muscle snatch."

2. Any lift caught with the hips above parallel is a "power" variant of that lift. For instance, "power clean".

3. Lifts received in a full squat are simply called the name of the lift (i.e. "hang clean". This might seem obvious, but sometimes you might hear someone refer to a "hang squat clean". Same thing).

4. A lift initiated from reset position (i.e., standing with knees and hips fully extended) is a "tall" variation, e.g., "Tall muscle snatch."

5. Any lift initiated from Position 4 (known to some as "pockets") is a "high hang" variant, e.g., "high hang power snatch", or "power snatch from the high hang."

6. Lifts initiated from Position 3 ("extend" in BtN) are "hang" versions, e.g., "hang snatch."

7. Lifts that start in Position 2 are "low hang", as in, "clean from the low hang," or "low-hang snatch."

Just to make things extra confusing, you'll often find that weightlifters will use the upper positions to help set them up to execute a hang variation. For instance, an athlete may deadlift the bar, reset, sit down into Clean Position 4 to set tension, then lower the bar down his leg. As soon as he hits Clean Position 3, he immediately rebounds and executes the lift, catching the bar in a full squat. That rebound is considered the initation of the lift, so he has done a "hang clean", not a "high hang clean." Get it? It's okay, you will.

Here are a few clean variants (barbell and dumbbell) you may find in MMGPP programming.

Clean Variants

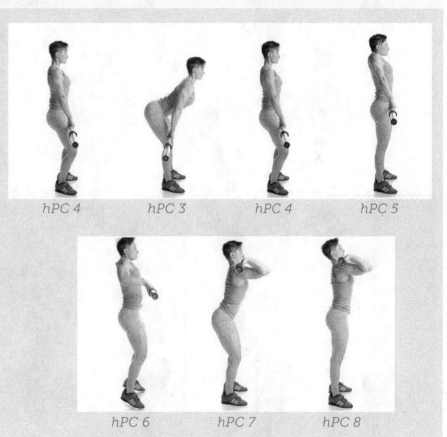

hPC 4   hPC 3   hPC 4   hPC 5

hPC 6   hPC 7   hPC 8

"Hang Power Clean. The positions of the hang power clean are identical to those of the power clean.

"Start by seting up in **Hang Power Clean Position Four (PC 4)**, setting your back and getting your weight back on your heels. Drop into **hPC 3,** and then aggressively re-bound. Pull under to receive the barbell in a partial front squat.

"In the clean, the hook grip is surrendered as the bar is received. Usually you'd reset your grip with the bar on the ground, but for multi-rep sets of a hang clean, you need to regrip without putting down the bar. To reset the hook grip between reps, lower the bar, then hinge back to tuck the bar into the crook of your hip. With the bar supported by your legs, you are free to reset your hook grip.

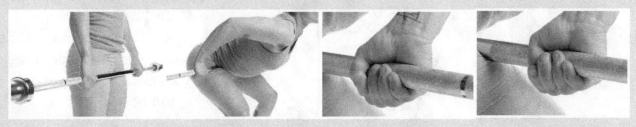

Reset, hinge to tuck bar into the crook of your hip, then switch from standard to hook grip.

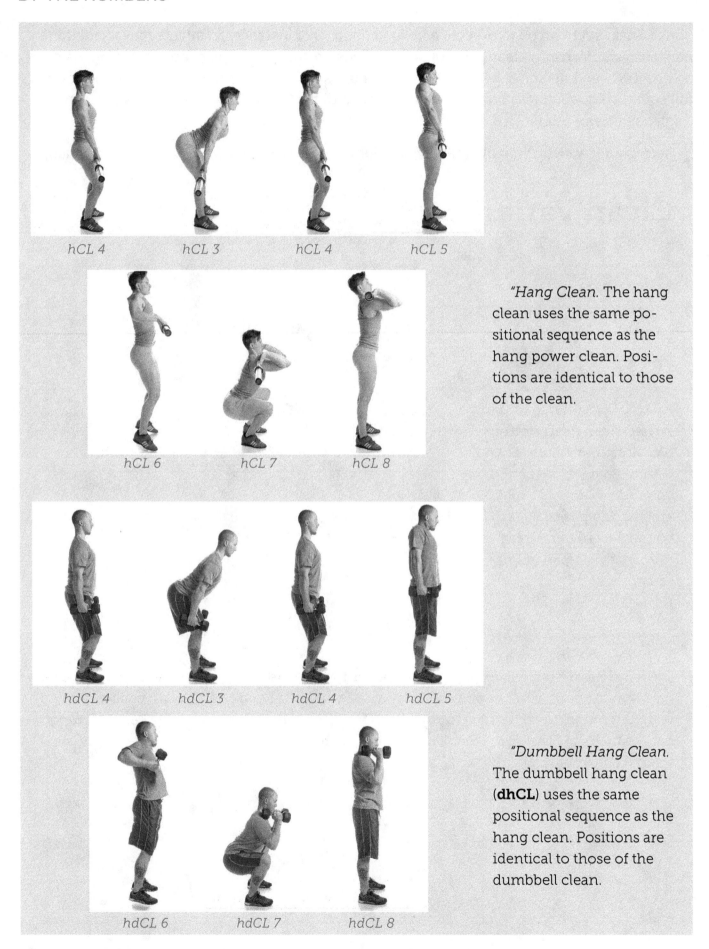

hCL 4   hCL 3   hCL 4   hCL 5

hCL 6   hCL 7   hCL 8

"Hang Clean. The hang clean uses the same positional sequence as the hang power clean. Positions are identical to those of the clean.

hdCL 4   hdCL 3   hdCL 4   hdCL 5

hdCL 6   hdCL 7   hdCL 8

"Dumbbell Hang Clean. The dumbbell hang clean (**dhCL**) uses the same positional sequence as the hang clean. Positions are identical to those of the dumbbell clean.

"Dumbbell Split Clean. The first six positions of the **dSC** are the same as the dumbbell clean, but the receiving position "rhymes" with Split Jerk Position 4. The lift is recovered by stepping the front foot back, then the rear foot forward."

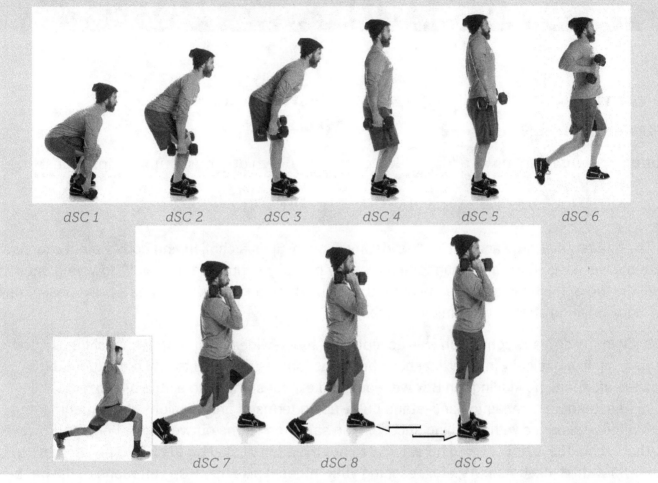

dSC 1   dSC 2   dSC 3   dSC 4   dSC 5   dSC 6

dSC 7   dSC 8   dSC 9

Hang Clean Variants Common Faults and Fixes, cont.

1. Knees come forward in hang.

Hang Power Clean Position 3 violation. Athlete shoves knees forward as she moves into hPC 3 from hPC 4. When an athlete is performing a correct hang power clean or hang clean, at the initiation of the lift, the shins should be vertical.

 "Knees back!" or "Shins vertical!"

 Demonstrate a correct CL 3.

 As the athete sets up for the hang power clean, block her knee with the back of your hand.

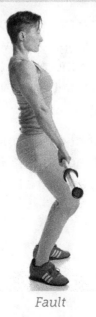

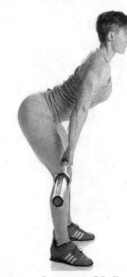

Fault   Correct CL 3

THE HANDSTAND PUSH-UP

Category: Push Away from Object (vertical, inverted, dynamic)

Movement screen: N/a

Ability screen: Push-up x 10 (down dog push-up), down dog push-up x 10 (pike push-up

The handstand (more accurately, "headstand") push-up is a challenging body weight exercise that involves kicking up into a handstand (usually partially supported by a wall), lowering oneself until the top of the head touches the ground, then pushing back up. It requires a great deal of upper body pushing strength and midline stability.

Back in the day, any contortion was acceptable (super-wide placement of hands, feet spread-eagled, midline basically in a vertical back bend), as long as the nose touched the ground (that was the standard, no kidding). In BtN we teach and expect something a little bit closer to the ideal freestanding gymnastic hand-stand push-up. In terms of progressions, I've experimented with band assistance with middling success; the safety concerns outweigh the benefits, however, so that technique is not covered here. I'm also not a big fan of scaling the HSPU by shortening the ROM with stacked Abmats, etc. Teaching your athletes pike push-up variations of the handstand push-up is safer, more practical, and provides as greater training effect, as they'll be working through a full range of motion.

HSPUs can be problematic as conditioning work because fatigue tends to cause form to break down, and when an athlete is upside down, that's potentially very dangerous. So it's important you give all of your athletes a thorough grounding in the HSPU movement hierarchy. That way, no matter how tired they may get, there will always be a HSPU option that will allow them to complete the workout safely.

If a trainee can't do 10 strict push-ups, he should not start on this progression. Have him perform dumbbell presses instead. Today, Harry, Amy, and Tim will all start with the Down Dog Pike Push-up, and then move on as their strength allows.

Handstand Push-up Teaching Script

"The handstand push-up is the calisthenic version of the barbell press.

"Set up with feet together. Brace your midline by squeezing your glutes and locking your abs down. Push both hands overhead as if pressing a barbell. A portion of your ears should be visible in front of your arms. This is a good approximation of the finish position of the press. With your hands in the frontal plane, from a bird's eye view, a shallow triangle can be drawn between the hands and the top of the head.

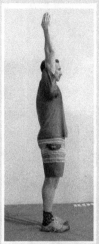
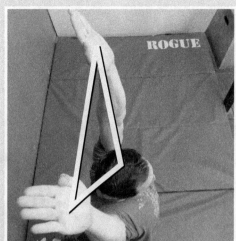

"Now mime bringing down the barbell. Stop when you reach an approximation of Press Position 2. Your hands should be anterior to your face. From above, the triangle between your hands and the top of your head is larger, and reversed.

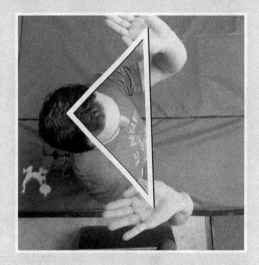

"This approximates the bottom position of the handstand push-up (HP). It's important to point out, because no matter which version of the HP you use, your hands and head should make a similar triangle shape on the ground.

"The extreme challenge of the HP is due to the fact that unlike the traditional push-up, which reduces the load that must be moved by the chest and arms by distributing your weight between your hands and feet, the HP forces you to support your body's entire weight on your hands—not to mention that the angle means you're relying on the triceps and deltoids, rather than triceps and the larger pectoral muscles of the chest, to do the work. So with that in mind, in order to make the HP accessible to more trainees, we need to figure out a way to reduce the load, while keeping the shoulders and arms the primary movers, which is the stimulus that must be preserved.

"We do it by changing the body's angle relative to the floor. Our first progression is the Down Dog Pike Push-up.

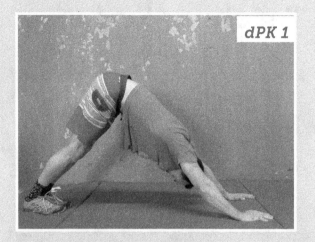

dPK 1

"Start in **Push-up Position 1**: feet to-gether, butt and abs locked tight, shoul-ders back and down, hands planted just outside the shoulders and screwed into the ground. Keeping your legs and arms straight, draw your hips up and back until your head is between your arms. This is **Down Dog Pike Push-up Position 1 (dPK 1)**.

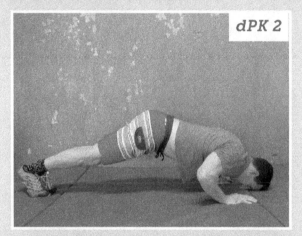

dPK 2

"From here, keeping your head neutral, lower yourself forward and down until your forehead touches the ground in front of your hands. This is is **Down Dog Pike Push-up Position 2 (dPK 2)**.

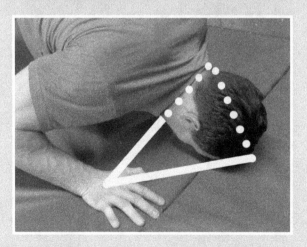

"Notice that Ramey's head and hands are in a tripod formation.

"Push back to **dPK 1**.

"A word of explanation: the action is not *up and down*, it's *forward and back*. The lowering of your head to the ground is a natural consequence of bending your elbows, and its rise in the return is due to the arms straightening. If you think 'up and down', you're going to do an incline push-up, loading the chest, and not the shoulders. Don't do this."

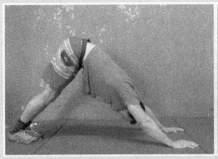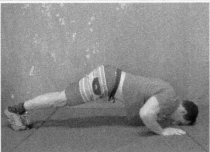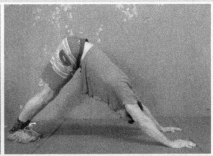

The down dog pike push-up. Trainees who cannot perform this simplified action should do dumbbell presses instead. Don't bother with reducing ROM by stacking Abmats.

"If this is too easy, you can elevate your feet on a box, so that you are supporting more and more of your body's weight on your hands.

"Set a box against the wall. Start modestly, with a 14" box. Later you can use the 20", 24", or 30".

"Get in a push-up position with your feet on the box. Set your feet against the wall. Keeping your knees bent, walk your hands back toward the box until the weight on your shoulders starts to feel challenging. Pushing your heels against the wall, straighten your legs to load your hamstrings. Ideally, your torso is perpendicular to the floor. This is **Pike Push-up from the Box Position 1 (bPK 1)**.

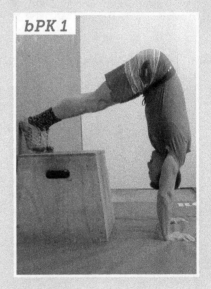

"Screw your hands into the ground as you would for a push-up. Then lower yourself forward so that the crown of your head touches the ground in front of your hands. Make sure your head and hands form a tripod. This is **Pike Push-up from the Box Position 2 (bPK 2)**.

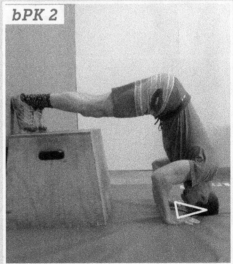

"Push your nose back toward the box to return to **bPK 1**. Again, don't think 'up and down', think 'forward and back.'

"The higher you set your feet, the more load on your shoulders and arms. When you run out of boxes you can keep walking your feet up the wall until you are starting from a nose-to-wall handstand.

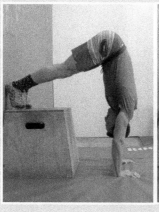 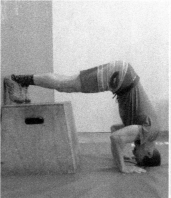 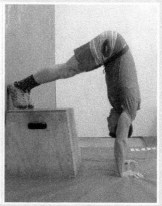

"Traditionally, though, the handstand push-up in CrossFit is executed with one's back to the wall. Generally speaking, this is the more practical approach: it's easier to get into position, and much easier to bail out of if something goes wrong.

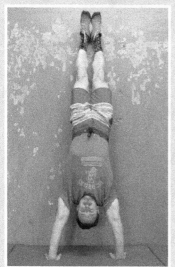 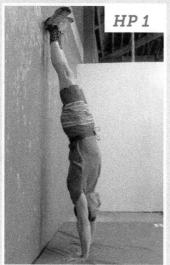

HP 1

"Set your hands just outside shoulder-width. Screw your hands into the ground and kick up to handstand. Your goal is a straight body position: feet stacked over knees over hips over shoulders over hands. To defeat the natural tendency to arch into a backbend, contract your abs to draw your pelvis toward your rib cage. This is **Handstand Push-up Position 1 (HP 1).**

"Continuing to try to screw your hands into the ground, and keeping your chin slightly tucked, lower yourself back and down such that the top of your head touches the ground between your hands and the wall. This is **Handstand Push-up Position 2 (HP 2).**

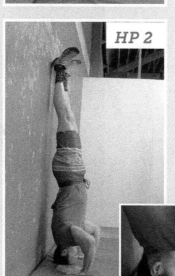

HP 2

"As you descend, imagine that you are winding your lats up tight. Use that tension to help drive you up out of the bottom position. Return to a strong, hollowed-out handstand, **HP 1**."

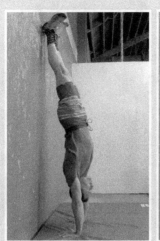
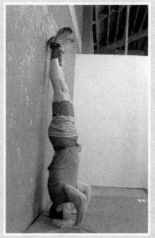
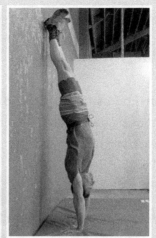

HP 1   *HP 2*   *HP 1*

Positional Drills

"1! 2! 1!" Practice the positions of the handstand push-up one at a time, with your trainees holding the pose while you make necessary corrections. Make sure your athletes maintain a neutral midline.

Handstand Push-up Common Faults and Fixes

1. Not maintaining a hollow body position.

Handstand Push-up Position 1 violation. Athlete arches from hands to heels. Following this fault to its logical conclusion leads to a nose-to-the-floor push-up. Discourage the trainee from trying to gain a mechanical advantage by turning the HP into an upside-down incline push-up. Lock the ribs down toward the pelvis.

 "Hollow out!" or "Six pack!" or "Head through!"

 Demonstrate a correct HP 1.

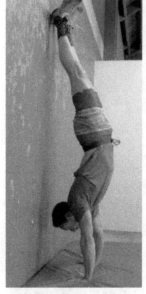

Fault

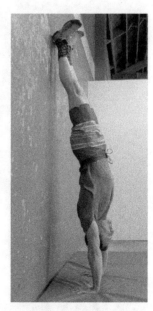

Correct HP 1

Handstand Push-up Common Faults and Fixes, cont.

2. Elbows flaring out.

Handstand Push-up Position 2 violation. Athlete's elbows rotate out as he descends. Cue him to screw hands into the deck to create stabilizing external rotation at the shoulder.

 "Screw your hands into the floor!" or "You need to see your elbows!"

 Demonstrate a correct transition from HP 1 to HP 2.

 Block elbows with boxes on either side of athlete.

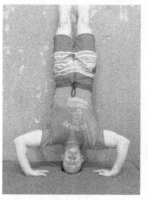 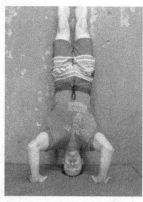

Fault   *Correct HP 2*

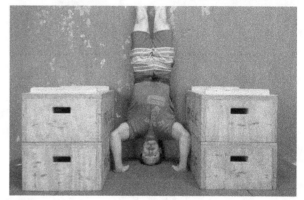

Orthosis

3. Hands set too wide.

Handstand Push-up Position 1 violation. Athlete sets hands too wide, shortening the range of motion and making the exericse easier. Unfortunately, the shoulders are less stable under load when hands are set wide. Hands should be push-up or press width.

 "Hands in closer!"

 Demonstrate a correct HP 1.

 Put down tape on the mat to to define correct distance (just outside hands in push-up position). Hands must remain inside tape.

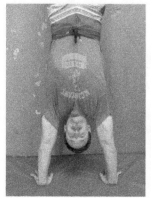

Fault

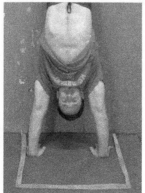

Correct HP 1   *Orthosis*

Handstand Push-up Common Faults and Fixes, cont.

4. Tripod fail.

Handstand Push-up Position 2 violation. In the bottom position of the handstand push-up, the head is in line with the hands, putting the shoulders in a disadvantageous position. The head and hands should form a tripod.

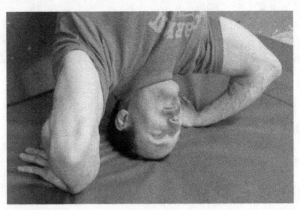
Fault

 "Head toward wall!"

 Demonstrate a correct HP 2.

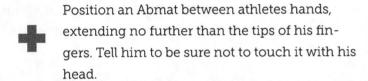 Position an Abmat between athletes hands, extending no further than the tips of his fingers. Tell him to be sure not to touch it with his head.

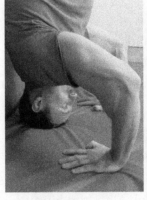
Correct HP 2

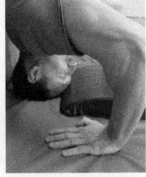
Orthosis

THE KIPPING HSPU

Category: Push Away from Object (vertical, inverted, dynamic)

Movement screen: N/a

Ability screen: Handstand push-up x 5

The kipping handstand push-up involves lowering oneself into a headstand, drawing the knees down to close the hip, then driving the heels violently up the wall to create an upward momentum that reduces demand on the arms and shoulders.

Kipping HP are a valuable tool for metcons, but are not a substitute for the strict movement. CAVEAT EMPTOR, etc. If your athlete is too tired or weak to push out of Headstand Push-up Position 2, once she's kicked up to Position 1, what are the odds she'll be strong enough to lower herself back down under control? The danger of coming down hard on one's head, causing injury to the neck/spine, is real. Also, the kipping handstand push-up has been known to aggravate lower back problems. Make sure your athlete understands the kipping HP is one of the riskier movements in the MMGPP arsenal. Unless she has serious competitive ambitions, there's probably a better training option.

Do not under any circumstance teach the kipping HP to anyone who does not have strict handstand push-ups! And even if they already know how to do kipping HP, don't let your athletes do them if they can't pass a strict HP test. Enforce the standard.

This one is a little advanced for most of the members of Team Space Monkey. Only Harry, who can do seven strict HP in good form, is ready for it. No big deal! I'm willing to be that within a year, Amy will be be allowed to try kipping HP as well. As for Tim, I think he'll be satisfied to keep working on his Down Dog Pike Push-ups.

The Kipping HSPU Teaching Script

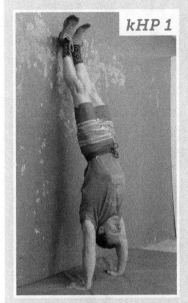

kHP 1

"Kick up into a handstand with your heels against the wall. This is **Kipping Handstand Push-up Position 1 (kHP 1).**

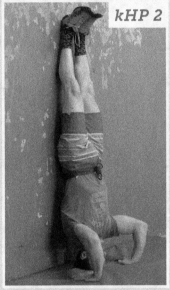

kHP 2

"Continuing to try to screw your hands into the ground, and with your head held neutral, lower yourself back and down such that the top of your head touches the ground between your hands and the wall. As you descend, imagine that you are winding your lats up tight. This is **Kipping Handstand Push-up Position 2 (kHP 2).**

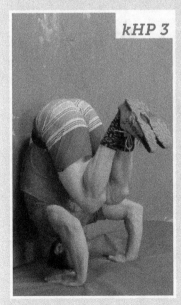

kHP 3

"Having assumed a strong tripod position (supported by hands and top of head), tuck your knees in to your chest. Keep your butt against the wall to keep your back straight. This is **Kipping Headstand Push-up Position 3 (kHP 3).**

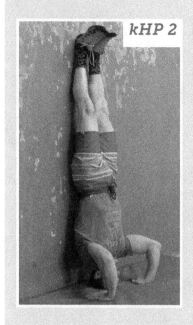

kHP 2

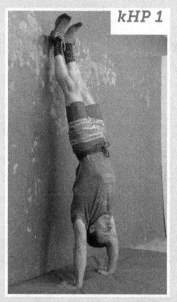

kHP 1

"Violently kick the heels up the wall. The driving extension of the hip creates momentum that makes it easier to press the arms to lockout. Once the legs straighten, but before the elbows extend, you're back in **kHP 2**.

"Press to lock out in **kHP 1**, a strong, hollowed-out handstand."

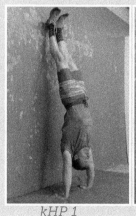

kHP 1

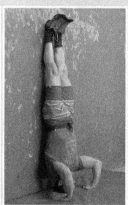

kHP 2

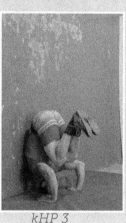

kHP 3

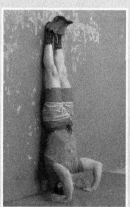

kHP 2

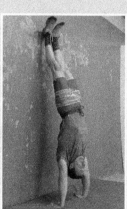

kHP 1

Positional Drills

"1! 2! 3! Go!" Have athlete lower to tripod support. Make sure he keeps his back against the wall as he draws his knees to his chest. After he kicks up, make sure both heels are in contact with the wall when he locks out in kHP 1.

Kipping HSPU Common Faults and Fixes

1. Heels come off wall too soon.

Kipping Handstand Push-up Position 1 violation. For the rep to count, the heels of both feet must be touching the wall when the arms lock out. In a competitive situation, the athlete must wait for the judge to count the rep. In training, the athlete should pause long enough to mentally count the rep number before descending.

 "Heels against the wall!"

 Demonstrate a correct kHP 1.

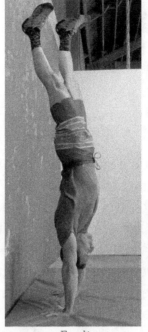

Fault

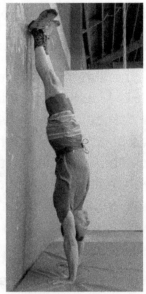

Correct kHP 1

2. Heels never touch wall.

Kipping Handstand Push-up Position 1 violation. From the tucked position of kHP 3, the athlete kicks up and out, rather than up and back (toward the wall). His legs extend without the wall's support, and he topples forward. NO REP!

 "Drive up and back!"

 Demonstrate a correct kHP 1.

Fault

Correct kHP 1

THE BUTTERFLY PULL-UP

Category: Pull to Object (kipping)

Movement screen: N/a

Ability screen: Chest-to-bar pull-up x 10

The butterfly pull-up is a kipping pull-up variant invented by James "OPT" Fitzgerald and Brent "AFT" Marshall sometime around 2006/2007. It's become the de facto standard for competitive MMGPP, as it has a faster cycle time than the traditional kipping pull-up. But that rapidity comes at a price: doing butterfly pull-ups, it's easy to miss a basic performance standard: the chin must rise above the bar for the rep to count. If you're going to allow athletes to do butterfly pull-ups, require them to make contact between chest and bar on every rep. Otherwise you're going to have a bunch of "firebreathers" with very sore necks, as they snap their heads up and back over and over, trying to eke out "chin over bar."

Only Harry will work on butterfly pull-ups today. But the big news is Amy just got to 5 strict pull-ups, which means I can teach her to kip. Tim will work on strict pull-ups. He's up to 3!

Butterfly Pull-up Teaching Script

"The kipping pull-up is built off of extension of the hip, but the butterfly pull-up is built off flexion of the hip. It's much harder to create productive force via hip flexion, so consequently the butterfly pull-up will require greater upper body strength and continuous momentum.

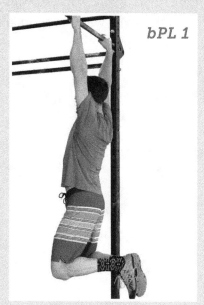

bPL 1

"**Butterfly Pull-up Postion 1 (bPL 1)** is a flexed knee hang with active, torqued shoulders.

"Come to a full body hang. Your hips and knees are straight. Keep your feet together. This is **Butterfly Pull-up Position 2 (bPL 2).**

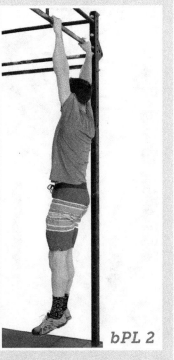

bPL 2

"Now pull your knees high. This is **Butterfly Pull-up Position 2 (BU 3).**

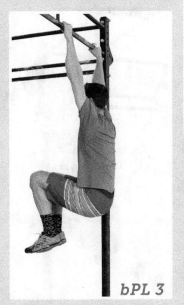

bPL 3

"The action of these three positions is a sort of 'reverse bicycle pedal.' From **bPL 1**, sweep your feet down through **bPL 2** before pulling your knees high in **bPL 3**. If you move agressively enough, you'll feel a moment of weightlessness just after arriving in **bPL 3**. Practice that sequence to get a feel for it."

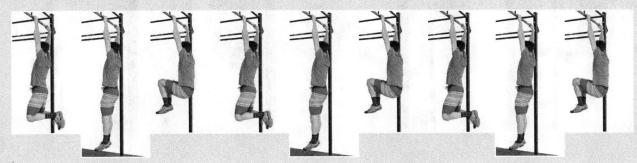

Positional Drills

"1! 2! 3!" Drill first three positions of the butterfly pull-up one at a time.

"1! Go!" Practice creating momentum and elevation through three positions.

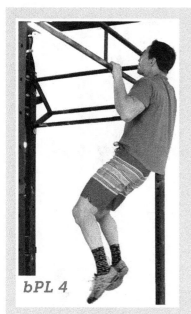

bPL 4

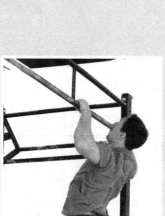

bPL 5

"The powerful flex of the hip in **bPL 3** generates upward momentum. Use this upward momentum to power pulling your chin over the bar.

"Repeat the sequence **bPL 1-bPL 2-bPL 3,** and then do a pull-up and hold with your chin over the bar. This is **Butterfly Pull-up Position 4 (bPL 4).**

"Come down and reset.

"In the traditional kipping pull-up, once your chin is over the bar, you push away to swing back to **kPL 1(e)**. In the butterfly pull-up, you instead allow yourself to fall foward.

"Repeat the sequence, and this time, at the top of the pull-up, allow yourself to fall forward, chest skimming the bar as you kick your feet back. This passing position is **Butterfly Pull-up Position 5 (bPL 5).**

"To cycle the movement, aggressively kick forward through **bPL 1**, **bPL 2**, and **bPL 3**."

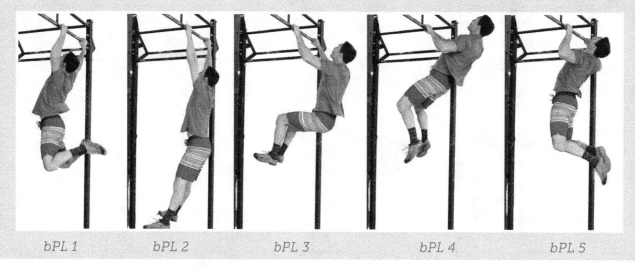

bPL 1   bPL 2   bPL 3   bPL 4   bPL 5

Positional Drills

"1! 2! 3! 4!" Drill positions of the butterfly pull-up one at a time. **bPL 5** is a passing position that occurs naturally in the transition from **bPL 4** to **bPL 1**.

"1! Go!" Practice creating momentum and elevation through four positions.

Butterfly Pull-up Common Faults and Fixes

1. Chin doesn't make it over the bar.

Butterfly Pull-up Position 4 violation. Athlete doesn't get enough elevation, so throws his head back in a wild bid to meet the standard of "chin over bar". Chin must rise clearly over the bar for rep to count, and head should be in a neutral position to make the rep legit.

 "Chin over bar!" or "Chest to bar!"

 Demonstrate a correct bPL 4.

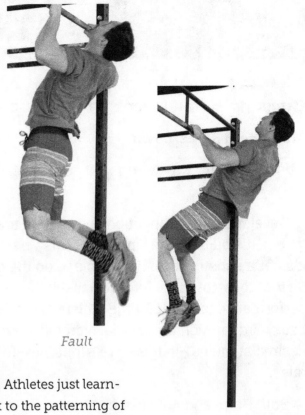

Fault

Correct bPL 4

2. Forward bicycle.

Butterfly Pull-up Positions 1, 2, 3 sequencing violation. Athletes just learning the butterfly pull-up will invariably, as they tire, revert to the patterning of the kipping pull-up, raising the knees and then kicking the feet back to drive up with extending hips.

 "Knees swoop up then pull!"

 Demonstrate a correct BU 1, 2, 3 sequence.

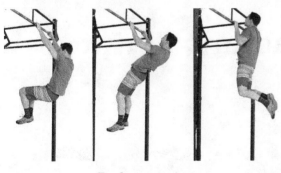

Faulty sequence

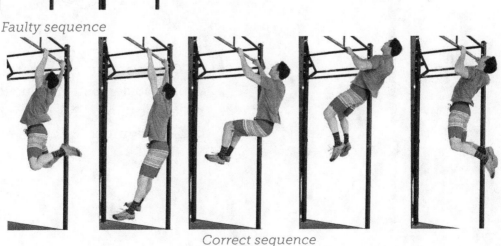

Correct sequence

THE KIPPING TOES-TO-BAR

Category: Hip and Trunk Flexion (hanging, straight-leg)

Movement screen: N/a

Ability screen: Kip swing x 10, toes-to-bar x 5

Developed for competition, the kipping toes-to-bar is a much faster version of the strict toes-to-bar. It's built off the kip swing. This version of toes-to-bar is appropriate for metcons, but it's not a substitute for being able to do the strict version. BtN requires athletes to be able to do 5 strict toes-to-bar before we'll teach them this movement. If and when fatigue impairs their performance to the point the athlete can no longer chain repetitions together, I have them default backward through the familial hierarchy of complexity to a simpler movement that preserves the desired stimulus—in this case, strict toes-to-bar, then the hanging leg raise, then the supine leg raise.

Both Harry and Amy can do at least 5 strict toes-to-bar, so they'll learn the kipping variation today. Tim will keep working on his hanging straight-leg raises. I doubt, given his age and flexibility issues, he'll ever do kipping toes-to-bar—so what? The important thing is he always does

Kipping Toes-to-Bar Teaching Script

"The kipping toes-to-bar is built off the kip swing.

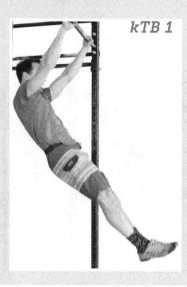

kTB 1

"Contract your lats to partially close your shoulder joint and put yourself into a hollow position. This is **Kipping Toes-to-bar Position 1 (kTB 1)**.

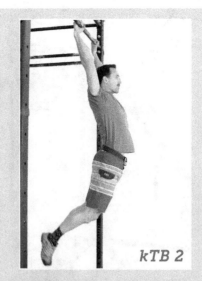

kTB 2

"Keeping your shoulders active, allow yourself to swing forward into an arch. Squeeze the bar tightly. The feet must be behind the plane of the bar. This is **Kipping Toes-to-bar Position 2 (kTB 2)**.

"Execute three kip swings by cycling between **kTB 1** and **kTB 2**. As you transition, allow your hands to relax as they rotate around the bar."

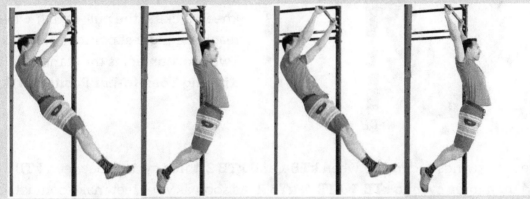

"Come down and rest.

"The next step is to tuck your knees to your chest while in **kTB 1**. We'll call this new position **Kipping Toes-to-bar Position 3 (kTB 3)**.

"If you bring your knees to your elbows rather than tucked in to the chest, this serves as a **Kipping Knees-to-Elbows**, useful for "Chuck Norris".

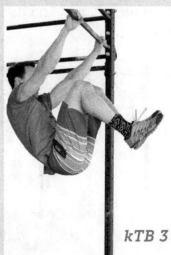

kTB 3

"As soon as your knees come high, drive your feet straight down and then back into **kTB 2**. If you don't arch strongly in the forward swing, you'll quickly begin to pendulum swing under the bar, defeating attempts to string reps together.

"Do three swings cycling between **kTB 1** and **kTB 2**, and then three more cycling between **kTB 3** and **kTB 2**. Then come down and rest."

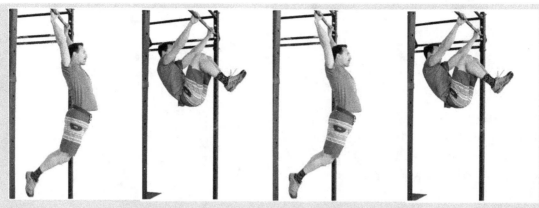

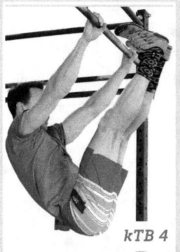

kTB 4

"From this knees-to-chest back swing, the final step is to powerfully extend the knees, kicking the pull-up bar when you reach the highest point of the back swing. Two foot contact is the standard. This is **Kipping Toes-to-bar Position 4 (kTB 4).**

"Do three kip swings cycling between **kTB 1** and **kTB 2**, three cycling between **kTB 3** and **kTB 2**, and then three cycling **kTB 3-kTB 4-kTB 2**. As soon as your feet make contact with the bar, drive them straight down and then back. If you start to pendulum swing under the bar, stop and reset."

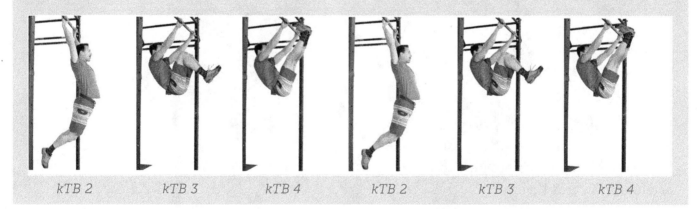

| kTB 2 | kTB 3 | kTB 4 | kTB 2 | kTB 3 | kTB 4 |

Positional Drills

"1! 2! 1! 2!!" Drill positions of the kip swing.

"2! 3! 2! 3!" Knees to chest as you push down on the bar (useful as kipping K2E).

"2! 3! 4! 2!" Kipping toes-to-bar.

Kipping Toes-to-bar Common Faults and Fixes

1. Pendulum swinging.

Kipping Toes-to-bar Positions 2 and 3 violations. The athlete must be able to consistently maintain the rhythm of the swing while remaining centered in the plane of the bar. Once the pendulum starts swinging, it can't be stopped, so have the trainee arrest the swing with a toe on a box, and then start again.

 "Stay in the plane of the bar!"

 Take athlete back to positional drills.

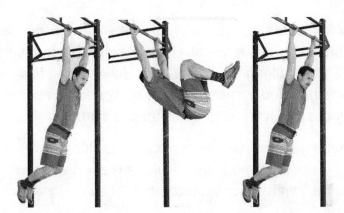

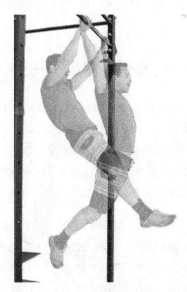

Fault: pivots around hands *Correct: pivots around shoulders*

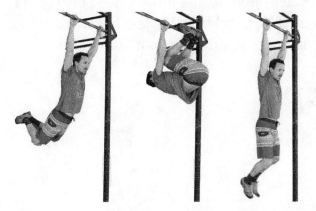

Faulty sequence

2. Unable to string reps together.

This usually this happens either when the athlete is not moving back swiftly enough into kTB 2, or because he is curling his trunk to get his feet to the bar, rather than elevating the entire body by pressing down on the bar in kTB 3, or because he has simply grown too fatigued to control the movement.

 "Arch back!" or "Push down on bar!" as appropriate.

 Demonstrate a correct kTB sequence.

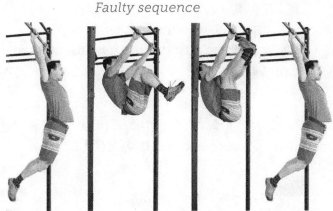

Correct sequence

Category: Push Away from Object (vertical, inverted, ambulatory)

Movement screen: Posterior tilt pelvic test

Ability screen: Push-up x 10 (inchworm), full inchworm/walkback x 5 (wallwalk)

The wallwalk is a gymnastic exercise that appears occasionally in MMGPP programming. The athlete begins in a push-up position with his feet against a wall. He then walks his feet up the wall, and when he can step no higher he begins walking his hands back until he is vertical with his nose pressed to the wall, all the while maintaining a strong, hollow body position. When he's ready to descend, he walks his hands back out and returns to push-up position.

I include the wallwalk because it's a great core exercise and confidence builder for the free-standing handstand, and also because I've visited too many gyms where the wallwalk was executed incredibly sloppily in metcon workouts. I want to emphasize that it has utility as a skill developer first, conditioning exercise second.

One of the cool things about the wallwalk is that it's self-limiting; the athlete need only go as high as feels safe. So Tim can give the wallwalk a whirl; if he only walks his feet halfway up, he'll still derive some training benefit. Harry and Amy should have no problem with this.

Wallwalk Teaching Script

"The best way to begin learning how to walk up the wall is to stay safely on the ground. This exercise is called the 'inchworm/walkback'.

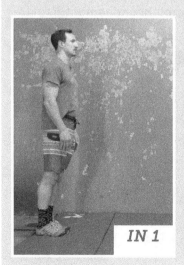 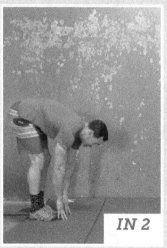

IN 1   IN 2

"Start in reset position: feet hip width, standing tall, midline braced, shoulders packed. This is **Inchworm/walkback Position 1 (IN 1)**.

"Unlock your knees, hinge back at the hips, and touch your toes. This is **Inchworm/walkback Position 2 (IN 2)**.

"Walk your hands out until you are in a well-organized plank position **(IN 3)**. If that's easy, continue to walk your hands out until your nose and trunk are just barely above the ground **(IN 4)**. As you stretch out, keep your abds strong contracted to maintain a posterior pelvic tilt. Wherever you end up, walk your hands back to your feet and then stand."

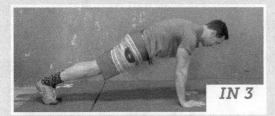 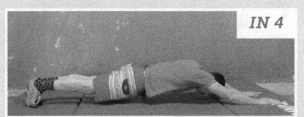

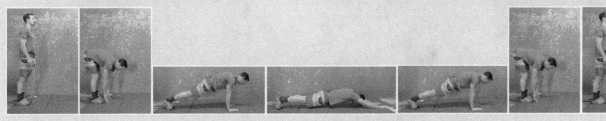

Walk your hands out as far as you can without losing tension, then walk your hands back.

"For many athletes, the inchworm will be challenging enough. Master it before attempting the wallwalk, and if you ever find exhaustion making wallwalks prohibitively difficult (and dangerous—remember, you're going to be getting upside down, and no workout is worth breaking your neck), you can always default back to the inchworm/walkback.

"To execute a wallwalk, start in a well-organized push-up position. This is **Wall Walk Position 1 (WW 1).**

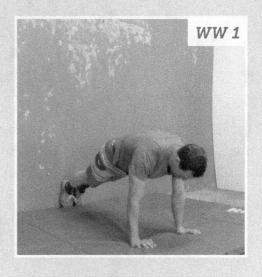

"Keeping your feet close together, initiate a walk up the wall, maintaining a strict hollow position. When your torso is at about 45 degrees relative to the ground, you are in **Wall Walk Position 2 (WW 2).**

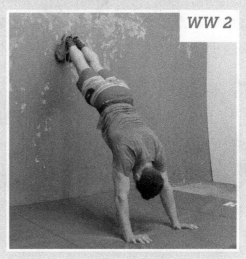

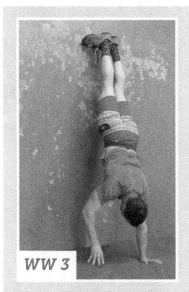

WW 3

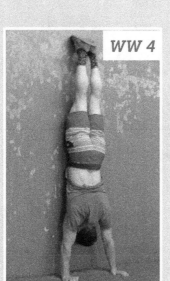

WW 4

"Begin walking your hands back toward the wall. Seesaw your weight back and forth between your arms as you go. When all of your weight is supported by one arm, and the other is moving into position, you're in **Wallwalk Position 3 (WW3).**

"Walk back until your entire torso is vertical against the wall. This is **Wall Walk Position 4 (WW 4).**

"At this point the athlete is in a **Nose-to-wall handstand**. Hands should be less than 4" from the wall, and under the shoulders. Fingers are splayed, hands screwed into the ground, and shoulders pressing as if trying to push the ground away. Abs, glutes, and quads should be maximally contracted, with feet together and toes pointed up along the wall.

"To descend, return to **WW 3** by walking your hands forward, shifting your weight back and forth between them. Keep your feet together and toes pointed as they slide down the wall.

"When your torso is again at 45 degrees, you are in **WW 2**. Your hands will remain in place as you tiptoe the rest of the way down to **WW 1.** Fight the urge to collapse to the floor."

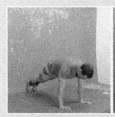 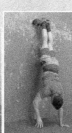 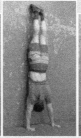 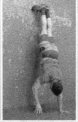 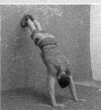 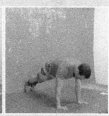

WW 1   WW 2   WW 3   WW 4   WW 3   WW 2   WW 1

Wallwalk Common Faults and Fixes

1. Failure to maintain hollow body position.

Wallwalk Position 3 violation. Athlete sags at the hips. One of the reasons to train the wallwalk is to learn how to maintain a straight body line while becoming inverted. Remind the athlete he must remain hollow at every stage of execution.

 "Hollow out!"

 Demonstrate a correct Wallwalk Position 3.

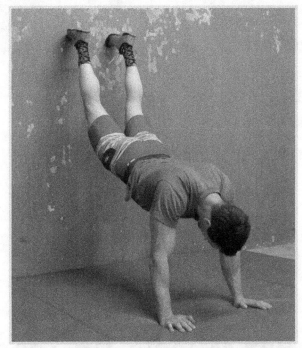

Fault

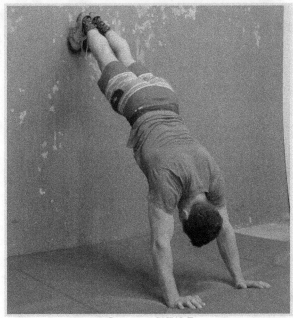

Correct WW 3

Category: Hybrid (pull to object [kipping], pull to object [horizontal], push away from object [vertical])

Movement screen: Posterior tilt pelvic test

    The bar muscle-up owes its burgeoning popularity to its regular inclusion in MMGPP competitions. It's built off of a tremendous kip swing, which can allow those with powerful hips, but lacking sufficient upper body strength, to get themselves into potentially dangerous positions. I won't let anyone who doesn't have a strict muscle-up try it, so this one's for Harry, only.

Bar Muscle-up Teaching Script

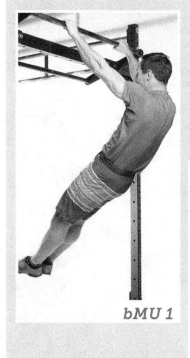

bMU 1

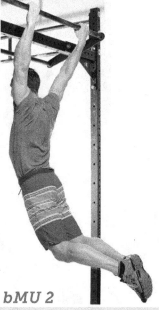

bMU 2

"The bar muscle-up begins with a basic kip swing: **Bar Muscle-up Position 1 (bMU 1)** is the hollow, with shoulders extending, and **Bar Muscle-up Position 2 (bMU 2)** is the arch, with the shoulders in flexion.

"Begin by cycling between **bMU 1** and **bMU2** a couple times to build momentum.

"On each back swing, increase the force with which you push down on the bar. The amplitude of your swing will grow, and as your elevation increases, your arms will eventually be almost parallel to the floor. At this point you are in **Bar Muscle-up Position 3 (bMU 3).**

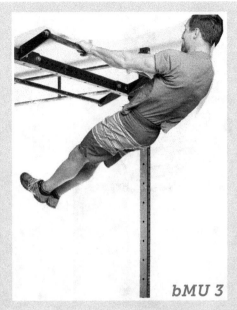

bMU 3

"At the top end of your highest swing, pull aggressively toward the bar. Because of the the angle of your body relative to the bar, this is a horizontal pull to just above the navel—**Bar Muscle-up Position 4 (bMU 4).**

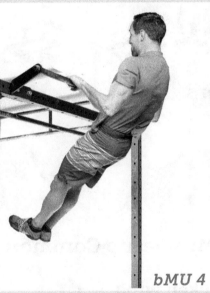

bMU 4

"As soon as your body makes contact with the bar, snap your torso forward from the hip so you 'sit up' over the bar while simultaneously flipping your elbows from below to above the bar. Stable and supported by your arms and your upper body resting on the bar, you are in **Bar Muscle-up Position 5 (bMU 5).**

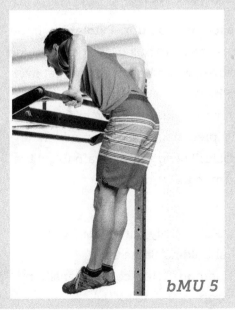

bMU 5

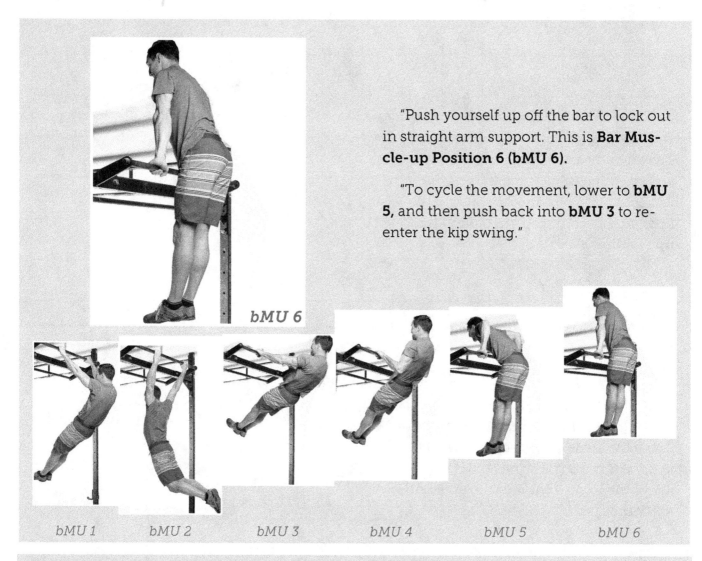

"Push yourself up off the bar to lock out in straight arm support. This is **Bar Muscle-up Position 6 (bMU 6)**.

"To cycle the movement, lower to **bMU 5,** and then push back into **bMU 3** to re-enter the kip swing."

bMU 6

bMU 1 *bMU 2* *bMU 3* *bMU 4* *bMU 5* *bMU 6*

Bar Muscle-up Common Faults and Fixes

1. Chicken wing.

Bar Muscle-up Position 4 violation. If the athlete isn't able to pull the bar low enough on his torso, when he attempts to get over the bar, he is only able to get one arm—usually his stronger one—over. This puts him in a precarious position in which he must basically wiggle and strain to get the other arm in positon.

 "Pull to belly button!" or "Both shoulders! Same time!"

 Demonstrate a correct transition from bMU 3 to bMU 4.

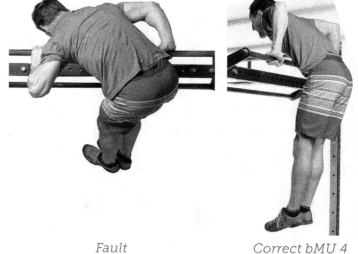

Fault *Correct bMU 4*

"TASTEE FREEZE"

Our last benchmark was named in honor of one of my favorite summertime treats:

"Tastee Freeze"

Three rounds for time of
49 Air squats
6 Muscle-ups
9 Hang power cleans 135/95lbs

But what I'd like to talk about is a famous video, easily found on YouTube, of three legendary athletes taking on a similar (but not identical!) workout way back when MMGPP was in its relative infancy. As I understand it, the workout featured in this video wasn't intended to be anything special. At the time, it didn't even have a name. In 2004, when the video was shot, the MMGPP community depended on internet videos for information about the workouts and the exercises that comprised them.

All three athletes were very strong and well-versed in the movements. For the first round, at least, they're all doing strict muscle-ups—something you hardly ever see these days! And when fatigue began to impede their performance, as experienced trainers, they knew what to do. For instance, toward the end of the second set of muscle-ups, one athlete begins self-assisting her muscle-ups by pushing off the ground with her feet.

The first athlete finishes in 9:50, the second around 10:20, but the third grinds on for another two-and-a-half minutes, obviously exhausted, crying in frustration, and ultimately collapsing under the barbell, before wrapping things up at 12:57.

While you have to admire this last athlete's gutsiness, this video is a perfect example of what *not* to do as a MMGPP coach: allow someone to risk serious injury by attempting movements they are too fatigued to perform properly. It's true that the athlete was very experienced, qualified to make an informed decision about risk. But really, was it worth it? In competition, it's accepted that athletes will go to any lengths to win. We admire competitors for their reckless bravery, their casual self-disregard in the face of potential danger. But this *wasn't* a competition—it was just another workout. And no workout is worth getting hurt for. Someone should have stepped in.

Prescribing the Correct Level of Movement Complexity

Harry will be doing muscle-ups today, but it'll probably be awhile before Amy can do them, and, realistically, Tim may never be able to. Muscle-ups present an interesting challenge as you attempt to find the stimulus-preserving exercise appropriate to each athlete. Traditionally, the substitution for muscle-ups was both pull-ups and dips, three of each for one muscle-up. But for our time-delimited efforts, that's impractical—it just takes too long. I suggest looking at the rest of the programming for the week, especially the day before and the day after: upper body pulling, or pushing? Whatever it is, take the opposite and use that for the muscle-up sub. In other words, if a WOD with lots of push-ups is scheduled for the following day, use pull-ups as the sole sub for muscle-ups. Use a 2:1 ratio—for today, that'll be 12 pull-ups per round. Amy just this week got her first kipping pull-ups. I'll let her start that way, but I'll keep a 1/2" band in reserve for band-assisted strict (no kipping on the band!) pull-ups. Tim will do piked ring rows, also 2:1.

Eight weeks in, the air squats of all three of our athletes are looking good! Tim may never be a speedster, but his mechanics are solid, and he rarely needs more than one cue to fix any problems that arise.

During the deliberate practice period, we determine that Harry and Amy should hang power clean. As with other barbell-centric workouts, we'll determine the loading for today's WOD with a strength training session.

Trial-and-error have taught me that for maximal intensity, 70% of 1RM is a workable load for "Tastee Freeze." That means a male athlete should have roughly a 100kg hang power clean to do "Tastee Freeze" as prescribed. Harry works his way up to a 200lbs hPC single; he'll use 120lbs today. Amy hang power cleans 83lbs for a good single, but fails on an attempted second rep. She'll use 50lbs.

Tim still isn't comfortable trying to front rack a barbell, but he's definitely getting stronger and better coordinated! He's learned the dumbbell hang power clean, so today he'll use that, with 20lbs in each hand.

Establishing Correct Volume

"Tastee Freeze" works well as a 12 minute effort.

"By the Numbers Testing 'Tastee Freeze'"

Three cycles of
AMRAP :80 Air squats. If you get to 49 before time is up, move on to...
AMRAP :80 Muscle-ups. If you get to 6 before time is up, move on to...
AMRAP :80 Hang power cleans. If you get to 9 before time is up, move back to air squats. If you're on your third round, you're done!

The 80 second increments make it a little awkward to know just when the intervals are expiring. You might want to jot down the times on the white board, or maybe just write it on your palm: "0:00 to 1:20, air squats. 1:21 to 2:40, muscle-ups. 2:41 to 4:00, hang power cleans." Etc. Just make sure you let your athletes know loud and clear when it's time to move on, whether or not they've completed the assigned work for the exercise they've been doing.

147 air squats is still too much volume for Tim, so I tell him to shoot for 35 squats each round.

"3...2...1...GO!"

Harry

As strong and fast as Harry was eight weeks ago, he's scary now. He fired off his air squats in :51, shooting up and down like a piston. That gave him almost 30 extra seconds on the muscle-ups. He strung together 3, then did a set of 2, and then a single. Over at the barbell, he did his 9 hPC unbroken, although after 5 he began tucking the bar into his hips to reset his hook grip before each subsequent rep. During cycle two he did have to set down the bar once to shake out his grip. Things got pretty tight in cycle three, when he basically had to do six muscle-up singles, but he got through them in time, and then proceded to knock out his final 9 hPC in a row. Time: 9:50! Outstanding!

Amy

Thanks to her newly developed kipping pull-ups, Amy was able to completely finish the work in cycle one. The hang power cleans gave her a problem, but not because of the weight. She caught her first two reps "limboing" under the bar—that is, leaning back, with her knees jammed forward. I cued her, "SIT BACK!" and "BARSTOOL!". Neither worked, so I brought her into Practice Mode and had her demonstrate for me the correct receiving position for Power Clean 7. That looked good, but when I let her start again, she reverted to her old movement pattern. At that point, I had her default to the next exercise down in the hierarchy: the muscle clean. These she performed correctly, and stuck with them for the rest of the workout.

By the third cycle, she was getting tired. As happens sometimes, exhaustion caused her to "forget" how do kip her pull-ups; suddenly, she was unable to generate any power from her hip, and wasn't able to get her chin over the bar after rep 6. Cueing "More hip drive!" didn't help, so I had her step into the red band to get three more pull-ups before time was up. In all, she got 140 air squats, 32 pull-ups and 22 muscle cleans. Nice work!

Tim

Just like mothers aren't supposed to have favorite children, instructors aren't supposed to have favorite clients, but Tim has earned a special place in my heart. His progress in the last eight weeks has been nothing short of remarkable. When he first started with our program, I thought of him as "The Tin Man" from *The Wizard of Oz*, because he was so slow and stiff. Watching him bang out 35 air squats in a minute flat today, you never would've guessed! Not only was he fluid, he was well-organized, with all three positions of the squat correct on every rep. Hot damn! He did his 12 piked ring rows and his 9 dumbbell hang power cleans with time to spare. And through the next two cycles he remained pretty consistent. After 35 squats in cycle two, he began to throw his hips forward in his piked ring rows—natural, as one grows tired—so I had him switch back to regular ring rows. Last cycle his numbers were 30 air squats, 10 ring rows, 7 dumbbell hPC. When time was called, he stepped out through the open garage door and peeled off his t-shirt.

"TIM!" I yelled. "YOU JUST DID 100 AIR SQUATS!"

"Next time," he said, opening his water bottle.

"Huh? Next time? This time! 100!"

He gulped water and then poured the rest over his head, grinning exultantly. "Next time, ONE HUNDRED FORTY-SEVEN!" And high fived me.

I could only grin back at him. Maybe not *next* time, but with an attitude like that, it won't be long!

PART THREE:

BY THE
NUMBERS

Supplemental Material

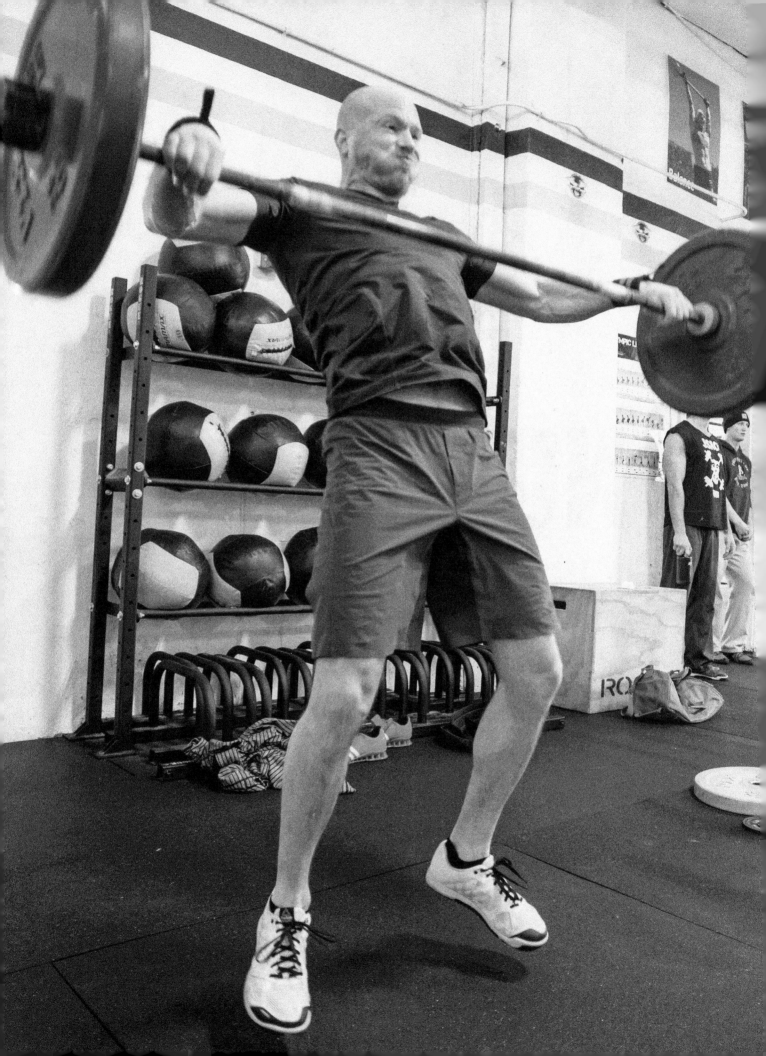

APPENDIX I

IMPLEMENTING BTN

As our group of archetypal athletes, Harry, Amy, and Tim, progressed from week to week, they got used to the classroom modes of instruction, practice, and performance. When new movements were introduced, they took it as a given that the basics needed to be mastered before a more complex exercise should be attempted, and if a variation was too challenging for their current abilities, they were content (for now) to continue using the version they could perform correctly.

If you're starting from scratch with a group of new athletes, teaching "By the Numbers" is a snap. Implementing BtN in an already established program can be a challenge, however.

It's possible you may get pushback from athletes who have been training MMGPP for awhile and have a certain amount of ego invested in their abilities. Such people often resent being asked to review the basics and to practice for mastery. Remember back in the Introduction when I said certain areas were outside the scope of this book? This is one of them. I'm no sports psychologist. What I will suggest is that if you get resistance from clients as you introduce new, more stringent standards for movements, *talk to them*. Let them know what you're doing, and why. Explain that you believe that this pose-by-pose approach to relearning movements, and the associated idea that conditioning work should only use exercise variations an athlete has mastered, will in the long run lead to much greater gains. Ask them to be patient and to have some faith. The benefits of careful, rigorous technique review ands practice sessions will soon be clear to them.

The challenge I *will* discuss is how to best structure your programming and run your classes to help your clients get the most from BtN.

There's No Time to Lose

Most MMGPP gyms run classes that last about an hour, and an hour goes by quickly when you've got to do some community building, get athletes warmed up, practice skills, supervise their strength training, administrate the high-intensity finisher, and then lead them through cooldown mobilizations.

With that in mind, I encourage you to minimize the amount of class time spent on warm-up activities that do not develop MMGPP-specific skills. I've visited many gyms where the first fifteen minutes or so of class was spent on dynamic warm-up exercises: jumping jacks, mountain climbers, etc. While the trainer performed the exercises, and the athletes imitated him as best they could, they shot the bull and generally had a pretty good time, which was fun, but no attempt was made to improve their execution, which was usually pretty sloppy. Other gyms I've seen have set warm-up routines of barbell exercises and calisthenics, but these were performed robotically, and again, without correction from the trainer. And don't get me started on leap frog and red rover and other kids' games-based activities. To me, it's all junk, because it represents missed opportunity.

At PVCF we taught our athletes a ten minute dynamic flexibility routine that they were supposed to do *before* class. Why? Because it frees up that much more time for warm-up activities designed to help our athletes become better at MMGPP training. Our coaches all have vast technical knowledge and experience, so why waste their time by having them lead a generic warm-up? I want them to apply their time to helping our clients get better *at the things that matter*. There's just too much to learn to waste any time.

Which brings me to my next point: especially for gyms transitioning to BtN, you can't allow your coaches to free-style the warm-ups. If you run eight classes a day, they should not vary wildly in content and quality depending on who is teaching. So I strongly suggest you program your warm-ups as carefully as you do the strength work and WODs, with a focus on developing MMGPP-specific movements and skills. What this looks like for a gym transitioning to BtN will be different than what it looks like in a gym that's been using the BtN model for a year or two.

You Don't Have to Teach Everything Every Day

The exercises commonly programmed in MMGPP training varying widely in complexity and technical challenge. Some, like the butterfly sit-up, need only be taught once. Others, like the snatch or Turkish get-up, which often take months for athletes to become even consciously competent with, must be taught and reviewed with great regularity.

The following table gives you a rough idea of how often to include a formal Technique Review for a given movement. A Technique Review puts you in Teaching Mode, while your group is in Learning Mode. You go over the positions of the exercise one-by-one, then lead the group through positional drills (as describing in the "Teaching and Coaching" section of the book). This process usually takes only about 5-10 minutes, because the members of your group should already have some familiarity with the material.

One and Done. You may occasionally review these exercises in the context of introducing a skills-based warm-up like the Standard Warm-up (Samson stretch, air squat, sit-up, etc.), but generally speaking initial instruction during fundamentals suffices. Thus, on "Cindy" day, there's no reason to re-teach the air squat and push-up (unless you think it's warranted). Use the time

One and Done	Once in a Blue Moon	Monthly	BiWeekly	Case-by-Case
Samson stretch	Deadlift	Overhead squat	Turkish get-up	Kipping pull-ups
Good morning	Back squat	Rowing	Muscle/power/full	Ring dips
Air squat	Front squat	Kettlebell swings	clean	GHD sit-up
Butterfly sit-up	Running	Pistol progressions	Muscle/power/full	Muscle-up
Ring row	Jumping mechan-	Toes-to-bar	snatch	progressions
Static hang	ics and box jumps	progressions		Bar muscle-up
Receiving heavy	Bench press set-	Press/push press/		Kipping handstand
push press	up and execution	push jerk		push-up
Push-up	Hip extension	Rope climbs		Handstand walk-
progressions	Dumbbell clean	Double-unders		ing progression
Kip swing	Dumbbell snatch	Handstand push-		Hip-and-back
Bailing out of back	Wallballs	up progressions		extension
squat	Burpees	Thruster		
Bailing out of a	Wallwalks	Rope climb		
front squat/missed	Back squat set-up	Double-unders		
clean	in rack	Handstand		
Bailing out of an	Front squat set-up	progression		
overhead squat/	in rack			
missed snatch	Press set-up in			
	rack			
	Dip progressions			
	L-sit progressions			
	Pull-up			
	progressions			
	Wallball			

for something more fun and productive.

Once in a Blue Moon. Some exercises are in this category because they're so basic (e.g., deadlifts), some because they are more esoteric (db snatch), and some because education will not necessarily make an immediate difference in execution (e.g, the burpee, which will only improve as athlete gains explosive strength). Review the exercises in this group once or twice a quarter (i.e., every 12 weeks), or more often if you think it necessary.

Monthly. These exercises are both commonly programmed in MMGPP and commonly performed poorly. These exercises *do* respond to strict attention to technical detail, so try to fit in a technique review for each about once a month. Usually it's most practical to schedule these on a day when the movements are programmed, so the positional drills can serve as part of the warm-up.

BiWeekly. The clean and the snatch take a long time to master, especially when athletes only get to practice them once or twice a week. Plan on teaching the clean and snatch on alternating weeks. If you have an athlete who can demonstrate superlative technique, then by all means send her off to warm-up on her own. But everyone else needs to work the positions one-at-a-time, then build then up into full movements.

The Turkish get-up I include in this group for lack of any other place to put it. Once every two weeks plan on teaching and drilling the 10 positions of the Turkish get-up. Again, any athlete who has a flawless get-up should be set free to work on her/his own, perhaps with a 10 min EMOM. More on that in a bit.

Case-by-case. These are movements that probably only the top 25% of your general population will ever qualify for (at least, by BtN standards). So there's really no point in teaching, say, the muscle-up to a whole group--not even the basic stuff like the false grip. Why bother, if most of them can't even do five strict pull-ups or a ring dip yet? As your athletes develop to the point when they are ready for a Case-by-case exercise, pull them aside for some one-on-one or two-on-one teaching.

When You Do Teach, Make Time for Practice

You can be the greatest teacher in the world, but if your students don't internalize the material you present and make it their own, you've failed. The only way they can "know it by heart" is by practicing. After each Technique Review session, make sure you set aside 5-10 minutes for Deliberate Practice. As described earlier (pg 46), deliberate practice in the context of BtN is simply moving mindfully through the positions of an exercise, often pausing at each new position to self-assess and correct. To make this a little more social, it can be helpful to have athletes team up, each taking turns as "athlete" or "coach". Solo or team deliberate practice can be performed as a follow up to a Technique Review session, or as a stand-alone warm-up.

On the follow page I offer a sample from a week's worth of programming I wrote recently for a gym that was converting to BtN. I'll show only the warm-ups and the enough of the day's work to give a flavor of why I made the warm-up choices I did.

If it seems like I'm scheduling a LOT of talking here, well... I am. The owners of this gym are intent on making the transition to a BtN-based pedagogy, and there's a lot of basic info they need to get to their clients as quickly and painlessly as possible. Even with all the gabbing, there's still 30-40 minutes of hard work scheduled for the athletes.

The programming should be self-explanatory; one thing I would like to clarify is that on Friday, when the CF Standard Warm-up is introduced, the instructor takes the group through it piece-by-piece, demoing an exercise's positions, then having the class try it. Same things goes for the explanation of the exercise progressions for the pistol later in class. As each more complex variant is introduced, the athletes make an attempt at it. If it's easy, they move on; if not, they stay with

Monday	Tuesday	Wednesday	Thursday	Friday
1. Dynamic warm-up (5 min) 2. Technique review: 3 positions of the back squat + positional drills (10 min) 3. Five minutes deliberate practice of the 3 positions of the back squat w/ "five in the hole" 4. Technique review: setting up for back squat success by creating maximal tension in the rack (10 min) 5. Back squat 5-5-5-5-5 (15 min) Etc...	1. Technique review: 7 positions of the muscle snatch, 8 positions of the power snatch (15 min) 2. Twenty minutes deliberate practice of the muscle or power snatch OR Power snatch 2-2-2-2-2-2-2 LIII: work up to your best double for the day LII and LI: W/ instructor permission, add weight in small increments, but ONLY if your positions are spot on. 4. Technique review: the midfoot strike + positional drills (10 min) 5. EMOM 10 100m sprint Etc...	1. Technique review: the hollow position (5 min) 2. Technique review: the wall walk (5 min) 3. Five minutes deliberate practice of the wall walk. (5 min) 4. Technique review: 3 positions of the press + positional drills (10 min) 5. Press 5-5-5-5-5 (15 min) Etc...	1. Dynamic warm-up (5 min) 2. Technique review: 3 positions of the deadlift + positional drills (10 min) 3. Five minutes deliberate practice of the 3 positions of the deadlift 4. Deadlift 5-5-5-5-5 (15 min) Etc...	1. Technique review: the CF Standard warm-up (simplified): Samson stretch X :15/side, air squat x 10, butterfly sit-up x 10, PVC good morning x 10, pull-ups x 10, push-ups x 10 (15 min—demo each exercise, then athletes do reps) 2. An additional round of the CFWU (5 min) 3. Technique review and deliberate practice: building the pistol. Box step-up, reverse lunge, hanging leg pistol from box, elevated leg pistol from box, pistol. (10 min) 4. "Cindy" AMRAP 20 5 Pull-ups 10 Push-ups 15 Squats Etc...

Sample practice schedule for beginning BtN program

the variant that challenged them.

What all this talking means is that roughly 50 min out of every hour class is scheduled; therefore it's vital that the trainer follow the time constraints written into the programming. There IS a lot to get done, and it will get done if they keep an eye on the clock.

Notes on Specific Days:

Monday. The gym I was programming for had a population that was used to doing a group dynamic warm-up, so rather than getting rid of it altogether to make more time for teaching (thus forcing them into one more adaptation), we compromised by reducing the "unskilled" stuff (pogo bounces, jumping jacks, leg swings, reverse lunges w/ hands raised, childpose-upward dog-downward dog-upward dog-child pose, mountain climbers, crash victims, scap pull-ups, kip swings) to five minutes at the beginning of class.

The technique review and positional drills are performed with the class set up as on page 53, with empty barbells. The trainer, in teaching mode, should explain what's about to happen, then demo the 3 positions of the back squat, talking through the finer points while the athletes, in learning mode, listen. Then the athletes pick up their barbells and the trainer leads them through positional drills ("1! 2! 3! 2! 1!", etc.), making corrections at each stage as necessary. All this time the athletes are still in learning mode, moving only at the trainer's direction. After that follows an additional 5 minutes od deliberate practice on their own as the trainer circulates and makes corrections.

Tuesday. Tuesday's snatch instruction follows a similar pattern. Athletes can work with PVC or light barbells. The 20 minute lifting session should see them adding weight ONLY when they can competently move through all assigned positions.

Wednesday. Wednesday follows a pattern of instruction, work, instruction, work. Generally speaking, don't front load your instruction. If you know you need to teach a couple different movements, review the first and supervise practice before moving on to the next. This way, the second skill review will still be fresh in the athletes' minds when they set to work.

Thursday. This idea of instruction, work, instruction, work is also evident on Thursday. Don't teach the deadlift and muscle clean back-to-back--spread them out.

Friday. On Friday the athletes are (re)introduced to the CF Standard warm-up. Many of these movements are in the "one-and-done" category, but it never hurts to review them once in a while; doing the trainer should bring the entire group through the warm-up, first introducing and demoing the Samson stretch, then having the athletes work on it, then reviewing the positions of the air squat, then having the athletes do reps for correction, etc.

Monday	Tuesday	Wednesday	Thursday	Friday
1. Warm-up B: three rounds of the parallette complex @ 5 reps plus 10 air squats. Accrue one minute of L-sit in three 20 second efforts. If you don't have strong push-ups, stay off the parallettes and do 10 strict push-ups per round, using assistance as required. (10 min) 2. Technique review: setting up for the bench press. (10 min) 3. Bench press 3-2-2-2-1-1-1-1 (15 min) Etc...	1. EMOM 10 Even minutes: 30 sec handstand hold, or 5 handstand push-ups Odd minutes: five air squats; on last rep hold AS 3 until :30 on the clock. Bonus points if you do this as elbows-up wall squat tests. (10 min) 2. Five minutes deliberate practice of the 3 positions of the front squat and the 4 positions of the push press. (5 min) 2. "Scotty J." Front squat 1-2-3-1-2-3-1-2-3 GHD sit-ups 3-6-9-3-6-9-3-6-9 Push press 1-2-3-1-2-3-1-2-3 Etc...	1. 100 double-unders or five minutes double-under practice. (5 min) 2. Technique review: 7 positions of the muscle snatch, 8 positions of the power snatch and snatch (5 min). 3. Five minutes to practice the eight positions of the snatch. Then review how to construct hang variations of the snatch. (5 min) 2. Warm-up for EMOM. (10 min) 3. EMOM 10 High hang snatch Hang snatch Snatch Etc...	1. Ten minutes deliberate practice of the 10 positions of the Turkish get-up, OR EMOM 10 Turkish get-up x 2 (alternate sides per minute) 3. Technique review: building the kipping pull-up. Kip swing, kipping pull-up progression, C2B pull-up. (10 min) 4. Five minutes deliberate practice to figure out which pull-up variation is appropriate for you today. (5 min) 4. "Helen's Tra-vest-y" Four rounds of AMRAP :60 10m shuttle runs AMRAP :60 Kettle-bell swings AMRAP :60 Pull-ups Rest one minute Etc...	1. Warm-up E: Reverse lunges x 5/side, 10 strict toes-to-bar, single-leg Romanian deadlifts x 5/side, kick up to hand stand x 5, 10 kip swings. Then two rounds of pistols x 5/side, kipping toes-to-bar x 10, contra-lateral dumbbell single-leg Romanian deadlifts x 5/side, 10 headstand push-ups, 10 chest-to-bar pull-ups (10 min) 2. Warm-up F: 3 rounds of deadlift x 3, power clean x 3, front squat x 3, press x 3, push press x 3, push jerk x 3. First round work position to position, then you can smooth and speed things up. (5 min) 3. "Blackwater" 10-8-6-4-2 reps for time of Deadlifts x2 Toes-to-bar

Sample practice schedule for established BtN program

A Spoonful of Sugar Helps the Medicine Go Down

On the preceding page, you'll find an excerpt from some programming I did for my old gym, Pioneer Valley CrossFit, which has been incorporating BtN for a couple of years.

At PVCF the athletes have been taught a dynamic flexibility warm-up that they are expected to go through before class. This frees up another 10 minutes of class time for more technical warm-ups and instruction. I would HIGHLY encourage you to consider teaching your athletes a simple dynamic warm-up they can before on their own (or better yet, in self-organized groups!) before the start of class. These movements tend to be dumbed down and low-skill, and honestly, I think supervising them day after day is a waste of your expertise. Use class time for stuff that requires your knowledge and expert eye.

This additional class time allows you to program skills-based warm-ups that keep the challenges fresh, even for experienced athletes.

Notes on Specific Days:

Monday. Monday's warm-up begins with the parallette complex. At this point, the majority of athletes in any class know the complex and roughly what level they should participate at. If we have a new person just out of Elements, or if we have a drop-in, the Assistant instructor (we always have two instructors on the floor, a Primary and an Assistant) will either quickly bring the athlete up to speed before we begin, or work with them separately while the rest of the class does the complex.

Following that, we spend 5-10 minutes going over the finer points of setting up for the bench press before having the athletes work to a best single for the day.

Tuesday. EMOMs are a way to disguise practice as additional exercise (athletes seem to always feel like they're getting more of their money's worth when they are breathing hard). Again, this assumes that everyone in the group is up to speed on the assigned movements. If someone is not, again, they work with the assistant.

Wednesday. Today we have a full technique review for the snatch. This usually unfolds as a quick review of the individual positions of the muscle snatch, followed by the catch position of the power snatch and squat snatch. The instructor takes the athletes through the positions one-by-one, then introduces the common positional drills ("4! Go!", "3! Go!" etc.) Notice that afterwards athletes are turned loose for a deliberate practice session; this can be done solo, or in teams as coaching pairs (see pg. 320).

Thursday. For the Turkish get-ups I leave the instructor some discretion: if she knows a particularathlete already has an excellent get-up, she ca give him permission to warm-up for the EMOM on his own. Otherwise the trainer takes the group through the ten positions of the TGU one-at-a-time. Generally speaking, we limit instruction of the kipping pull-up to athletes who have strict pull-ups. But today I wanted to reinforce good mechanics on the kip swing and to give athletes a chance to practice, so I scheduled it like this.

Friday. PVCF's "Warm-up E" is a kind of advanced version of the CFWU, with exercises that demand greater strength, balance, and flexibility. Again, during this ten minute period the class can be broken into groups. Some athletes will be free to go work on their own, only needing an occasional cue from a trainer to help them refine their technique. Other athletes, though, may need to be taken through this sequece step by step. If so, no problem! We can roll instruction and deliberate practice into an organic whole. This warm-up was selected in part because it includes the toes-to-bar, which will allow us to help athletes decide which exercise in Hip and Trunk Flexion (hanging, straight leg) Movement Hierarchy is going to be appropriate for them today.

I include 5 minutes deliberate practice of the deadlift as both task-specific warm-up and as a chance to hammer home fundamentals. Every athlete, no matter how experienced or accomplished, can learn something by moving slowly with a barbell and really paying attention to what their body is doing!

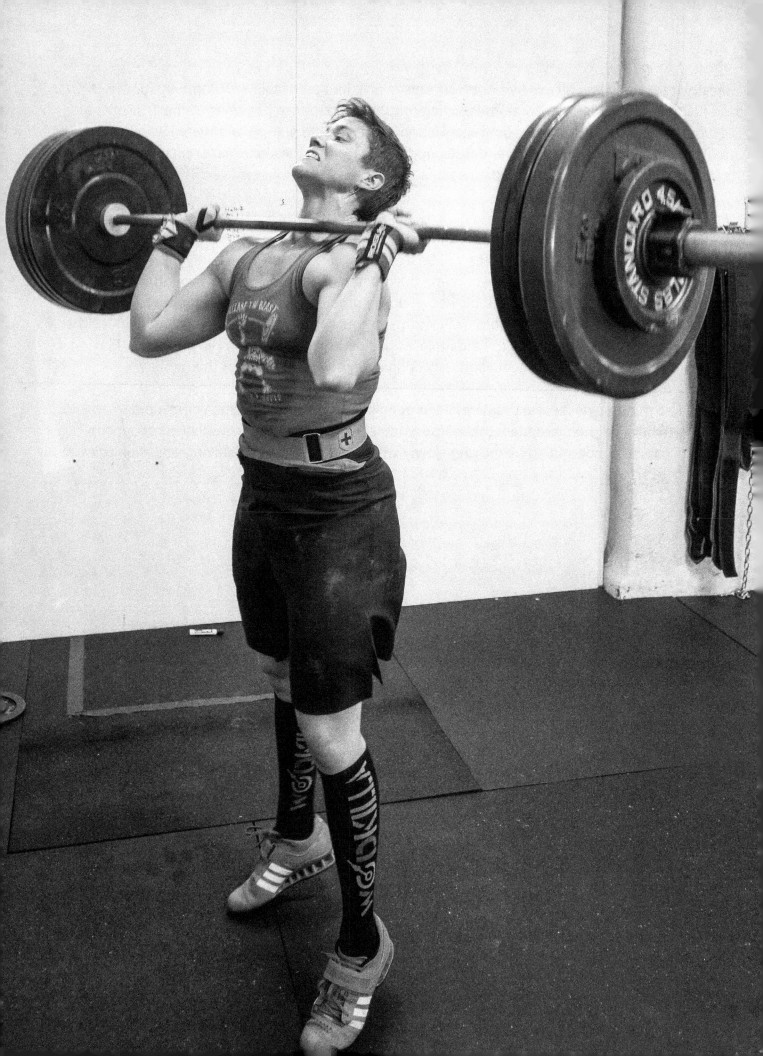

SKILLS-BASED WARM-UPS

Here are some ideas to get you started with programming BtN-style skills practice sessions. Feel free to spin endless variations. Remember, the format is just there to keep some novelty in the training; hidden in the fun is the relentless, absolutely necessary grind of careful, deliberate practice. Don't allow your trainees turn practice into an auxiliary metcon, either. Teach them the only thing more important than getting it right when practicing is to stop immediately when they make a mistake, figure out what went wrong, and then fix it.

Skills-based warm-ups should be part of every single class. Keep their appearances constantly varied, as you might the elements in the WOD, but over a seven day microcycle, try to make sure at least four days include deliberate practice sessions. And there's nothing wrong with doubling up, combining, say, a calisthenic WU and deliberate practice, or deliberate practice, and then an EOMOM. Twenty minutes of warm-up and dedicated skill work, twenty minutes of strength work, a ten minute ass-whupping finisher, ten minutes of cool down mobility techniques...now that's a class!

CALISTHENIC/GYMNASTICS-BASED

1) Three rounds of the parallette complex @ 5 reps : push-up, shoot through, dip, swing back. If you don't have strong push-ups, stay off the parallettes and do 10 strict push-ups per round, using assistance as required. After five reps of the complex, "shoot the duck" 10 sec/side. After three rounds, accrue one minute of L-sit in three 20 second efforts. (10 min)

2) Two rounds of 10-15 reps: Samson stretch, overhead squats, GHD sit-ups (sub: butterfly sit-ups), back extensions (sub: good mornings), pull-ups, and dips (10 min)

3) Reverse lunges x 5/side, 10 strict toes-to-bar, single-leg Romanian deadlifts x 5/side, kick up to handstand x 5, 10 kip swings. Then two rounds of pistols x 5/side, kipping toes-to-bar x 10, contralateral dumbbell single-leg Romanian deadlifts x 5/side, 10 handstand push-ups, 10 chest-to-bar pull-ups. Choose version of each movement appropriate to your level of development. (10 min)

4) Two rounds: 3 scapular pull-ups, 3 strict pull-ups, 3 kipping pull-ups. 3 down dog push-ups, 3 pike push-ups from box, 3 handstand push-ups. 3 hanging leg raise, 3 strict toes-to-bar, 3

kipping toes-to-bar. 3 hands-up wall squats, 3 elbows-ups wall squats, 3 hands overhead wall squats. If the advanced element is too challenging, repeat the version you can perform correctly.

5) Three rounds: 10 ring push-ups, 10 horizontal ring rows, 10 pistol into single-leg Romanian deadlift (alternating), 10 L-sit knee extensions

EMOMs and EOMOMs

1) EMOM 10, 2 x Turkish get-ups. Alternate hands.

2) EOMOM 10. Even minutes: handstand x 30s. Odd: two pistols (alternating), with "three in the hole".

3) EOMOM 8. Even: 1 wall walk or 10' handstand walk. Odd: 8 kettlebell swings (Russian or American).

4) EOMOM 8. Even: 10 thrusters (45/33lbs). Odd: 15 sec L-sit on even. If you beat 15 seconds last time, try 20.

5) EOMOM 8. Even: 3 hang clean. Odd: 30 second handstand hold.

6) EOMOM 10. Even: 2 wall walks. Odd: 3 strict toes-to-bar.

7) EOMOM 10. Even: 10 chin-ups. Odd: 15 sec L-sit.

BABY BENCHMARKS

1) 21-15-9 reps of thrusters and pull-ups.

2) 15-10-5 of cleans and ring dips.

3) 15-10-5 of deadlifts and handstand push-ups.

4) 21-15-9 of overhead squats and 3-2-1 slow muscle-ups.

5) 21-15-9 of calorie row and GHD sit-ups.

6) 15-10-5 of power snatch and toes-to-bar.

7) 15-10-5 of hang squat cleans and 30-20-10 seconds handstand hold.

DELIBERATE PRACTICE

1)Take ten minutes to practice the barbell squat of your choice: back squat, front squat, overhead squat. Use the simpler versions to warm up to the exercise appropriate for your level of development. Drill three positions, spending 5-10 seconds hanging out in "the hole." If you have mobility issues affecting your front or overhead squats, address them between sets.

2) Take ten minutes to practice the Single-leg Squat of your choice: reverse lunge, hanging leg pistol from box, elevated leg pistol from box, pistol. Use the simpler versions to warm up to the exercise appropriate for your level of development.

3) Take ten minutes to practice the Hip and Trunk Flexion (hanging, bent knee) exercise of your choice: supine knee draw, hanging knee raise, knees-to-elbows, skin-the-cat. Use the simpler versions to warm up to the exercise appropriate for your level of development.

4) Take ten minutes to practice the Hip and Trunk Flexion (hanging, straight leg) exercise of your choice: supine leg raise, hanging leg raise, strict toes-to-bar, kipping toes-to-bar, glide kip. Use the simpler versions to warm up to the exercise appropriate for your level of development.

5) Take ten minutes to practice positions of the Pull Object (ground to shoulder) exercise of your choice: muscle clean, power clean, power clean + front squat, clean. Use the simpler versions to warm up to the exercise appropriate for your level of development.

6) Take ten minutes to practice positions of the Pull Object (ground to overhead) exercise of your choice: muscle snatch, power snatch, power snatch + overhead squat, snatch. Use the simpler versions to warm up for the exercise appropriate for your level of development.

7) Take ten minutes to practice positions of the Push Object (vertical) exercise of your choice: press, push press, push jerk, split jerk. Use the simpler versions to warm up to the exercise appropriate for your level of development.

8) Ten minutes of deliberate practice of the ten positions of the Turkish get-up.

9) Take ten minutes to practice the Pull to Object (vertical, strict) exercise of your choice: scapular pull-up, piked ring row, pull-up, weighted pull-up. Use the simpler versions to warm up to the exercise appropriate for your level of development.

10) Practice the Push Away from Object (vertical, inverted, static) exercise of your choice for ten minutes: down dog hold, pike hold from box, handstand against wall, nose-to-wall handstand, partner-spotted handstand, handstand. Try to accumulate 3 full minutes upside down.

11) Choose one Push Away from Object (vertical, inverted, dynamic) exercise and practice for ten minutes: down dog pike push-up, pike push-up from box, handstand push-up, kipping handstand push-up, deficit handstand push-up, freestanding handstand push-up. Use the simpler versions to warm up to the exercise appropriate for your level of development.

APPENDIX III
POSITIONAL DIAGRAMS

When teaching movements, I've found it very helpful to sketch on the whiteboard stick figure representations of the positions I'm explaining. It's useful for illustrating certain points of about leverage and efficiency I like to make, and once I've completed my demos, the drawings remain on the board for athletes to study as they practice. Here are a selection of my go-to stick figure diagrams; I hope you can find them useful.

Air Squat

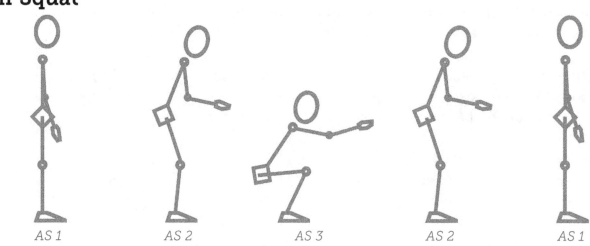

AS 1   AS 2   AS 3   AS 2   AS 1

Front Squat

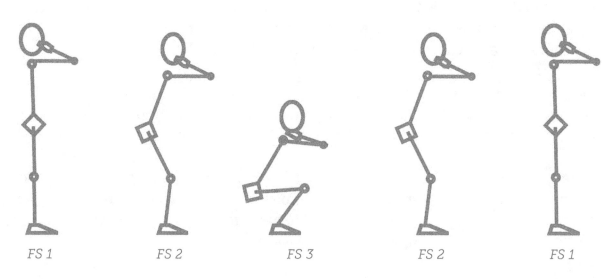

FS 1   FS 2   FS 3   FS 2   FS 1

Overhead Squat

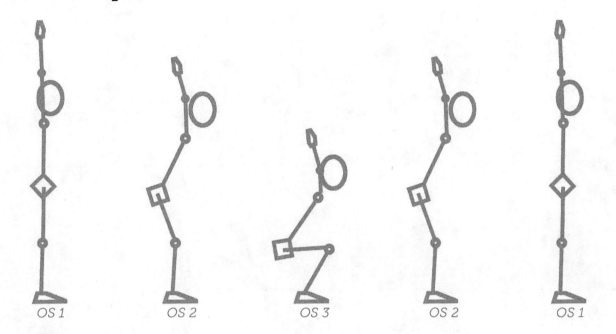

OS 1   OS 2   OS 3   OS 2   OS 1

Deadlift

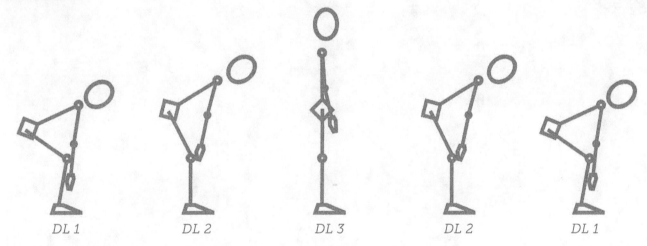

DL 1   DL 2   DL 3   DL 2   DL 1

Russian and American Kettlebell Swings

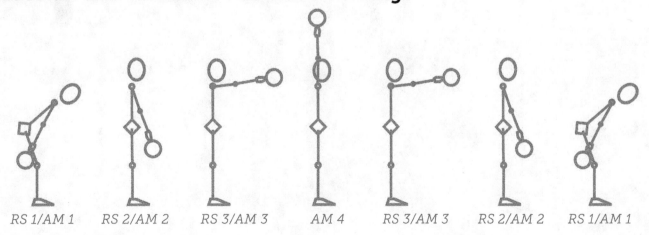

RS 1/AM 1   RS 2/AM 2   RS 3/AM 3   AM 4   RS 3/AM 3   RS 2/AM 2   RS 1/AM 1

Row

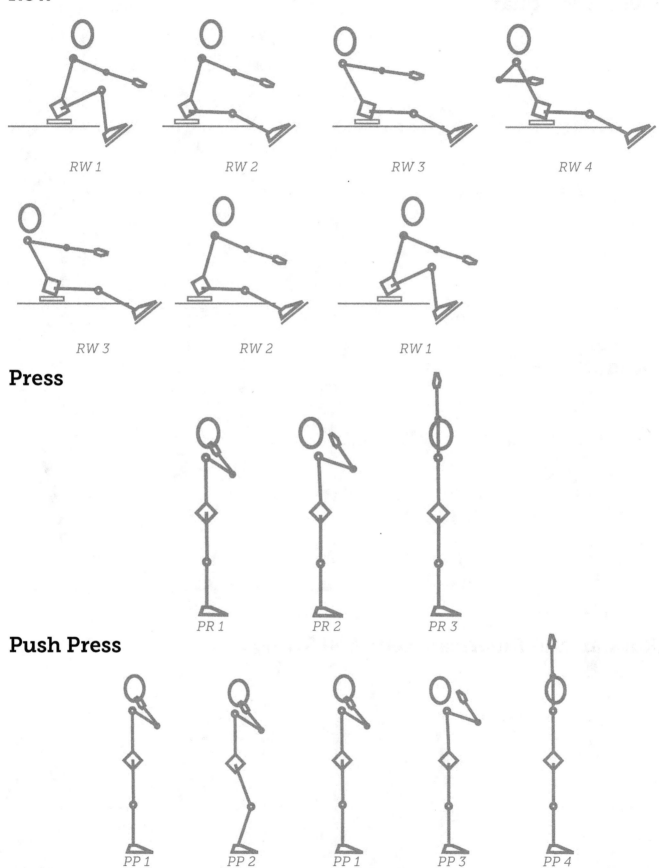

RW 1   RW 2   RW 3   RW 4

RW 3   RW 2   RW 1

Press

PR 1   PR 2   PR 3

Push Press

PP 1   PP 2   PP 1   PP 3   PP 4

Push Jerk

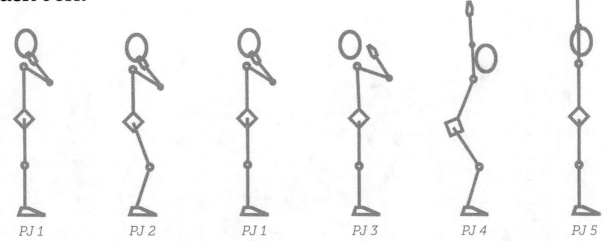

PJ 1   PJ 2   PJ 1   PJ 3   PJ 4   PJ 5

Split Jerk

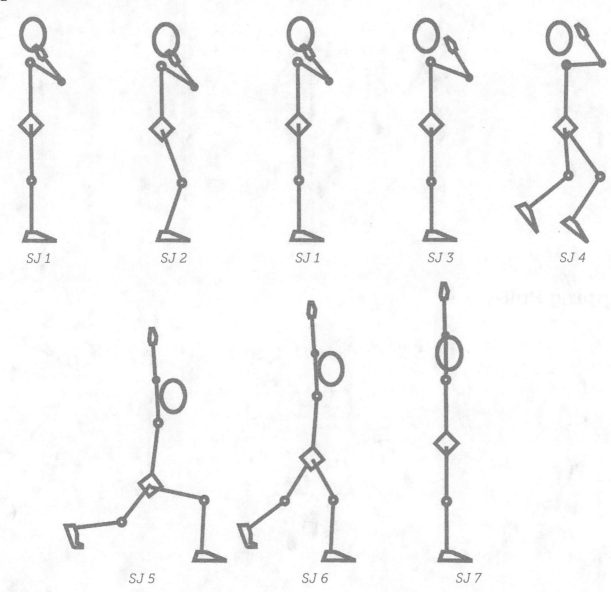

SJ 1   SJ 2   SJ 1   SJ 3   SJ 4

SJ 5   SJ 6   SJ 7

Thruster

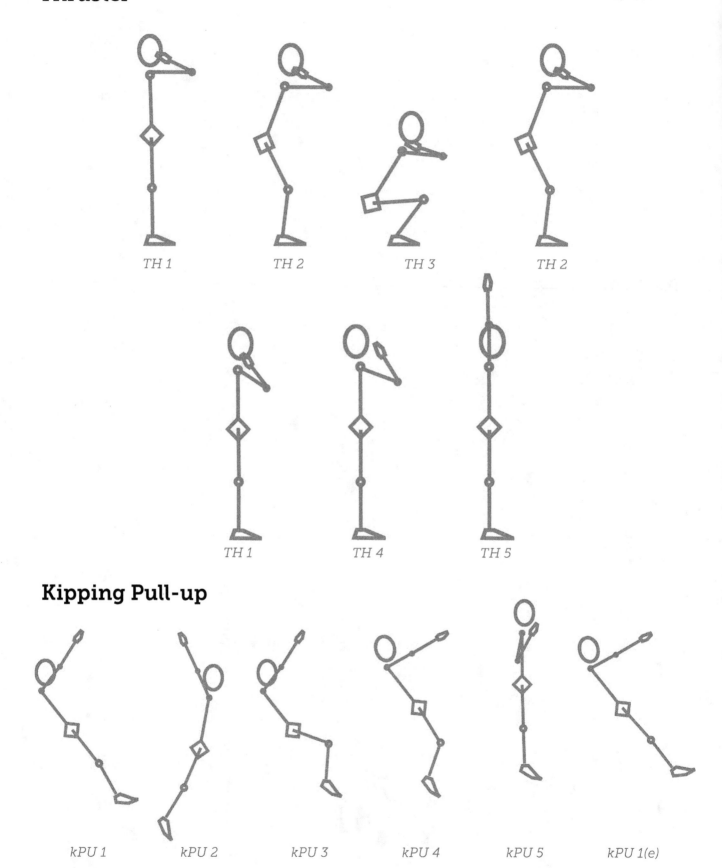

TH 1   TH 2   TH 3   TH 2

TH 1   TH 4   TH 5

Kipping Pull-up

kPU 1   kPU 2   kPU 3   kPU 4   kPU 5   kPU 1(e)

Pistol

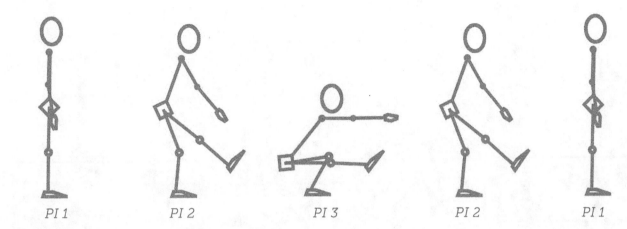

PI 1   PI 2   PI 3   PI 2   PI 1

Dip

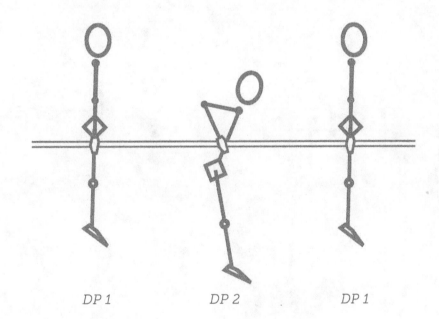

DP 1   DP 2   DP 1

Running

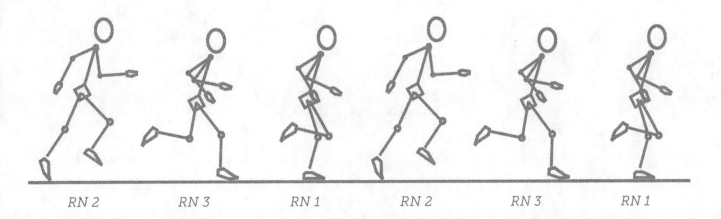

RN 2   RN 3   RN 1   RN 2   RN 3   RN 1

Clean (front view)

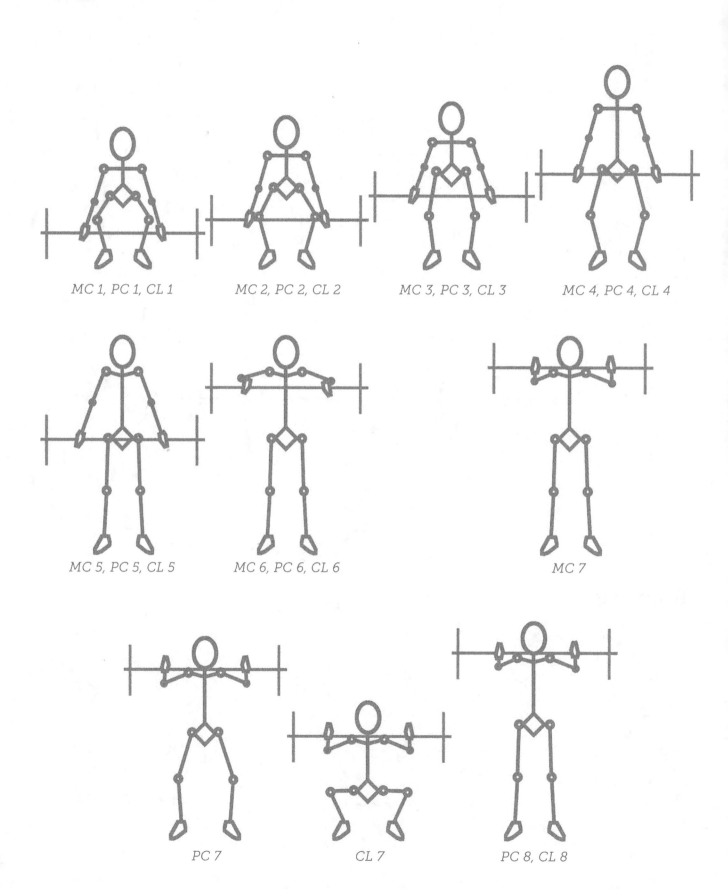

MC 1, PC 1, CL 1 MC 2, PC 2, CL 2 MC 3, PC 3, CL 3 MC 4, PC 4, CL 4

MC 5, PC 5, CL 5 MC 6, PC 6, CL 6 MC 7

PC 7 CL 7 PC 8, CL 8

Clean (side view)

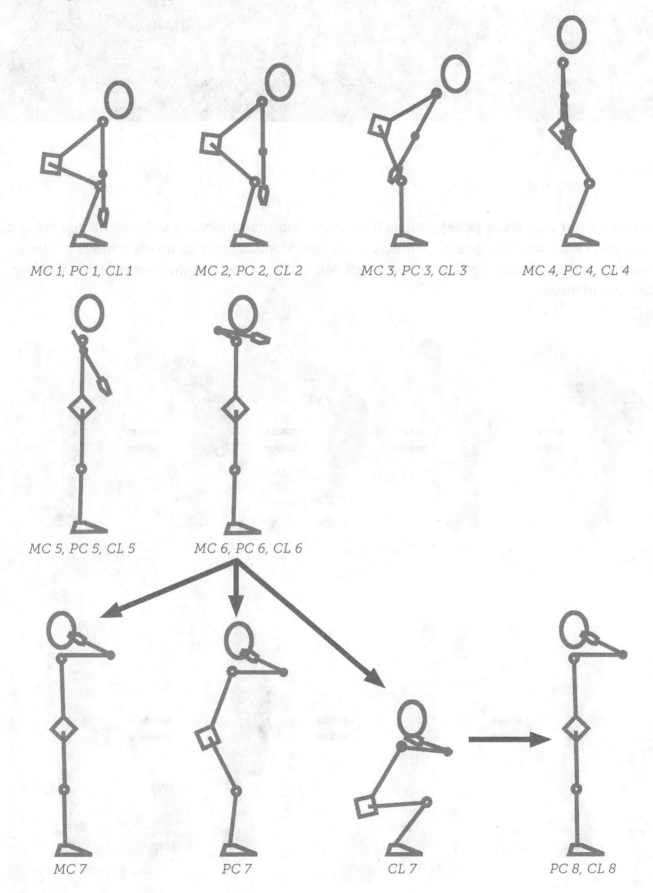

MC 1, PC 1, CL 1   MC 2, PC 2, CL 2   MC 3, PC 3, CL 3   MC 4, PC 4, CL 4

MC 5, PC 5, CL 5   MC 6, PC 6, CL 6

MC 7   PC 7   CL 7   PC 8, CL 8

Certain movements share poses, and as they arise these commonalities should be pointed out to expedite the learning process. Some positions are identical, and some are more like "slant rhymes"—merely similar. Here are a few to get you started. In what other exercises do you see correspondences?

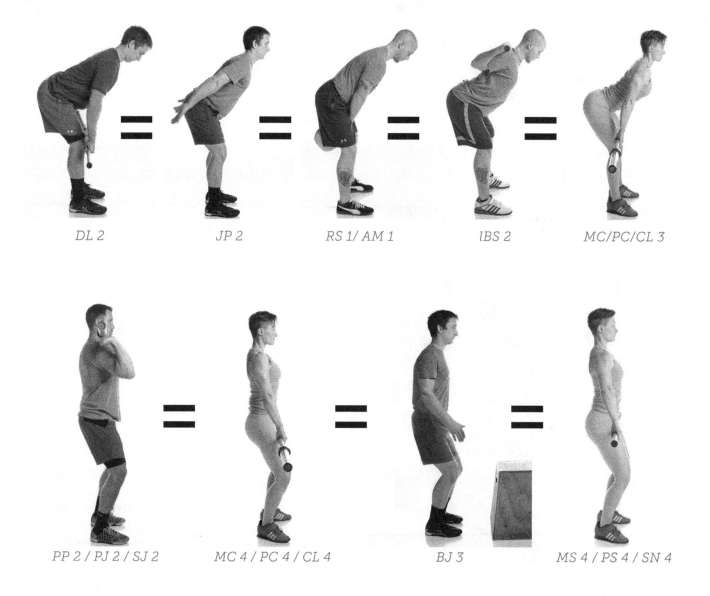

DL 2　　JP 2　　RS 1/ AM 1　　IBS 2　　MC/PC/CL 3

PP 2 / PJ 2 / SJ 2　　MC 4 / PC 4 / CL 4　　BJ 3　　MS 4 / PS 4 / SN 4

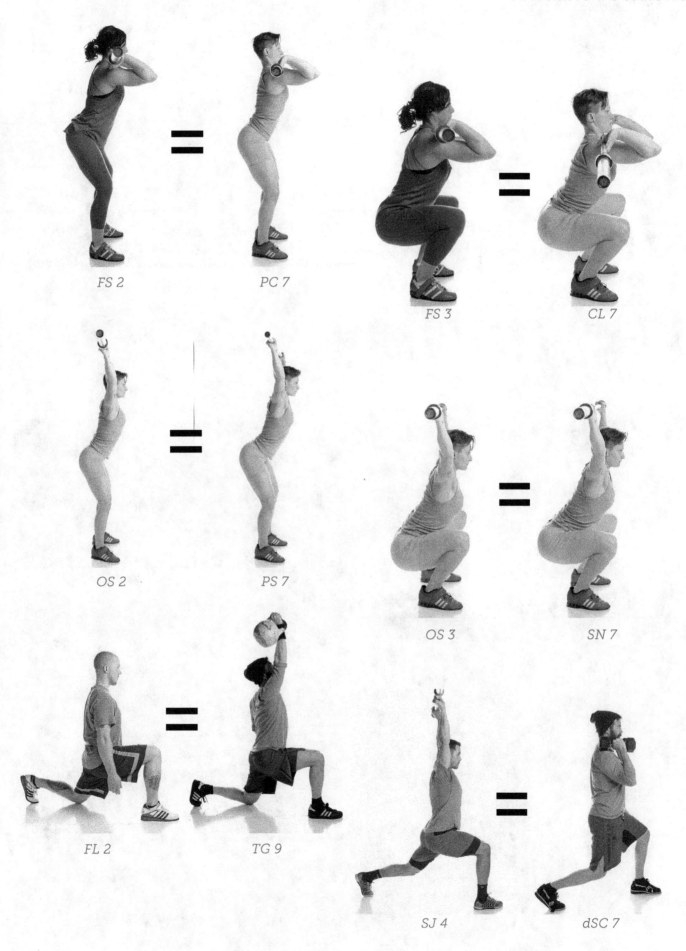

FS 2 = PC 7

FS 3 = CL 7

OS 2 = PS 7

OS 3 = SN 7

FL 2 = TG 9

SJ 4 = dSC 7

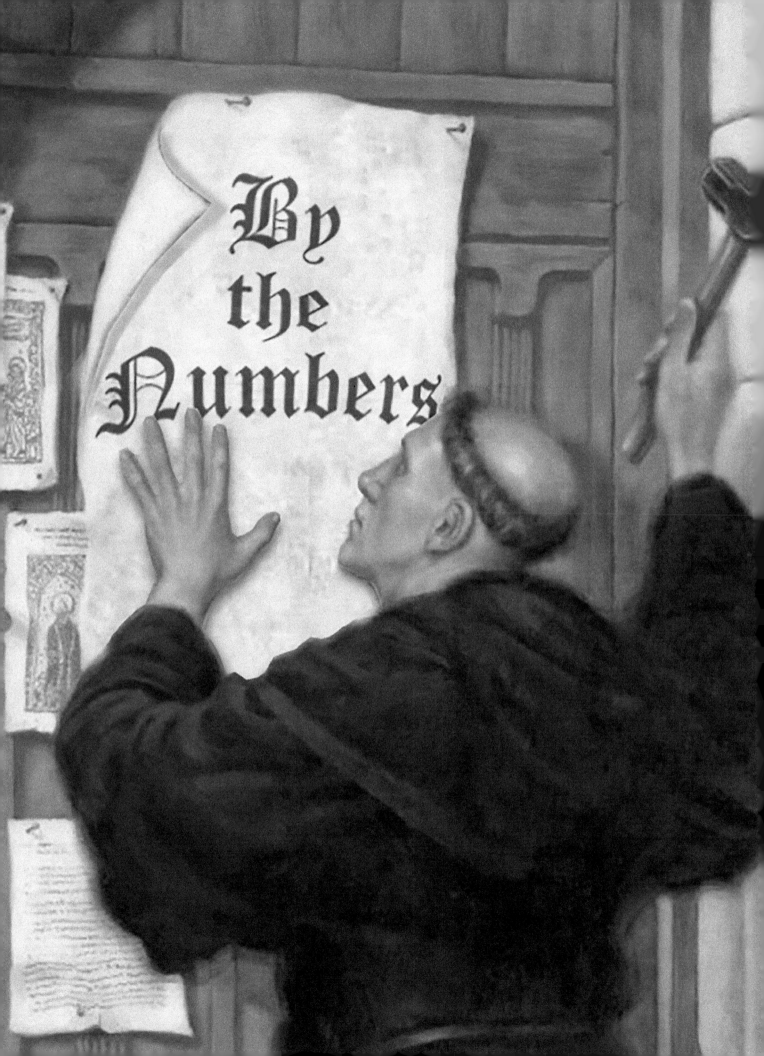

I think every gym should program benchmark workouts regularly, both to provide their clients with regular tests of their (hopefully increasing) capacities, and to familiarize them with MMGPP history and culture.

Traditionally, coaches try to make MMGPP workouts accessible to newer athletes using a "top down" model: the workout is written on the whiteboard with prescribed movements, loads, and repetitions, with athletes encouraged to scale (that is, reduce load and/or volume) as necessary. However, assigning scales is largely a matter of guesswork, and even worse, certain Type A personalities will take what's written on the whiteboard as a personal challenge, and will insist on attempting movements and loads for which they're not ready, sometimes necessitating a *mana*-draining contest of wills as you try to rein them in.

I believe these issues can be obviated by structuring the benchmark WODs for logical progression, as detailed at the end of each "week" in the previous section. In this Appendix, I offer more benchmark WODs, arranged BtN style.

Benchmarks should show up regularly in programming, about every 3-4 months. The idea is that athletes first make the acquaintance of these workouts with light weights and simplified movements. Each time they "beat" the workout (that is, accomplish the desired volume of work in the assigned time domain), they can add weight and/ or complexity on their next outing. **BtN prioritizes movement quality, time domain, volume, and load, in that order.**

Getting strong and fit takes time. Help your athletes to understand *there is no rush*. If they approach these WODs with respect, if they move with integrity, and improve incrementally, they'll reach their goals, and after multiple dates with the benchmarks, when your athletes finally jot "as Rx'd" next to their times, they'll have truly earned it.

"The Art of Asking"
8-6-4 reps for time of
Muscle-ups
Snatch 135/95lbs
Score is time to completion.

"Mrs. Bowie"
For time:
99 Pull-ups, 99 Push-ups,
99 Sit-ups, 99 Squats
Score is time to completion.

"BtN Testing 'The Art of Asking'"

AMRAP :75 Muscle-ups. If you get to 8 before time is up, move on to...
AMRAP :75 Squat snatches. If you get to 8 before time is up, move on to...
AMRAP :60 Muscle-ups. If you get to 6 before time is up, move on to...
AMRAP :60 Squat snatches. If you get to 6 before time is up, move on to...
AMRAP :45 Muscle-ups. If you get to 4 before time is up, move on to...
AMRAP :45 Squat snatches. If you get to 4 before time is up, you're done!

Total time: 6:00.

1. Use rx'd weight or 60-70% of your snatch 1RM, depending on which is lighter.
2. If you use rx'd loads and movements and complete 18 muscle-ups and 18 snatches in
< 6:00, record your time.
3. If you used a reduced load and simpler movements and completed 18 Hybrid (pull to object [vertical], push away from object [vertical]) and 18 Pull Object (ground to overhead) in < 6:00, record your time, and next time, add weight and complexity.
4. If you used a 2:1 sub of pull-ups or dips for muscle-ups, record total Hybrid (pull to object [vertical] or push away from object [vertical])/total Pull Object (ground to overhead). Next time, repeat at same level of challenge.

"BtN Testing 'Mrs. Bowie'"

AMRAP 4 Pull-ups. If you get to 99 before time is up, move on to...
AMRAP 4 Push-ups. If you get to 99 before time is up, move on to...
AMRAP 4 Sit-ups. If you get to 99 before time is up, move on to...
AMRAP 4 Squats. If you get to 99 before time is up, you're done!

Total time: 16:00.

1. If you completed 99 PL, 99 PU, 99 SU, and 99 SQ to standard, record your time.
2. If you used movements of reduced complexity, record total reps of Pull to Object (vertical)/Push Away from Object (horizontal)/Hip and Trunk Flexion (seated)/Squats. Next time, repeat at the same level of challenge.

Note: a lot of people will not be able to complete 99 pull-ups in four minutes! That's okay. Four minutes of intense effort is more productive in terms of maximizing power output than 8 minutes of grinding.

"St. Vincent"

49-39-29-19-9 reps for time of
Double-unders
Sit-ups
Score is time to completion.

"BtN Testing 'St. Vincent'"

AMRAP :90 Double-unders. If you get to 49 before time is up, move on to...
AMRAP :90 Sit-ups. If you get to 49 before time is up, move on to...
AMRAP :75 Double-unders. If you get to 39 before time is up, move on to...
AMRAP :75 Sit-ups. If you get to 39 before time is up, move on to...
AMRAP :60 Double-unders. If you get to 29 before time is up, move on to...
AMRAP :60 Sit-ups. If you get to 29 before time is up, move on to...
AMRAP :45 Double-unders. If you get to 19 before time is up, move on to...
AMRAP :45 Sit-ups. If you get to 19 before time is up, move on to...
AMRAP :30 Double-unders. If you get to 9 before time is up, move on to...
AMRAP :30 Sit-ups. If you get to 9 before time is up, you're done!

Total time: 10:00

1. If you completed 145 double-unders and 145 sit-ups in < 10:00, record your time.
2. Otherwise, record total reps of Mono-structural (jump rope)/Hip and Trunk Flexion (seated). Next time, repeat at the same level of challenge.

"Streisand"

For time: 19 Pull-ups, 29 Push-ups, 39 Sit-ups, 49 Squats
Rest exactly three minutes and repeat for a total of five cycles.
Score is time to completion.

"BtN Testing 'Streisand'"

AMRAP :30 Pull-ups. If you get to 19 before time is up, move on to...
AMRAP :40 Push-ups. If you get to 29 before time is up, move on to...
AMRAP :50 Sit-ups. If you get to 39 before time is up, move on to...
AMRAP :60 Squats. If you get to 49 before time is up, rest.

Rest exactly three minutes and then start again. Total of five cycles.

Total time: 27:00.

1. If you use the prescribed movements and can stay ahead of the clock to complete all five rounds < 27:00, record your time to completion.
2. Otherwise record total reps of Pull to Object/Push Away from Object (horizontal)/Hip and Trunk Flexion (seated)/Squats. Next time, repeat at the same level of challenge.

"Mrs. Clinton, Jr."

Every minute on the minute for 30 minutes,
4 Pull-ups, 8 Push-ups, 12 Squats
When you can no longer start on the minute, complete as many rounds as possible before time is up. Record your score as total rounds on the minute/total rounds.

Ideally, a round of work for "Mrs. Clinton, Jr." takes somewhere between 30-45 seconds. However, many of your trainees will not be able to handle 4-8-12 of pull-ups, push-ups, and squats in anything like that time frame. What to do? Stage a time trial, a test to determine what kind of volume they can do in that approximate time domain. Before the WOD, run something like this (it's 45 seconds, for ease of administration, and athletes use whatever level of movement complexity they plan to use in the workout):

AMRAP :10 Pull-ups.
AMRAP :15 Push-ups
AMRAP :20 Squats

Athlete A got 5 ring rows, 6 push-ups on a box, and 11 squats. Round down to an easily remembered sequence. In this case, 4 ring rows, 6 push-ups on the box, 10 squats. That's her assignment for each round. It might seem nit-picky, but that represents a 30% reduction in volume for the push-ups and a little over 26% for the squats. Over the course of the workout, that will make a big difference, in terms of not hitting muscle failure and grinding to a halt.

You can use this time trial to establish proper volume for a round of "Mrs. Clinton, Jr.", as well. Push-ups in particular seem to be the sticking point for many athletes; reducing the volume per round will allow for

"BtN Testing 'Mrs. Clinton, Jr.'"

EMOM 30
x Pull-ups, *y* Push-ups, *z* squats

When you can no longer start on the minute, complete as many rounds as possible before time is up. Record your score as total rounds on the minute/total rounds.

1. If you perform 4 pull-ups, 8 push-ups, 12 squats each round, record total number of rounds.
2. If you used a reduced volume or simplified version of the movements, record your volume per round of Pull to Object/Push Away from Object (horizontal)/Squat, and how many rounds. Next time, either test out, or repeat at the same level of

"Sin City"

As many rounds as possible in 20 minutes of
4 Pull-ups, 8 Push-ups, 12 Squats

"BtN Testing 'Sin City'"

AMRAP 20
x Pull-ups, *y* Push-ups, *z* squats

Score is total number of rounds, or total pull-ups/push-ups/squats.

1. If you perform 4 pull-ups, 8 push-ups, 12 squats each round, record total number of rounds.
2. If you used a reduced volume or simplified version of the movements, record your volume per round of Pull to Object/Push Away from Object (horizontal)/Squat, and how many rounds. Next time, either test out, or repeat at the same level of

"Arbus"
20-15-10 reps for time of
Deadlifts 225/155lbs
Handstand Push-ups
Score is time to completion.

"BtN Testing 'Arbus'"

AMRAP :75 Deadlifts. If you get to 20 before time is up, move on to...
AMRAP :75 HSPU. If you get to 20 before time is up, move on to...
AMRAP :60 Deadlifts. If you get to 15 before time is up, move on to...
AMRAP :60 HSPU. If you get to 15 before time is up, move on to...
AMRAP :45 Deadlifts. If you get to 10 before time is up, move on to...
AMRAP :45 HSPU. If you get to 10 before time is up, you're done.

Total time: 6:00.

1. Use rx'd weight or 50-60% of your DL 1RM, depending on which is lighter.
2. If you use rx'd loads and movements and complete 45 deadlifts and 45 HSPU in < 6:00, record your time.
3. If you used a reduced load and simpler movements and completed 45 deadlifts and 45 HSPU in < 6:00, record your time, and next time, add weight and complexity.
4. Otherwise record total deadlifts/total HSPU. Make sure you note weight used for Pull Object (ground to hip) and what version of Push Away from Object (vertical, inverted) you used. Next time, repeat at same

"Taylor"
20-15-10 reps for time of
Cleans 135/95lbs
Ring Dips
Score is time to completion.

"BtN Testing 'Taylor'"

AMRAP 2 Cleans. If you get to 20 before time is up, move on to...
AMRAP 2 Ring dips. If you get to 20 before time is up, move on to...
AMRAP 1:30 cleans. If you get to 15 before time is up, move on to...
AMRAP 1:30 ring dips. If you get to 15 before time is up, move on to...
AMRAP 1 cleans. If you get to 10 before time is up, move on to...
AMRAP 1 ring dips. If you get to 10 before time is up, you're done!

Total time: 9:00.

1. Use rx'd weight or 50-60% of your CL 1RM, depending on which is lighter.
2. If you use rx'd loads and movements and complete 45 cleans and 45 ring dips in < 9:00, record your time.
3. If you used a reduced load and simpler movements and completed 45 Pull Object (ground to shoulder) and 45 Push Away from Object (vertical) in < 9:00, record your time, and next time, add weight and complexity.
4. Otherwise record total Pull Object (ground to shoulder)/total Push Away from Object (vertical). Make sure you note weight used for Pull Object (ground to shoulder) and what version of Push Away from Ob-

Note: High-level competitors who regularly finish "Arbus" in about two minutes still take a little over five to complete a full (not power!) "Taylor". That's why this BtN "Arbus" is 6 minutes, while the BtN "Taylor" is 9. Feel free to adjust the time limits on all of these WODs as you see fit.

"Kukla"
20-15-10 reps for time of
Thrusters 95/65lbs
Pull-ups
Score is time to completion.

"BtN Testing 'Kukla'"

AMRAP :75 Thrusters. If you get to 20 before time is up, move on to...
AMRAP :75 Pull-ups. If you get to 20, move on to...
AMRAP :60 Thrusters. If you get to 15, move on to...
AMRAP :60 Pull-ups. If you get to 15, move on to...
AMRAP :45 Thrusters. If you get to 10, move on to...
AMRAP :45 Pull-ups-ups. If you get to 10, you're done!

Total time: 6:00.

1. Use rx'd weight or 40-50% of your thruster 1RM, depending on which is lighter.
2. If you use rx'd loads and movements and complete 45 thrusters and 45 pull-ups in < 6:00, record your time.
3. If you used a reduced load and simpler movements and completed 45 Hybrid (squat, push object [vertical]) and 45 Pull to Object in < 6:00, record your time, and next time, add weight and complexity.
4. Otherwise record total Hybrid (squat, push object [vertical])/total Pull to Object. Make sure you note weight used for Hybrid (squat, push object [vertical]) and what version of Pull to Object you used. Next time, repeat at same level of challenge.

"Miss Jones"
For time:
29 Clean & jerks 135/95lbs
Score is time to completion.

"BtN Testing 'Miss Jones'"

AMRAP 4 Pull Object (ground to shoulder) & Push Object (vertical). If you get to 29 before time expires, you're done.

Total time: 4:00.

1. Use rx'd weight, or 70% of your push jerk 1RM, whichever is lighter.
2. If you use prescribed load and movements and complete 29 reps in < 4:00, record your time.
3. If you used reduced load and complete 29 reps in < 4:00, add weight next time.
4. If you failed to complete 29 reps in < 4:00, next time repeat at the same weight.

"Hell's Bells"
Three rounds for time of
Run 400m, 20 Kettlebell swings (1.5/1 pood)
11 Pull-ups

"Reina de España"
For time:
29 Snatches 135/95lbs
Score is time to completion.

"BtN Testing 'Hell's Bells'"

Three cycles of
AMRAP 2 Run 400m. If you complete the run in < 2:00, move immediately to
AMRAP 1 Kettlebell swings. If you get to 20 before 1 minute is up, move on to...
AMRAP :30 Pull-ups. If you get to 11 before thirty seconds is up, head out on the next run. If, during the third cycle, you get to 11 before 1 minute is up, you're done.

Total time: 10:30.

1. If you use prescribed loads and movements and complete 3 x 400m runs, 60 kettlebell swings, and 33 pull-ups in < 10:30, record your time.
2. If you use reduced loads and simpler movements and complete 3 x 400m runs, 60 kettlebell swings, and 33 pull-ups in < 10:30, record time, and add weight/movement complexity next time.
3. If you failed to complete 3 x 400m runs, 60 kettlebell swings, and 33 pull-ups in < 10:30, record total kettlebell swings/total pull-ups, and next time, repeat at the same level of challenge.

Note: if you have an athlete you believe will have difficulty running 400m in 2 minutes, reduce run to 300m, or assign them a 200m walk.

"BtN Testing 'Reina de España'"

AMRAP 4 Pull Object (ground to overhead). If you get to 29 before time expires, you're done.

Total time: 4:00.

1. Use rx'd weight or 70% of your Pull Object (ground to overhead) 1RM.
2. If you use prescribed load and movements and complete 29 reps in < 4:00, record your time.
3. If you used reduced load and complete 29 reps in < 4:00, add weight next time.
4. If you failed to complete 29 reps in < 4:00, next time repeat at the same weight.

"Mrs. Kennedy"
For time:
Row 1000m, 49 thrusters (45/33lbs), 29 Pull-ups
Score is time to completion.

"BtN Testing 'Mrs. Kennedy"

AMRAP 4 Row for total meters. If you get to 1k before 4:00 is up, move on to...
AMRAP 3 Thrusters. If you get to 49 before time is up, move on to...
AMRAP 2 Pull-ups. If you get to 29 before time is up, you're done!

(Note: if desired, push row out to 5:00 for female athletes.)

Total time: 9:00.

1. If you completed the assigned work with prescribed movements and loads in < 9:00, record your time.
2. If you used reduced loads and simpler movements and completed a 1000m row, 49 thrusters, and 29 pull-ups in < 9:00, record your time, and next time increase load and/or complexity.
3. If you failed to complete a 1000m row, 49 thrusters, and 29 pull-ups in < 9:00, record total meters rowed/total thrusters/total pull-ups, and next time, repeat at the same level of challenge.

"Mrs. Henry Hill"
For time:
149 Wallballs (20/14lbs to 10/9' target)
Score is time to completion.

"BtN Testing 'Mrs. Henry Hill'"

AMRAP 7 Wallballs. If you get to 149 before time is up, you're done!

If you complete 149 wallballs in < 7:00, record your time. Otherwise, record total number of wallballs completed.

Note: athletes' first exposure to "Mrs. Henry Hill" should be with a medicine ball one degree lower than rx'd, e.g., men should use 14lbs, women should use

Total time: 7:00.

1. If you completed the assigned work with prescribed movements and loads in < 7:00, record your time.
2. If you used a reduced load and completed 149 wallballs < 7:00, record your time, and next time increase load.
3. If you failed to complete 149 wallballs < 7:00, record total wallballs, and next time, repeat at the same level of challenge.

"Regan"
10-8-6-4-2 reps for time of
Bench Press (@ body weight), deadlift (1.5 x body weight), clean (.75 x body weight)
Score is time to completion.

"BtN Testing 'Regan'"

AMRAP 5:00 Bench press x 10, deadlifts x 10, cleans x 10. If you complete all 30 reps before time is up, move on to...
AMRAP 4:00 Bench press x 8, deadlifts x 8, cleans x 8. If you complete all 24 reps before time is up, move on to...
AMRAP 3:00 Bench press x 6, deadlifts x 6, cleans x 6. If you complete all 18 reps before time is up, move on to...
AMRAP 2:00 Bench press x 4, deadlifts x 4, cleans x 4. If you complete all 12 reps before time is up, move on to...
AMRAP 1:00 Bench press x 2, deadlifts x 2, cleans x 2. If you complete all 6 reps before time is up, you're done!

Recommended load for each exercise is 60% of your 1RM. If you complete 30 bench press, 30 deadlifts, and 30 cleans in < 15:00, record your time. Otherwise, record total number of bench press/deadlift/cleans.

Total time: 15:00.

1.Use rx'd weight or 50-60% of your bench press, deadlift, and clean 1RMs, whichever is lighter.
2. If you completed the assigned work with prescribed movements and loads in < 15:00, record your time.
3. If you used a reduced loads and simpler movements and completed 30 bench press, 30 deadlifts, and 30 cleans <15:00, record your time, and next time increase loads.
4. If you failed to complete 30 bench press, 30 deadlifts, and 30 cleans < 15:00, next

Note: if you want to expand the volume of this workout (say, to 55 reps of each exercise), figuring an average of 10 seconds/ rep allows for decreases of :30 from round to round. I'll let you do the math.

"Queen of Scots"

As many rounds as possible in 20 minutes of
4 Handstand push-ups, 8 pistols (alternating), 12 pull-ups

Sometimes athletes, getting bored with "Sin City" after their third or fourth exposure, want to give "Queen of Scots" a whirl before they're actually ready for her. Here's a simple test you can administer to determine if they're ready to take on "Queen of Scots" as prescribed:

AMRAP :10 Handstand push-ups
AMRAP :20 Pistols (alternating)
AMRAP :30 Pull-ups

If they score at least 4 hPU, 8 Pl, 12 PL, they can do "Queen of Scots" as rx'd. Otherwise, scale the volume (assuming they are technically proficient in the movements).

"BtN Testing 'Queen of Scots'"

AMRAP 20
x Handstand push-ups, *y* Pistols (alternating), *z* pull-ups

Score is total number of rounds, or total handstand push-ups/pistols/pull-ups.

Total time: 20:00.

1. If you perform 4 hPU, 8 Pl, 12 PL each round, record total number of rounds.
2. If you used a reduced volume or simplified movements, record your volume per round of Push Away from Object (vertical, inverted, dynamic)/Single-leg Squat/Pull to

"Sluggo"

Five rounds for time of
Run 400m
14 Overhead Squats 95/65lbs
Score is time to completion.

"BtN Testing 'Sluggo"

Five cycles of three minutes of
Run 400m
AMRAP Overhead squats. If you get to 14 before 3 minutes is up, immediately head out on your next run. If you finish 14 OS before time is up in the last 3 minute cycle, you're done.

Total time: 15:00.

1. If you completed the assigned work with prescribed movements and loads in < 15:00, record your time.
2. If you used a reduced loads and simpler movements and completed 70 overhead squats < 15:00, record your time, and next time increase loads.
3. If you failed to complete 70 overhead squats in < 15:00, next time, repeat at the same level of challenge.

AFTERWORD
EVERY ATHLETE IS A COACH

If your clients train with you for long enough, there will come a time when you have taught them virtually all there is to know about MMGPP training. It's inevitable; in terms of MMGPP per se, there are a finite amount of exercises with which one needs to be competent, and only a double-handful of standardized benchmark workouts to conquer. So how do you keep them progressing?

You turn them into coaches—not by insisting they get certified and teach classes, but by encouraging them to look after and mentor new members. One of the unfortunate side effects of the rise of competitive MMGPP is that more experienced athletes are abandoning group MMGPP classes in favor of specialized training. I think there's room for that, but I also believe that when a gym's most accomplished athletes segregate themselves, they're missing out on a wonderful opportunity to improve both as athletes and human beings.

There's a (possibly aprocryphal) quote from Albert Einstein that goes, "If you can't explain it to a six year old, you don't understand it yourself." I'll slightly alter that to "You don't really understand something until you can teach it". That's why, once an athlete has learned how to train MMGPP, one important way he can continue developing as an athlete is by sharing his hard-won knowledge with his less experienced classmates. Trying to articulate what he knows how to do will force him to think it through logically, sharpen his understanding, and ultimately make him a better athlete. It's just one more way that working out as part of a community creates a superior brand of fitness.

So as your newbies grow into salty MMGPP athletes, do everything you can to keep them involved with your general training population. Encourage your experienced athletes to give generously of themselves, to make the path their more junior classmates must tread a little smoother, and to help them feel a little bit less lost and intimidated. Helping others can not only make us better athletes, it can help us become better people. Ultimately, isn't that what all this is about?

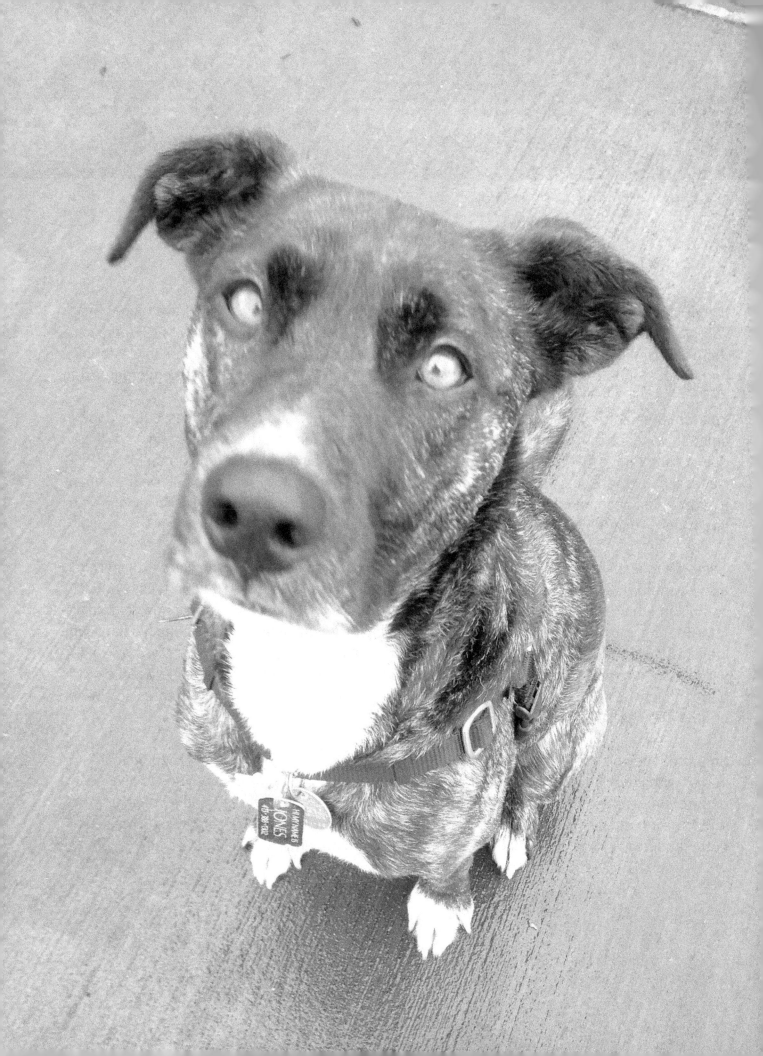

MOVEMENT INDEX

Acknowledgements

"By the Numbers" turned out to be an enormous project. Thank God I had no idea what I was letting myself in for, or I never would've had the courage to start! It would not have been possible without the efforts and support of the following people, so THANK YOU to...

Brian Poon, a remarkably talented photographer who was willing to slash his rates for an impecunious writer. Brian, your hard work made this book ten times better than it could have been without you! Also Greg Saulmon, who contributed the cover photo, and who along with Liz Greene shot the many beautiful full-page photos that grace these pages.

Tyler Friedenrich, who taught me the basics of InDesign and created the template for the teaching sections. Without you, I would've had a bunch of blurry iPhone photos displayed in a Word doc.

Cheryl Masukawa of Torrance Training Lab for her work on the BtN Movement Index. Thanks Cheryl!

Thanks to my hardworking demo models: Ramey Harris, Emily Sigard, Rory Coyne, Sam Douglas, Kristina Lum, Laura Mohler, Chris Garceau, Vanessa Dickens, Rob Kerruish, and Mariah Lombard. Couldn't have done it without you, kids.

Special thanks go to Colin Broadwater and the rest of the Madlab Business Group for taking BtN under your wing. Your support and enthusiasm have been invaluable!

Who else? Lindsey Dion and Ryan Calkins at CrossFit The Lab, and Dave Werner at Level Four/CrossFit Seattle, for being such gracious hosts.

Also a huge thanks to Dr. Kelly Starrett, who's probably been my biggest influence as an instructor, beginning with his coaching at my CrossFit L1 cert in 2007 and extending through the publication of *Becoming a Supple Leopard*.

Everyone who read early drafts of this material: Eric Horne, Donna Spraggon, Adele Burke, Simon Halliday, Brian Zagata, Jill Boski, Jeff Gnatek, Ryan Calkins, Mael Walkowiak, Sally White, Kelly Starrett, Chip Conrad, Matthew Quinn, Rob Miller, and especially Kurt Roderick, for additional cues and trenchant criticism. Thank you.

And last but not least, all those on the home front: Jones, my trans-continental copilot; my mom and dad, for unflagging support; my partners at PCVF, Perrin Hendrick and Liz Greene; Sarah Tyrell, our controller and voice of reason; PVCF's incredible training cadre: Ayn Toppin, Ryan Katz, Mael Walkowiak, Ari Kasal, Brian Kazak, Heather Hamel, Jovan James, Matt Tudryn, Eric Horne, Sarah Gillio, and Paul Gillio; Huey Sun, who was there at the beginning; Sally White, who alternated between cheerleading and cracking the whip. While we're at it, thanks to each and every one of the couple thousand or so athletes that have come through PVCF's doors since 2007. This book wouldn't exist without them. And of course you, dear reader! I hope you found this book helpful.

For more information about the methodology described in this book, or to purchase a full-color poster of the BtN Movement Hierarchies, follow us on Facebook!

www.facebook.com/ BytheNumbersMethod

CPSIA information can be obtained
at www.ICGtesting.com
Printed in the USA
BVHW011930010520
579061BV00010B/1495